Advancements in Companion Animal Cardiology

Editor

JOSHUA A. STERN

VETERINARY CLINICS OF NORTH AMERICA: SMALL ANIMAL PRACTICE

www.vetsmall.theclinics.com

November 2023 • Volume 53 • Number 6

ELSEVIER

1600 John F. Kennedy Boulevard • Suite 1800 • Philadelphia, Pennsylvania, 19103-2899
http://www.vetsmall.theclinics.com

**VETERINARY CLINICS OF NORTH AMERICA: SMALL ANIMAL PRACTICE Volume 53, Number 6
November 2023 ISSN 0195-5616, ISBN-13: 978-0-443-18380-5**

Editor: Stacy Eastman

Developmental Editor: Varun Gopal

Veterinary Clinics of North America: Small Animal Practice (ISSN 0195-5616) is published bimonthly by Elsevier Inc., 360 Park Avenue South, New York, NY 10010-1710. Months of issue are January, March, May, July, September, and November. Business and Editorial Offices: 1600 John F. Kennedy Blvd., Ste. 1800, Philadelphia, PA 19103-2899. Customer Service Office: 3251 Riverport Lane, Maryland Heights, MO 63043. Periodicals postage paid at New York, NY and additional mailing offices. Subscription prices are $387.00 per year (domestic individuals), $844.00 per year (domestic institutions), $100.00 per year (domestic students/residents), $488.00 per year (Canadian individuals), $1049.00 per year (Canadian institutions), $528.00 per year (international individuals), $1049.00 per year (international institutions), $100.00 per year (Canadian students/residents), and $220.00 per year (international students/residents). To receive student/resident rate, orders must be accompanied by name of affiliated institution, date of term, and the *signature* of program/residency coordinator on institution letterhead. Orders will be billed at individual rate until proof of status is received. Foreign air speed delivery is included in all *Clinics* subscription prices. All prices are subject to change without notice. **POSTMASTER:** Send address changes to *Veterinary Clinics of North America: Small Animal Practice*, Elsevier Health Sciences Division, Subscription Customer Service, 3251 Riverport Lane, Maryland Heights, MO 63043. Customer Service (orders, claims, online, change of address): Elsevier Periodicals Customer Service, Elsevier Health Sciences Division Subscription **Customer Service 3251 Riverport Lane Maryland Heights, MO 63043. Tel: 1-800-654-2452 (U.S. and Canada); 314-447-8871 (outside U.S. and Canada). Fax: 314-447-8029. E-mail: journalscustomerservice-usa@elsevier.com (for print support); journalsonlinesupport-usa@elsevier.com (for online support).**

Reprints. For copies of 100 or more of articles in this publication, please contact the Commercial Reprints Department, Elsevier Inc., 360 Park Avenue South, New York, NY 10010-1710. Tel.: 212-633-3874; Fax: 212-633-3820; E-mail: reprints@elsevier.com.

Veterinary Clinics of North America: Small Animal Practice is also published in Japanese by Inter Zoo Publishing Co., Ltd., Aoyama Crystal-Bldg 5F, 3-5-12 Kitaaoyama, Minato-ku, Tokyo 107-0061, Japan.

Veterinary Clinics of North America: Small Animal Practice is covered in *Current Contents/Agriculture, Biology and Environmental Sciences, Science Citation Index, ASCA, MEDLINE/PubMed (Index Medicus), Excerpta Medica, and BIOSIS.*

Contributors

EDITOR

JOSHUA A. STERN, DVM, PhD
Diplomate, American College of Veterinary Internal Medicine (Cardiology); Associate Dean for Research and Graduate Studies, Professor of Cardiology, Department of Clinical Sciences, College of Veterinary Medicine, North Carolina State University, Raleigh, North Carolina, USA; Department of Medicine and Epidemiology, School of Veterinary Medicine, University of California, Davis, Davis, California, USA

AUTHORS

DARCY B. ADIN, DVM
Diplomate, American College of Veterinary Internal Medicine (Cardiology); University of Florida, College of Veterinary Medicine, Gainesville, Florida, USA

MARISA K. AMES, DVM
Diplomate, American College of Veterinary Internal Medicine (Cardiology); Department of Medicine and Epidemiology, School of Veterinary Medicine, University of California, Davis, Davis, California, USA

POPPY BRISTOW, BVetMeD, MVetMeD, PGCertVetEd, FHEA, MRCVS
Diplomate, European College of Veterinary Surgery; Head of Cardiac and Soft Tissue Surgery, Dick White Referrals, Linnaeus and Mars Veterinary Health, Station Farm, Cambridgeshire, United Kingdom

DAVID J. CONNOLLY, BSc, BVetMed, PhD, CertVC, Cert SAM, MRCVS
Diplomate, European College of Veterinary Internal Medicine (Cardiology); Department of Clinical Science and Services, Royal Veterinary College, Hertfordshire, Hatfield, United Kingdom

TERESA C. DeFRANCESCO, DVM
Diplomate, American College of Veterinary Internal Medicine (Cardiology); Diplomate, American College of Veterinary Emergency Critical Care; Professor, Department of Clinical Sciences, College of Veterinary Medicine, North Carolina State University, Raleigh, North Carolina, USA

RYAN FRIES, DVM
Assistant Professor, Department of Veterinary Clinical Medicine, University of Illinois at Urbana-Champaign, Urbana, Illinois, USA

ALLISON L. GAGNON, DVM, MS
Diplomate, American College of Veterinary Internal Medicine (Cardiology); Department of Medicine and Epidemiology, School of Veterinary Medicine, University of California, Davis, Davis, California, USA

WEIHOW HSUE, DVM
Diplomate, American College of Veterinary Internal Medicine (Cardiology); Department of Clinical Sciences, College of Veterinary Medicine, Cornell University, Ithaca, New York, USA

JOANNA L. KAPLAN, DVM
Diplomate, American College of Veterinary Internal Medicine (Cardiology); Department of Medicine and Epidemiology, School of Veterinary Medicine, University of California, Davis, Davis, California, USA

SAMANTHA KOVACS, DVM, PhD
Anatomic Pathology Service, School of Veterinary Medicine, University of California, Davis, UC Davis VMTH, Davis, California, USA

RONALD H.L. LI, DVM, MVETMED, PhD
Diplomate, American College of Veterinary Emergency and Critical Care; Associate Professor, Department of Clinical Sciences, College of Veterinary Medicine, North Carolina State University, Raleigh, North Carolina, USA

LAUREN E. MARKOVIC, DVM
Diplomate, American College of Veterinary Internal Medicine (Cardiology); Assistant Professor of Cardiology, Department of Small Animal Medicine and Surgery, University of Georgia, College of Veterinary Medicine, Athens, Georgia, USA

JOSE NOVO MATOS, DVM, PhD, AFHEA, MRCVS
Diplomate, European College of Veterinary Internal Medicine (Cardiology); Teaching Professor of Small Animal Cardiology, Principal Clinical Cardiologist, Department of Veterinary Medicine, University of Cambridge, Cambridge, United Kingdom

JESSIE ROSE PAYNE, BVetMed, MvetMed, PhD
Langford Vets Small Animal Referral Hospital, University of Bristol, Langford, United Kingdom

VICTOR N. RIVAS, MS
Department of Medicine and Epidemiology, School of Veterinary Medicine, University of California, Davis, Davis, California, USA; Department of Clinical Sciences, College of Veterinary Medicine, North Carolina State University, Raleigh, North Carolina, USA

LUÍS DOS SANTOS, DVM, PhD
Diplomate, American College of Veterinary Internal Medicine (Cardiology); Department of Veterinary Clinical Sciences, Purdue University, College of Veterinary Medicine, West Lafayette, Indiana, USA

BRIAN A. SCANSEN, DVM, MS
Diplomate, American College of Veterinary Internal Medicine (Cardiology); Professor and Service Head, Cardiology and Cardiac Surgery, Department of Clinical Sciences, Colorado State University, Fort Collins, Colorado, USA

MEG SHAVERDIAN, BS, PhD Candidate
Department of Surgical and Radiological Sciences, School of Veterinary Medicine, University of California, Davis, Davis, California, USA; Department of Clinical Sciences, College of Veterinary Medicine, North Carolina State University, Raleigh, North Carolina, USA

JOSHUA A. STERN, DVM, PhD
Diplomate, American College of Veterinary Internal Medicine (Cardiology); Associate
Dean for Research and Graduate Studies, Professor of Cardiology, Department of Clinical
Sciences, College of Veterinary Medicine, North Carolina State University, Raleigh, North
Carolina, USA; Department of Medicine and Epidemiology, School of Veterinary
Medicine, University of California, Davis, Davis, California, USA

YU UEDA, DVM, PhD
Diplomate, American College of Veterinary Emergency Critical Care; Department of
Clinical Sciences, College of Veterinary Medicine, North Carolina State University,
Raleigh, North Carolina, USA

ASHLEY L. WALKER, DVM
William R. Pritchard Veterinary Medical Teaching Hospital, University of California, Davis,
Davis, California, USA

JESSICA L. WARD, DVM
Diplomate, American College of Veterinary Internal Medicine (Cardiology); Associate
Professor, Department of Veterinary Clinical Sciences, College of Veterinary Medicine,
Iowa State University, Iowa, USA

JAMES WOOD, DVM
Department of Medicine and Epidemiology, School of Veterinary Medicine, University of
California, Davis, Davis, California, USA

Contents

Preface: Exciting Advancements and Compelling Future Directions in Companion Animal Cardiology xiii

Joshua A. Stern

The Role of Personalized Medicine in Companion Animal Cardiology 1255

Victor N. Rivas, Joshua A. Stern, and Yu Ueda

> Cardiomyopathies remain one of the most common inherited cardiac diseases in both human and veterinary patients. To date, well over 100 mutated genes are known to cause cardiomyopathies in humans with only a handful known in cats and dogs. This review highlights the need and use of personalized one-health approaches to cardiovascular case management and advancement in pharmacogenetic-based therapy in veterinary medicine. Personalized medicine holds promise in understanding the molecular basis of disease and ultimately will unlock the next generation of targeted novel pharmaceuticals and aid in the reversal of detrimental effects at a molecular level.

Predicting Development of Hypertrophic Cardiomyopathy and Disease Outcomes in Cats 1277

Jose Novo Matos and Jessie Rose Payne

> Echocardiography is the gold standard imaging modality to diagnose hypertrophic cardiomyopathy (HCM) in cats. Echocardiographic features can predict both cats at an increased risk of developing HCM and cats with HCM at an increased risk of developing cardiovascular events or experiencing cardiac death. Left atrial dysfunction seems to be an important feature of HCM, as it is an early phenotypic abnormality and is also associated with worse outcome.

Advancing Treatments for Feline Hypertrophic Cardiomyopathy: The Role of Animal Models and Targeted Therapeutics 1293

Joanna L. Kaplan, Victor N. Rivas, and David J. Connolly

> Feline HCM is the most common cardiovascular disease in cats, leading to devastating outcomes, including congestive heart failure (CHF), arterial thromboembolism (ATE), and sudden death. Evidence demonstrating long-term survival benefit with currently available therapies is lacking. Therefore, it is imperative to explore intricate genetic and molecular pathways that drive HCM pathophysiology to inspire the development of novel therapeutics. Several clinical trials exploring new drug therapies are currently underway, including those investigating small molecule inhibitors and rapamycin. This article outlines the key work performed using cellular and animal models that has led to and continues to guide the development of new innovative therapeutic strategies.

Preventing Cardiogenic Thromboembolism in Cats: Literature Gaps, Rational Recommendations, and Future Therapies   1309

Meg Shaverdian and Ronald H.L. Li

Cardiogenic arterial thromboembolism (CATE) is a devastating complication in cats with cardiomyopathies with significant morbidity and mortality. Despite recent advances in the diagnosis and treatment of CATE, its recurrence and mortality remain high. This highlights the urgent need for a greater understanding of CATE pathophysiology so that novel diagnostic tests and therapeutics can be developed. This comprehensive review aims to summarize existing literature on pathophysiology, clinical diagnosis, and current recommendations on the prevention and treatment of CATE. It also identifies and describes knowledge gaps and research priorities in the roles of immunothrombosis and procoagulant platelets in the pathogenesis of CATE.

Hypertrophic Cardiomyopathy–Advances in Imaging and Diagnostic Strategies   1325

Ryan Fries

 Video content accompanies this article at http://www.vetsmall. theclinics.com.

Hypertrophic cardiomyopathy (HCM) is the most important and prevalent cardiac disease in cats. Due to the highly variable nature of HCM, a multimodal approach including physical examination, genetic evaluation, cardiac biomarkers, and imaging are all essential elements to appropriate and timely diagnosis. These foundational elements are advancing rapidly in veterinary medicine. Newer biomarkers such as galectin-3 are currently being researched and advances in tissue speckle-tracking and contrast-enhanced echocardiography are readily available. Advanced imaging techniques, such as cardiac MRI, are providing previously unavailable information about myocardial fibrosis and paving the way for enhanced diagnostic capabilities and risk-stratification in cats with HCM.

Mitral Valve Repair–The Development and Rise of Options in the Veterinary World   1343

Poppy Bristow and Lauren E. Markovic

 Video content accompanies this article at http://www.vetsmall. theclinics.com.

Both open surgical repair and a hybrid-interventional option are now available for mitral valve repair (MVR) at select veterinary centers worldwide, making the need for awareness of options and the intricacies around case selection of increasing importance. This article will overview both options currently available and their current stages of progress.

Beyond Angiotensin-Converting Enzyme Inhibitors: Modulation of the Renin–Angiotensin–Aldosterone System to Delay or Manage Congestive Heart Failure   1353

Marisa K. Ames, Darcy B. Adin, and James Wood

The renin–angiotensin–aldosterone system (RAAS) consists of bioactive angiotensin peptides, enzymatic pathways, receptors, and the steroid hormone aldosterone. The RAAS regulates blood pressure, sodium, and electrolyte homeostasis and mediates pathologic disease processes. Within this system is an alternative arm that counterbalances the vasoconstrictive, sodium and water retentive, and pro-fibrotic and inflammatory effects of the classical arm. Improved biochemical methodologies in RAAS quantification are elucidating how this complex system changes in health and disease. Future treatments for cardiovascular and kidney disease will likely involve a more nuanced manipulation of this system rather than simple blockade.

The Role of Autoantibodies in Companion Animal Cardiac Disease   1367

Luís Dos Santos and Ashley L. Walker

Clinical studies exploring the role of autoimmune diseases in cardiac dysfunction have become increasingly common in both human and veterinary literature. Autoantibodies (AABs) specific to cardiac receptors have been found in human and canine dilated cardiomyopathy, and circulating autoantibodies have been suggested as a sensitive biomarker for arrhythmogenic right ventricular cardiomyopathy in people and Boxer dogs. In this article, we will summarize recent literature on AABs and their role in cardiac diseases of small animals. Despite the potential for new discoveries in veterinary cardiology, current data in veterinary medicine are limited and further studies are needed.

The Genetics of Canine Pulmonary Valve Stenosis   1379

Samantha Kovacs, Brian A. Scansen, and Joshua A. Stern

There have been recent advancements in understanding the genetic contribution to pulmonary valve stenosis (PS) in brachycephalic breeds such as the French Bulldog and Bulldog. The associated genes are transcriptions factors involved in cardiac development, which is comparable to the genes that cause PS in humans. However, validation studies and functional follow up is necessary before this information can be used for screening purposes.

Advances in the Treatment of Pulmonary Valve Stenosis   1393

Brian A. Scansen

 Video content accompanies this article at http://www.vetsmall. theclinics.com.

Pulmonary valve stenosis represents the most common congenital heart defect of dogs and appears to be increasing in prevalence due to the growing popularity of brachycephalic breeds. Current treatments include beta-blockade and balloon pulmonary valvuloplasty, though evidence-based approaches to this disease are lacking. Balloon pulmonary valvuloplasty is most effective for fused, doming valves leaving a large population of dogs with thick, dysplastic valves that fail to respond adequately to balloon dilation. Transpulmonary stent implantation is an emerging therapy to consider for dogs with valve dysplasia or who have failed balloon pulmonary valvuloplasty; current experience with transpulmonary stent implantation is provided.

Treating Stubborn Cardiac Arrhythmias—Looking Toward the Future   1415

Weihow Hsue and Allison L. Gagnon

  Video content accompanies this article at http://www.vetsmall.
theclinics.com.

As animals can develop significant side effects or remain refractory while
on antiarrhythmic medical therapy for tachyarrhythmias, interventional
therapies are progressively being explored. This review will highlight the
principles and utilities of implantable cardioverter-defibrillators, electrophysiological mapping and catheter ablation, three-dimensional electroanatomical mapping, and stereotactic arrhythmia radiotherapy. In
particular, three-dimensional electroanatomical mapping is emerging as
an adjunct electrophysiology tool to facilitate activation, substrate, and
pace mapping for intuitive analysis of complex tachyarrhythmias. Unlike
antiarrhythmic medications, these modalities offer potential for decreasing
risk of sudden death and even permanent termination of tachyarrhythmias.

The Role of Point-of-Care Ultrasound in Managing Cardiac Emergencies   1429

Jessica L. Ward and Teresa C. DeFrancesco

Point-of-care ultrasound (POCUS) is a useful imaging tool for the diagnosis
and monitoring of cardiac emergencies. Unlike complete echocardiography, POCUS is a time-sensitive examination involving a subset of targeted
thoracic ultrasound views to identify abnormalities of the heart, lungs,
pleural space, and caudal vena cava. When integrated with other clinical
information, POCUS can be helpful in the diagnosis of left-sided and
right-sided congestive heart failure, pericardial effusion and tamponade,
and severe pulmonary hypertension and can help clinicians monitor resolution or recurrence of these conditions.

VETERINARY CLINICS OF NORTH AMERICA: SMALL ANIMAL PRACTICE

FORTHCOMING ISSUES

January 2024
Canine and Feline Behavior
Carlo Siracusa, *Editor*

March 2024
Practice Management
Peter Weinstein, *Editor*

May 2024
Small Animal Oncology
Craig A. Clifford and Philip J. Bergman, *Editors*

RECENT ISSUES

September 2023
Small Animal Theriogenology
Bruce W. Christensen, *Editor*

July 2023
Rehabilitation Therapy
Molly J. Flaherty, *Editor*

May 2023
Diabetes Mellitus in Cats and Dogs
Chen Gilor and Thomas K. Graves, *Editors*

SERIES OF RELATED INTEREST

Veterinary Clinics: Exotic Animal Practice
https://www.vetexotic.theclinics.com/
Advances in Small Animal Care
https://www.advancesinsmallanimalcare.com/

THE CLINICS ARE NOW AVAILABLE ONLINE!
Access your subscription at:
www.theclinics.com

Preface

Exciting Advancements and Compelling Future Directions in Companion Animal Cardiology

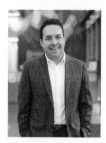

Joshua A. Stern, DVM, PhD,
DACVIM (Cardiology)
Editor

It is a great privilege to curate a collection of articles that highlight groundbreaking advancements in companion animal cardiology. Veterinary cardiology has recently seen incredible advancements due in part to the research teams, clinician scientists, and translational cardiology breakthroughs of authors in this collection. Authors of this collection range from graduate students and cardiology residents to full professors and represent the current and future of impactful research and clinical prowess that define our present and future standards of care.

Through this collection, we examine breakthroughs in the most common and troubling cardiovascular diseases, such as feline hypertrophic cardiomyopathy and canine myxomatous mitral valve degeneration. We see the impact of novel therapeutics informed by molecular pathology and the promise of interventional and surgical successes. The authors of this collection challenge the status quo for the betterment of cats and dogs.

A feature of this collection that I'm most proud of is the authors' ability to distill basic science and benchtop research in ways that demonstrate their clear impact on clinical practice. What we've learned from a molecular and mechanistic perspective about diseases, like hypertrophic cardiomyopathy, arrhythmogenic cardiomyopathy, and pulmonary valve stenosis, is paving the way for novel clinical trials and development of first-in-class compounds that will help move the needle on future therapies. The role of precision medicine and cardiovascular genetics is also featured; if we take notes from our human cardiology colleagues, these areas will soon give way to breakthrough therapies and become essential practice in canine and feline cardiology.

Vet Clin Small Anim 53 (2023) xiii–xiv
https://doi.org/10.1016/j.cvsm.2023.08.009
0195-5616/23/© 2023 Published by Elsevier Inc.

I'm proud to serve as the editor for this special issue and hope that, as you read the collection, you appreciate the depth and breadth of skill and foresight presented by the authors. I'm confident these works will serve as exceptional references in clinical companion animal cardiology.

Joshua A. Stern, DVM, PhD, DACVIM (Cardiology)
Department of Clinical Sciences
North Carolina State University College
of Veterinary Medicine
1060 William Moore Drive
Raleigh, NC 27607, USA

E-mail address:
jastern@ncsu.edu

The Role of Personalized Medicine in Companion Animal Cardiology

Victor N. Rivas, MS[a,b],
Joshua A. Stern, DVM, PhD, DACVIM (Cardiology)[a,b],
Yu Ueda, DVM, PhD, DACVECC[b,*]

KEYWORDS

- Hypertrophic cardiomyopathy (HCM) • Dilated cardiomyopathy (DCM)
- Arrhythmogenic right ventricular cardiomyopathy (ARVC) • Cats • Dogs
- Pharmacogenetics • Pharmacogenomics • Genetics

KEY POINTS

- Only a handful of pathogenically confirmed mutations leading to common cardiomyopathies have been described in dogs and cats.
- Whole-genome association studies remain the gold-standard approach for cardiovascular genetic studies, however, their utility is limited for complex and heterogenous cardiovascular diseases.
- Precision medicine and pharmacogenetic-guided therapy holds promise for increasing drug development, improving efficacy, and reducing adverse drug reactions in patients with cardiovascular disease.
- Revolutionizing the prevention and treatment of cardiovascular disease in veterinary patients requires the availability of datasets overarching various -omic disciplines and health record data; having such a system in place could facilitate the discovery and understanding individual differences in genotypes and exposures that account for specific cardiac phenotypes of each individual veterinary patient.
- Incorporation of personalized medicine into veterinary practice could result in early treatment and preventative recommendations for individual patients and/or a small population of individuals sharing similar disease and molecular profiles.

[a] Department of Medicine and Epidemiology, School of Veterinary Medicine, University of California-Davis, One Shields Avenue, Davis, CA 95616, USA; [b] Department of Clinical Sciences, College of Veterinary Medicine, North Carolina State University, 1038 William Moore Drive, Raleigh, NC 27606, USA
* Corresponding author.
E-mail address: yueda@ncsu.edu

Vet Clin Small Anim 53 (2023) 1255–1276
https://doi.org/10.1016/j.cvsm.2023.05.016

INTRODUCTION

Cardiomyopathies remain as one of the most common inherited cardiac diseases in both human and veterinary patients.[1–3] These adult-onset cardiac disorders are characterized by aberrant myocardial composition and structure which ultimately lead to impaired cardiac function causing a variety of clinical signs. The most common subtypes of cardiomyopathies include hypertrophic cardiomyopathy (HCM), dilated cardiomyopathy (DCM), and arrhythmogenic right ventricular cardiomyopathy (ARVC) in both human and animal populations, with HCM being the most pervasive. In the absence of phenocopies, the etiology of such primary cardiomyopathies are largely considered genetic and have been extensively studied over the preceding 20 years. To date, well over 100 mutated genes are known to cause cardiomyopathies in humans with a handful known in cats and dogs (**Fig. 1**, **Table 1**), commonly of sarcomeric, z-disk, and calcium handling ontology.[4] Despite this wealth of human genetic advancement, this number mostly represents case series of familial cardiomyopathies, where ~40% of population-based studies report failure to identify causal mutations. This is mostly due to the inherent heterogenous nature and allelic architecture of these complex diseases.[5,6] With the average cost of whole-genome sequencing (WGS) decreasing over the years, and as standardized pipelines for WGS analyses are becoming more accessible, whole-genome association studies (WGAS) have remained the gold-standard approach for genetic studies of the past decade, specifically for rare and simple mendelian traits.[7–9] While comparably few, simple, Mendelian inherited diseases remain for discovery in human and veterinary cardiology, the use of WGS still provides important information on genotype-phenotype relationships. This reduced cost and increased experience has led to a respective increase in the

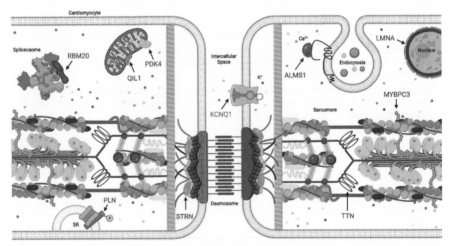

Fig. 1. Known pathogenic mutations of HCM, DCM, ARVC, and LQTS in companion animals. The protein products of genes with known pathogenic mutations in cats or dogs for HCM (*red*: MYBPC3, ALMS1), DCM (*blue*: PDK4, TTN, RBM20, PLN, and LMNA), ARVC (*green*: STRN), and LQTS (*purple*: KCNQ1) are illustrated with respect to protein function and localization within cardiomyocytes. ALMS1, Alström Syndrome-1; Ca²⁺, calcium; K⁺, potassium; KCNQ1, potassium voltage-gated channel subfamily Q member-1; LMNA, lamin-A; MYBPC3, myosin binding protein-C; P, phosphorus; PDK4, pyruvate dehydrogenase kinase-4; PLN, phospholamban; QIL1, MICOS complex subunit; RBM20, RNA-binding motif protein-20; SR, sarcoplasmic reticulum; STRN, striatin; TTN, titin.

Table 1
Known pathogenic mutations for common cardiovascular disease in companion animals

Disease	Gene Name	Protein/DNA Change	Mutation Type	Species	Breed	MOI	Proposed Pathogenesis
HCM	MYBPC3	A31P	Missense	Cat	Maine Coon	Autosomal dominant	Altered actin/myosin interaction, sarcomere hypercontractility
	MYBPC3	R820W	Missense	Cat	Ragdoll	Autosomal dominant	Altered myosin interaction, sarcomere hypercontractility
	ALMS1	G3376R	Missense	Cat	Sphynx	Autosomal dominant	Increased myocyte nuclear activity, compromised myocyte cell cycle arrest
DCM	PDK4	16-bp 5′ intron 10 deletion	Splice site deletion	Dog	Doberman	Autosomal dominant	Reduced metabolic flexibility, increased reliance on glycolytic energy production
	TTN	G8898R	Missense	Dog	Doberman	Autosomal dominant	Myofiber disarray, z-disk streaming, decreased protein springing
	RBM20	22-bp exon 11 deletion	Missense	Dog	Standard Schnauzer	Autosomal recessive	Abnormal intracellular calcium handling, altered cardiac transcript splicing
	PLN	R9H	Missense	Dog	Welsh Springer Spaniel	Autosomal dominant	Decreased myocardial calcium uptake
	QIL1	G109S	Missense	Dog	Rhodesian Ridgeback	Autosomal dominant	Hyperplastic mitochondria, irregular cristae formation, mitochondrial destabilization
	LMNA	D576T	Frameshift	Dog	Nova Scotia Duck Tolling Retriever	Autosomal recessive	Soft myocardial nuclear structures, altered chromatin organization, ventricular arrhythmogenesis
ARVC	STRN	8-bp 3′ UTR deletion	3′ UTR deletion	Dog	Boxer	Autosomal dominant	Myocardial infiltration of adipocytes and fibrosis, ventricular arrhythmogenesis
	ARVC2[a]	-	Missense	Dog	Boxer	Autosomal dominant	-
LQTS	KCNQ1	T377K	Missense	Dog	English Springer Spaniel	Autosomal dominant	Prolonged QT interval, ventricular arrhythmogenesis

Abbreviations: ALMS1, Alström Syndrome-1; ARVC, arrhythmogenic right ventricular cardiomyopathy; DCM, dilated cardiomyopathy; HCM, hypertrophic cardiomyopathy; KCNQ1, potassium voltage-gated channel subfamily Q member-1; LMNA, lamin-A; LQTS, long QT syndrome; MOI, mode of inheritance; MYBPC3, myosin binding protein-C; PDK4, pyruvate dehydrogenase kinase-4; PLN, phospholamban; QIL1, MICOS complex subunit; RBM20, RNA-binding motif protein-20; STRN, striatin; TTN, titin; UTR, untranslated region.
[a] Boxer ARVC2 mutation specifications not published.

use of personalized one-health approaches to cardiovascular case management in both human and veterinary medicine. Personalized medicine capitalizes on a priori knowledge of a patient's own genomic and/or proteomic profile to guide decisions for a more effective therapeutic intervention. The hope is that understanding the molecular basis of disease and the genetic architecture of the patient will unlock the next generation of targeted novel pharmaceuticals and aid in the reversal of detrimental effects at a molecular level. This review provides an updated understanding of the genetics and prognostication of the most common inherited cardiomyopathic disorders, as well as the most well-investigated pharmacogenetic discoveries in medications used for common cardiovascular diseases in dogs and cats.

INHERITED CARDIOMYOPATHIES
Hypertrophic Cardiomyopathy

Hypertrophic cardiomyopathy is the single most common inherited cardiac disorder with a prevalence of up to 0.29% and 15% in the human and cat population, respectively.[3,10–12] Cases of primary dog HCM are rare, yet disease incidence is thought to be one-tenth that of human and higher in smaller breeds such as terriers.[13,14] The disease is largely considered a disorder of the cardiac sarcomere, the single most basic unit of cardiac contraction, and is characterized by aberrant myocardial hypertrophy of the left ventricle (LV), diastolic dysfunction, and variably identifiable LV outflow tract obstruction. Hallmark pathologic features of HCM include hypertrophied LV cardiomyocytes, myofiber disarray, increased interstitial fibrosis, and structural alterations of intramural coronary arteries leading to regional myocardial ischemia. In humans, over 1500 HCM-associated genetic mutations have previously been reported; the majority harbored within 20 sarcomeric genes, although calcium-handling, z-disk, and lysosomal storage gene mutations have also demonstrated HCM pathogenicity. Despite cats having the greatest frequency of HCM diagnosis of any mammalian species, the total number of known pathogenic mutations remains markedly low. Currently, the only known causal mutations for HCM in cats remain breed-specific and do not explain the disease in the greater cat population. A candidate gene-led study revealed the first HCM mutation of any domestic animal species in Maine Coon cats. This mutation, referred to as A31P, is due to the substitution of a single nucleotide base which causes the amino acid to be altered from alanine to proline in the C0-C1 domain of myosin binding protein-C3 (MYBPC3) protein.[15–19] An R820W missense mutation in this same gene was later discovered exclusively in Ragdoll cats with HCM; genetic screening efforts in humans have identified this identical mutation in patients with HCM and LV non-compaction, making it the only reported, naturally occurring, shared HCM mutation between at least two mammalian species.[20,21] A recent study identified a novel Sphynx-specific guanine-to-cytosine missense mutation in the Alström syndrome-1 (ALMS1) gene via WGS. The mutation results in a highly conserved nonpolar glycine to substituted for a positively charged arginine amino acid. Albeit, the role of ALMS1 is not fully understood, particularly in HCM pathogenesis, Sphynx cats with the G3376R mutation exhibit increased myocyte nuclear activity, suggestive of compromised myocyte cell cycle arrest.[22] To date, genetic mutations underlying HCM in the general cat population, or in dogs with HCM, have yet to be reported.

The median survival time of cats affected by subclinical HCM in the general cat population is reported at 709 days.[23] In a recent retrospective study, the median survival times at the time of diagnosis for dogs with HCM ranged from one day to 114 months across 28 different breeds.[24] Maine Coon, Ragdoll, and Sphynx HCM mutations present in an autosomal dominant mode of inheritance (MOI) with incomplete and age-related penetrance. Penetrance is defined as the proportion of mutation positive individuals that express disease. Although cats only require one mutated allele to express the HCM phenotype, patients expressing two mutated allele copies commonly present with earlier disease onset and increased disease morbidity and mortality, therefore, decreasing their disease prognosis. In the general population, heterozygotes are more common than homozygotes for a given HCM mutation, perhaps due to earlier removal from the breeding population due to increased risk of the sudden cardiac death (SCD) and congestive heart failure (CHF) disease outcomes in homozygous patients.[25–27] Cat patients sharing the same HCM genotype can also express varying disease severity, regardless of similar diet, exercise, and environmental factors, for reasons that have yet to be explained.[25] Modifying variants, which alone do not cause an HCM phenotype, are thought to modulate disease severity and may explain a significant amount of the disease heterogeneity observed within cardiomyopathies.[28,29] Because mixed-bred and other pure-bred cats are also at high risk of developing HCM, researchers have attempted to elucidate shared and other breed-specific HCM mutations, though have not yet been successful.[25,30,31]

Dilated Cardiomyopathy

Primary DCM, not to be confused with nutritionally-mediated DCM, is the most common cardiomyopathy and the second most prevalent cardiac disease in dogs with a reported overall incidence of 0.5% to 10% in the general dog population, with higher rates reported in predisposed breeds.[32–39] The disease affects roughly one in 2500 humans and is rare in cats accounting for less than 5% of the total cardiomyopathies reported.[40–42] Primary DCM is caused by genetic mutations in genes of sarcomeric, calcium binding, cytoskeletal, and protein/receptor binding ontology that have a pathologic consequence of sarcomeric hypocontractility, a hallmark pathophysiologic feature of this disease. Characteristically, DCM-affected hearts show a dilated LV phenotype with reduced LV systolic function and subsequently reduced cardiac output. Histologically, two forms of DCM are described in dogs: fatty infiltration-degenerative and attenuated wavy fiber DCM.[43] More than 250 genes spanning greater than 10 gene ontologies have been associated with human DCM; in dogs, a total of seven individual mutations or genetic loci across five breeds have been identified.[44,45] An autosomal dominant splice site and missense mutation in *pyruvate dehydrogenase kinase-4* (*PDK4*) and *titin* (*TTN*) have been discovered in the Doberman breed (DCM1 & DCM2 mutations, respectively).[46,47] These variants are commonly employed in breed screening practices of Dobermans and may be used in tandem with 24-h ambulatory electrocardiogram and echocardiographic screening practices. An autosomal recessive 22 base-pair deletion mutation in a master cardiac splicing regulator gene, *RNA-binding motif protein-20* (*RBM20*), has been identified in Standard Schnauzers.[48] A variety of *de novo* mutations, which appear to be restricted to small families, have been described and are not currently considered a risk for the general breed population. Briefly, an R9H *phospholamban* (*PLN*) variant resulted in a large litter of Welsh Springer Spaniel puppies with severe, juvenile DCM.[38] In Rhodesian Ridgebacks, a mutation in *MICOS complex subunit* (*QIL1*) is associated with inherited ventricular arrythmias and SCD; this may represent a purely arrhythmic form of DCM or a separate disease category all together.[49] Dogs harboring this *QIL1* mutation display early onset of ventricular and/or supraventricular tachycardia and atrioventricular block, usually within seven to 12 months of age. A recently discovered frameshift mutation in the *lamin-A* (*LMNA*) gene results in severe myocardial fibrosis and DCM in Nova Scotia Duck Tolling Retrievers; this mutation is recessive in pattern of inheritance and results in severe juvenile DCM, variable cardiac arrhythmias, fulminant myocardial fibrosis, and most commonly SCD.[50] The extent of this mutation and disease in the general Nova Scotia Duck Tolling Retriever Population is unknown. In a genome-wide association study (GWAS) interrogating DCM-associated variants in a population of 190 Irish Wolfhounds, a total of six distinct single nucleotide polymorphisms (SNPs) were highly associated with the disease, but no causal variant has been determined: three of these SNPs identified are harbored within the *rho GTPase activating protein-8* (*ARHGAP8*), *follistatin-5* (*FSTL5*), and *phosphodi-esterase-3B* (*PDE3B*) genes, the other three reported SNPs are positioned within inter-genic regions of the dog genome.[51] The homozygous genotype of a deletion mutation in the 3′ untranslated region (UTR) of the *striatin* (*STRN*) gene is highly associated with a DCM phenotype in the boxer breed, although the primary disease is considered to be another type of cardiomyopathy (see "*Arrhythmogenic Right Ventricular Cardiomy-opathy*").[52] In German Shorthair Pointers, a spontaneous homozygous 3′ UTR muta-tion in the *Duchenne muscular dystrophy* (*DMD*) gene has been identified in two male littermates with non-primary DCM.[53] Similar to canine HCM, studies aimed to interrogate DCM-associated mutations in cats have yet to reported, likely because they are infrequently observed in veterinary clinical settings.[40]

Breed is an influential variable when prognosticating disease and survival times for a DCM-affected patient. DCM prognosis in veterinary patients remains poor; the average median survival time for symptomatic DCM in Doberman's and cats is 329 and 49 days, respectively, despite clinical intervention, representing the importance of early patient diagnosis.[54,55] Roughly 40% of humans with primary DCM are bearers of at least one copy of a DCM mutation; in cats and dogs with primary DCM, the inci-dence of disease-positive and genotype-negative dog patients have yet to be re-ported, although it is thought to closely recapitulate that of the human population.[56] In one study of DCM-positive Doberman Pinschers, 13% of the subjects were nega-tive for the reported *PDK4* and *TTN* gene mutations, suggesting at least one other cause of DCM in Dobermans exists within the population. That study highlighted that compound mutations were common (21%) and that those with the *PDK4* variant alone had the youngest reported age of presentation.[57] Ultimately, a given DCM mu-tation is dependent on the type of mutation and its effect on canonical protein func-tion.[58] Changes in protein amino acid charge, polarity, protein-protein binding, and 3D-folding result from changes in coding genetic sequences and can lead to a protein with null or hypomorphic function. The type of mutation will determine how much of the original proteins' function will be affected. For example, large structural mutations in a protein coding sequence, such as insertions and deletions, usually result in greater protein sequence alterations, therefore, the likelihood that the protein function will be altered increases. For smaller point mutations, their impact on wild-type protein func-tion is usually less severe, although, type of point mutation (ie, missense or nonsense), mutation position (ie, exon or intron), and conservations of the affected amino acids are considered when assessing its propensity at altering normal function.

Arrhythmogenic Right Ventricular Cardiomyopathy

Arrhythmogenic right ventricular cardiomyopathy is an autosomal dominant cardiac disorder with reduced penetrance that almost exclusively affects Boxers and English Bulldogs, and less commonly other dog breeds and cats. In humans, the disease is explained in 60% of patients harboring mutations that affect desmosomal and/or extra-desmosomal ontology. Given the low number of ARVC cases in dogs and cats, true estimates of the disease are lacking in the literature. In dogs, clinical man-ifestations of the disease are commonly reported by the age of five to seven years. The disease primarily affects the right ventricle (RV) and is characterized by the aberrant replacement of the myocardium with fatty fibrotic tissue. This aberrant compositional change alters myocardial electrical stability and results in patients experiencing ventricular arrhythmias such as ventricular premature complexes (VPCs) and ventricular tachycardia which may cause syncope and SCD events.[59] Histopathologically, ARVC is characterized by fibrofatty infiltrates where cardiomyocytes are substituted for mature adipocytes and mild interstitial fibrosis frequently extending from the epicardium to the endocardium.[60,61] Although incomplete penetrant, the only reported causal mutation for ARVC in companion animals is the previously mentioned *STRN* 3' UTR deletion in Boxers. This autosomal dominant mutation is inherited with incomplete and age-related penetrance. Like several other veterinary cardiomyopathies, the mutation in its homozygous form is associated with vastly more severe forms of the disease including higher number and more complex ventricular arrhythmias as well as structural changes to the left and right ventricles.[52] Boxers with a homozygous genotype of the *STRN* mutation frequently progress into developing a DCM phenotype (termed type III ARVC), albeit the primary disease is in fact ARVC.[52] Heterozygotes, on the other hand, do not progress into the more severe DCM phenocopy of ARVC as frequently, instead only display canonical histopathological features of the disease with no identifiable structural changes on echocardiography.[52] This suggests that genotyping Boxers for the *STRN* mutation may provide valuable information that impacts when cardiac screening via 24-h ambulatory electrocardiogram (ECG) and echocardiogram should be instituted (earlier for homozygous positive individuals). This degenerate interaction observed in Boxers is a great example of allelic architecture and demonstrates its importance in discerning the basic mechanisms responsible for common progressive cardiomyopathies in companion animals. Despite disease outcomes as severe as SCD, Boxers that are heterozygous for the *STRN* mutation and are treated for their ventricular arrhythmias have a normal life expectancy when compared to apparently healthy Boxers.[62] Finally, *STRN* mutation-negative Boxers have been described with clinical and/or histopathological evidence of ARVC suggesting the presence of at least one other mutation responsible for this disease in the breed. To that end, a second mutation (termed ARVC2) is now commercially tested, but not yet reported in the literature, limiting critical review of its association.

Arrhythmogenic right ventricular cardiomyopathy has been shown to affect a handful of cats in an autosomal dominant MOI with no reported breed overrepresentation as well as Bulldogs, where disease manifestations are similar. In cats and Bulldogs, common clinical features are owed to the significant structural change to the RV and include right-sided CHF characterized by caval and hepatic vein distention, abdominal effusion, and hepatosplenomegaly. Gross pathologic features of ARVC in cats and Bulldogs closely resemble those observed in human patients, including right heart enlargement, segmental or diffuse RV dilation, abnormal RV trabeculation, and aneurysm formations with apparently normal left heart features. Similar to Boxers, the hallmark histopathological feature associated with ARVC in cats and Bulldogs involves RV myocardial replacement with either fibrous or fibrofatty infiltrates. Reported patient median survival times range anywhere from two days to four months in cats after the first episode of CHF, and 12.4, 4.9, 8.3 months for subclinical, syncopal, and CHF-afflicted Bulldog cases, respectively.[63,64]

Long QT Syndrome

In a family of English Springer Spaniels, a mutation in *potassium voltage-gated channel subfamily Q member-1* (*KCNQ1*) results in long QT syndrome (LQTS) and arrhythmic sudden death.[65] This mutation appears to be de novo in this single extended family and is not currently recommended for testing in the dog population.

PHARMACOGENETICS IN CARDIOLOGY AND CARDIOVASCULAR THERAPY

It is well described that interindividual and breed-specific variability in drug response occurs in veterinary patients.[66] The intrinsic and extrinsic causes of these variabilities include altered bioavailability, drug-to-drug interactions, poor owner compliance, and pharmacogenetic effects. Pharmacogenetic research has principally focused on identifying and evaluating genetic polymorphisms in genes related to drug metabolism, drug transport systems, and drug targets. The potential benefits of pharmacogenetic-guided therapy include identifying individuals who benefit from a specific drug therapy, and who develop adverse drug reactions to a particular drug therapy. With an improved understanding of genetic variability among individuals and ethnicities, the concept of pharmacogenetics has been translated into clinical practice guiding the treatment of cardiovascular diseases in human patients.[67] Advancement in pharmacogenetic-based therapy in veterinary medicine has been outpaced by our human counterparts. Nevertheless, altered pharmacokinetics and pharmacodynamics, due to genetic polymorphisms, have been reported in various cardiovascular drugs in dogs and cats (**Fig. 2**).

Clopidogrel and P2RY1 polymorphism in cats

Clopidogrel is commonly used for preventing the development of thromboembolic complications in patients with various cardiac diseases. Once metabolized to its active

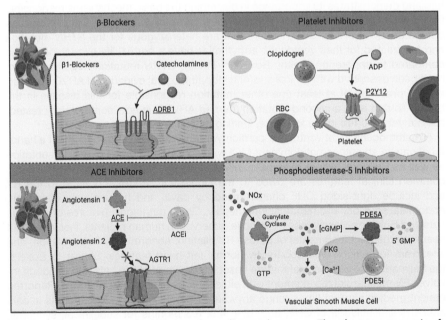

Fig. 2. Common pharmacologic targets in cardiovascular genes. The pharmacogenomic effects between consequential mutated proteins (*underlined*) and commonly used cardiovascular drugs in companion animals are illustrated. 5′ GMP, 5′ guanosine monophosphate; ACE, angiotensin-converting enzyme; ACEi, angiotensin-converting enzyme inhibitor; ADP, adenosine diphosphate; ADRB1, adrenoceptor beta-1; AGTR1, angiotensin II receptor type-1; Ca²⁺, calcium; cGMP, cyclic guanosine monophosphate; GTP, guanosine triphosphate; NOx, nitrous oxide; P2Y12, purinergic receptor; PDE5A, phosphodiesterase-5A; PDE5i, phosphodiesterase-5 inhibitor; PKG, protein kinase-G; RBC, red blood cell.

metabolite by the cytochrome P450 enzyme, it irreversibly inhibits a platelet adenosine diphosphate (ADP) receptor called P2Y12.[68] In humans, several clinical trials demonstrate that clopidogrel reduces incidence of thromboembolic complications.[69–71] A recent clinical study in cats with cardiomyopathy and arterial thromboembolism demonstrated a reduced risk of developing recurrent thromboembolic events by treating with clopidogrel, compared to aspirin.[72] However, various studies demonstrated that thromboembolic events frequently occur with variable responses to clopidogrel therapy.[72–74] Besides various causes of interindividual variability of drug responses as described above, genetic variants in the cytochrome P450 enzyme (CYP) and platelet ADP receptor genes have been investigated as possible causes of clopidogrel resistance in both humans and cats.[68,75–77] CYP2C19 polymorphisms have been investigated most frequently as a cause of clopidogrel resistance in people.[78] Individuals with two loss-of-function alleles in CYP2C19 are considered poor metabolizers (PMs) and have significantly reduced CYP2C19 enzymatic activity compared to normal metabolizers (NMs).[79] Intermediate metabolizers (IMs) have a single no-function allele and less enzymatic activity compared to NMs, but more activity than their PM counterparts. Multiple clinical trials have shown an increased risk of cardiovascular death, myocardial infarction, or stroke after percutaneous coronary intervention in IMs and PMs, compared to NMs when treated with appropriate doses of clopidogrel.[80,81] In cats with HCM, variable responses to clopidogrel treatment were also investigated by analyzing platelet function.[73] As in human patients, several non-synonymous polymorphisms in the CYP2C, P2RY1, and P2RY12 genes were identified.[77,82] Among these variants, a single genetic variant in the CYP2C41 gene was reported to associate with increased concentration of the clopidogrel active metabolite after administration in healthy cats.[82] In a subsequent clinical trial, the pharmacogenetic impact of the polymorphisms found in the cytochrome P450 and platelet ADP receptor genes (P2RY1 and P2RY12) on response to clopidogrel therapy was investigated in cats with HCM.[68] This study revealed that one of the polymorphisms in the P2RY1 gene (A236 G) was associated with significant reduction of platelet inhibition by clopidogrel therapy. Clopidogrel active metabolites inhibit P2Y12 but not the P2Y1, however, activation of the P2Y1 on the platelet surface induces a shape change of the platelet surface membrane and signals activation of P2Y12.[83,84] Therefore, a gain-of-function mutation of P2RY1 may reduce clopidogrel efficacy and explains why some cats do not respond as expected to clopidogrel therapy. These pharmacogenetic findings suggest that clinicians should seek alternative or additional antithrombotic agents in cats with the P2RY1 polymorphism, particularly when they have a high risk of developing thromboembolic complications.

Angiotensin-converting enzyme inhibitors and angiotensin-converting enzyme polymorphism in dogs

Angiotensin-converting enzyme (ACE) converts angiotensin I to angiotensin II, the primary enzyme for aldosterone synthesis and release. Angiotensin II and aldosterone are the key hormones for stimulating sodium and water retention and vasoconstriction, but also result in pathologic remodeling of vascular, cardiac, and renal tissues. ACE inhibitors are, therefore, commonly used drugs for managing heart disease in both human and veterinary patients.[85,86] Albeit, the effects of ACE inhibitors vary among individuals.[87] Also, the long-term administration of an ACE inhibitor sometimes fails to suppress aldosterone synthesis and release, and plasma concentration may even exceed the pre-treatment level. This phenomenon is called aldosterone breakthrough, which could result from enhanced ACE activity in response to chronic suppression of the renin angiotensin aldosterone system (RAAS) or increased levels of angiotensin II or aldosterone via alternative pathways independent of ACE activity.[88,89] In addition, *ACE* polymorphisms are proposed to contribute to interindividual variability of response to ACE inhibitors and development of aldosterone breakthrough.[87,90,91] In humans, an intronic *ACE* polymorphism has been demonstrated to increase basal ACE activity and increased angiotensin II levels.[92] Patients with the *ACE* polymorphism require a higher dose of ACE inhibitors to achieve therapeutic target. In dogs, a genetic polymorphism was identified in the same intron of the *ACE* gene.[93] This polymorphism further demonstrated breed predilections.[94,95] Three studies investigated the impact of *ACE* polymorphisms on ACE activity level.[94,96] Two of these studies found that dogs with the homozygous *ACE* variant had a lower ACE activity level than wildtype dogs.[94] However, the most recent study failed to demonstrate similar changes in the ACE activity level in dogs with *ACE* variants.[96] The discrepancy in the study findings could result from the different methodologies used for measuring ACE activity levels. Alternatively, the upregulation of other enzymes may counterbalance decreased ACE activity with *ACE* polymorphisms. Interestingly, the latter study also demonstrated that dogs with the *ACE* gene polymorphism had a significantly higher aldosterone level after the administration of the ACE inhibitor, enalapril, compared to wildtype dogs.[96] This finding implies that aldosterone breakthrough occurs more frequently in dogs harboring the *ACE* gene polymorphism compared to wildtype dogs. Additionally, an aldosterone to angiotensin II ratio after treatment with enalapril was higher in dogs with the *ACE* polymorphism, than in wildtype dogs, indicating the aldosterone breakthrough may not be due to enhanced angiotensin II synthesis with an increased ACE activity.[96] These findings suggests that the *ACE* polymorphism may influence the angiotensin II-independent pathway of aldosterone synthesis and release from the adrenal cortex, and that *ACE* polymorphism positivity may mediate an enhanced alternative route of aldosterone synthesis and release. These findings may underscore a need to consider alternative RAAS pathway mediation in dogs with the *ACE* polymorphism to limit the negative impacts of aldosterone breakthrough.

Adrenoceptor Beta-1 Antagonists and Adrenoceptor Beta-1 Polymorphisms in dogs and cats

β-adrenergic receptor antagonists, such as atenolol, are widely utilized for managing various cardiac diseases in both human and veterinary patients.[97–99] They have been demonstrated to increase ventricular diastolic filling time and reduce myocardial systolic wall stress.[100] Although various studies described the beneficial effects of β-blocker therapy, subgroups of patients with cardiac diseases do not respond as expected or even develop adverse drug reactions.[101] Two *adrenoreceptor-1 (ADRB1)* gene polymorphisms encoding the β-adrenergic receptors have been identified and are believed to be clinically relevant in humans.[102] These *ADRB1* gene polymorphisms are both gain-of-function variants augmenting the activity of β1-adrenergic receptors with increased heart rate, blood pressure, and left ventricular ejection fraction.

In dogs, two deletion polymorphisms were identified within *ADRB1* in various dog breeds with a high prevalence of cardiac diseases.[103] The structural and functional significance of these polymorphisms were investigated in clinically healthy dogs with the *ADRB1* polymorphisms.[104] In this study, the protein structure was altered at the cytoplasmic tail of the β1-adrenergic receptor. In a subsequent study, clinically healthy dogs with the *ADRB1* variants were evaluated for phenotypic differences in response to atenolol administration, compared to control dogs without the mutation. Lower heart rate was observed in dogs with thege *ADRB1* double deletion polymorphism for both pre- and post-atenolol administration. Because these polymorphisms occur commonly in canine breeds with a high prevalence of cardiac diseases, and these dogs may be more frequently treated with β1-adrenergic receptor antagonists, a pharmacogenetic approach to treatment may provide us beneficial effects with better management of these cardiac diseases.[66] In cats, three *ADRB1* polymorphisms have been identified.[105] One of these polymorphisms alters the amino acid sequence and computer modeling predicts an altered protein structure due to the genetic variants. Further studies are warranted to determine if this polymorphism changes response to β-blocker therapy or baseline disease characteristics.

Sildenafil with pulmonary hypertension and PDE5A polymorphism in dogs

Sildenafil is a selective phosphodiesterase-5 (PDE5) inhibitor used to treat patients with pulmonary hypertension (PH).[106,107] It exerts its main therapeutic effect by reducing pulmonary arterial (PA) pressure through cyclic guanosine monophosphate (cGMP) accumulation in the pulmonary vascular smooth muscle cells via inhibiting cGMP metabolism by phosphodiesterase.[108,109] Sildenafil also decreases PA resistance by preventing the proliferation of the pulmonary arterial wall.[110] Several experimental and clinical studies investigated the response to sildenafil therapy as a part of PH management in dogs.[111–113] Both experimental and clinical studies demonstrated that sildenafil therapy reduces PA pressure and improves clinical signs associated with PH.[111,114–116] Despite the overall positive response to sildenafil in PH patients, clinically significant interindividual variability, in response to sildenafil therapy, has been reported.[117] In humans, sildenafil is metabolized by the CYP3A and CYP2C9 isoenzymes, and genetic variants in genes encoding these isoenzymes appear to alter the effect of sildenafil therapy.[118–120] For example, one clinical study in human patients with heart failure demonstrated that genetic variants in *CYP3A4* were associated with decreased peak concentrations of sildenafil in the subpopulation of patients with heart failure.[120] Other investigators also identified and studied polymorphisms in the *PDE5A* gene encoding the PDE5 enzyme, where these variants in humans cause a reduced response to sildenafil with reduced nitric oxide and altered levels of cGMP concentrations.[121] Another mutation in *PDE5A* was also found to decrease the binding affinity of phosphodiesterase inhibitors to its receptor.[122]

A *PDE5A* gene polymorphism has also been identified in dogs.[123] The preliminary study reported lower basal cGMP concentrations in clinically healthy dogs homozygous for the *PDE5A* variant when compared to wildtype dogs.[123] The subsequent clinical trial investigated naturally occurring PH in dogs with *PDE5A* variants.[124] In this study, dogs with the *PDE5A* variant had a significantly worse quality of life (QOL) score than the wildtype group after four weeks of sildenafil treatment. The simple and multiple regression analyses also revealed that plasma cGMP levels and *PDE5A* variant status significantly predicted the reduction in QOL score after sildenafil treatment. This study demonstrated that the *PDE5A* variants blunt the therapeutic response to sildenafil in terms of QOL improvement after sildenafil therapy likely due to altered plasma cGMP level. This finding highlights the importance of investigating genetic mutations to better understand the interindividual variation of the efficacy of cardiovascular drugs.

CLINICAL APPLICATION OF PHARMACOGENETIC-GUIDED PHARMACOTHERAPY

Pharmacogenetic-guided therapy holds promise for increasing the efficacy of drugs, reducing adverse drug reactions in patients with cardiovascular diseases, and improving the outcome for these patients.[67] For example, clinical studies in human patients with cardiovascular diseases support improved outcomes with pharmacogenetic-guided therapies for *CYP2C19* gene polymorphisms in response to clopidogrel therapy.[125] Some hospitals perform genetic testing for the *CPY2C19* gene in patients with a high risk of cardiovascular events after the percutaneous coronary procedure, whereas other hospitals perform the genetic testing for most patients undergoing the procedure.[67] Nevertheless, most hospitals recommend alternative antiplatelet therapy for IMsS and PMsSms. Although the implementation of genetic testing in clinical settings is logistically challenging since it generally takes time to obtain the genetic test results, point-of-care or pre-emptive testing may overcome these challenges. In veterinary medicine, pharmacogenetics could also offer the possibility of implementing therapy-altering precision medicine for companion animals.[66,125] However, to establish pharmacogenetic-guided therapy, it is imperative to expand our genetic database in veterinary patients. Although there are only a few genetic tests related to pharmacogenetics currently available, recent advancements are likely to increase the availability of novel tests for companion animals. Additionally, studies have been performed with a whole genome-based approach, investigating the full spectrum of genetic variants from a pharmacogenomic approach. It is thus reasonable to anticipate that many new pharmacogenomic variants involved in various cardiovascular drug responses will be discovered, and the genetic database will be expanded for future clinical application. Ultimately, animals intended to receive the drugs discussed in this review for long-term therapy may benefit from the genetic screening of the aforementioned genetic variants and subsequent tailored therapy with alternative or additional therapeutic considerations.

FUTURE DIRECTIONS

In the past 20 years, animal genetics research has propelled the field of veterinary cardiology, primarily by elucidating the precise genetic and molecular pathogeneses of commonly acquired cardiomyopathies in companion animals. With better understanding of the molecular etiology of some cardiomyopathies, new treatment strategies aimed to target specific genes and/or proximal downstream pathways that mediate disease is possible. Albeit, the lack of clear genetic knowledge of many companion animal cardiovascular disease limits current direct treatment strategies for addressing the primary cause of disease. The continued gaps in knowledge behind the genetics of these cardiomyopathies in cats and dogs underscores the potential for improved understanding and the development and use of novel drug compounds aimed to reduce disease morbidity and premature mortality.

With advancements in disease identification and improved gene delivery techniques, enhanced veterinary cardiomyopathic treatment is more promising today than ever. The treatment of cardiomyopathies can be subdivided into two: direct pharmacologic or gene therapy intervention. Pharmacologic intervention refers to the administration of pharmaceutical compounds for direct or indirect disease prevention and/or treatment. In the case of cardiomyopathies, pharmacologic intervention remains the most common practice for disease treatment and mitigation of disease outcomes. In animals, direct pharmacologic intervention is lacking in the clinical setting. To date, there are no known pharmaceutical drugs that target the genetic etiology or molecular pathway of primary cardiomyopathies in veterinary patients. Instead, positive inotropic, antiarrhythmic, natriuretic, and antithrombotic drugs have been developed to target disease features and outcomes rather than the primary cause.[126–128]

Gene therapy refers to the medical approach for the treatment and prevention of disease by correcting the underlying genetic problem. Gene therapy for cardiac disorders in veterinary medicine are in their infancy, but hold promise at definitively targeting the genetic cause of HCM, DCM, and ARVC. The type of suitable gene therapy approach is dependent on the type of mutation. For single point mutations, like many described in veterinary cardiomyopathies, the most promising gene therapy approach is the utilization of CRISPR/cas9 techniques. CRISPR/cas9 is an adapted gene therapy mechanism from bacteria; researchers have modified this naturally occurring gene editing system in a way that allows for direct gene modification of a mutated gene.[129] Because all mammals are born with a fixed number of cardiomyocytes, to be effective in cardiology, CRISPR/cas9 gene editing would have to be performed at a very early stage of development in order to revert a mutated gene to its wildtype allele. Despite this scientific breakthrough, CRISPR/cas9 gene editing is in its early stages of development and has significant disadvantages due to its required early intervention, high risks of off-target effects which have the propensity of introducing random mutations throughout the genome, and requirement for use in point or small insertion/deletion mutations. A rather less invasive gene therapy method is gene replacement therapy, and it refers to the substitution of a known gene harboring a mutation with either complete or partial loss-of-function of its encoded protein product. Similar to CRISPR/cas9, in-utero utilization of gene replacement therapy has the potential to treat genetic cardiomyopathies before the onset of irreversible pathology. Gene replacement therapy requires the silencing of target endogenous mRNA expression for the administration of the wildtype gene sequence and its protein product. Two of the most understood methods of gene silencing are RNA interference (RNAi) and antisense oligonucleotides (ASOs), both of which use similar techniques for depleting endogenous expression of target genes via mRNA binding, subsequently inhibiting translation for protein synthesis.[130] Replacement of a null gene can be performed by coupling with CRISPR/cas9 methods, although other replacement methods involving viral and non-viral vectors exist. Robust, specific, and persistent delivery of viral and non-viral vectors expressing the exogenous wildtype allele to cardiomyocytes without generating a local or systemic toxicity continues to be a challenge in cardiovascular research. In adult human patients, delivery can be performed via direct myocardial injection, but can cause unnecessary acute myocardial degeneration, infarction, and fibrosis; this limits the use of this novel therapy in patients with more severe disease, therefore, making early identification of disease crucial.[131] A safer, less invasive, percutaneous catheter-based delivery method can be performed, but have yet to provide reliable results, specifically in patients with advanced disease.[132]

Pharmaceutical and gene therapy one-health approaches require the discovery of the genetics causing cardiomyopathies in patients. With only a handful of confirmed pathogenic mutations identified in veterinary patients with either HCM, DCM, or ARVC, the development of such therapies for use in the clinical setting remains limited and represents the primary challenge of contributing to a better understanding of these disorders. Commonly, genetic studies employ WGAS approaches for identifying causal genetic mutations, and although these methods serve as a powerful tool for genetic discovery, results are most high yielding when dealing with simple monogenic and homogenous disease traits. In terms of identifying cardiomyopathy variants in veterinary patients, case-control-based studies inherently introduce population admixture, disease-positive individuals with pathogenic mutations that are not shared across all affected individuals, and apparently unaffected controls that have yet to express disease phenotypes, all of which inevitably decrease study statistical power and success. To reduce the effects of this unforeseen variability, we encourage veterinary researchers to adopt robust phenotyping methods: the use of large population sizes, tight phenotype cut-off values, and adult/age-appropriate control individuals only. Because breeds exhibit their own genetic profile, gene-disease linkage, gene interactions, and environmental variables (ie, exposures, lifestyle, and health factors), allowing for only one breed in initial genetic studies can increase the success of identifying true casual mutations. Screening candidate mutations in larger validation populations comprised of multiple at-risk breeds as a subsequent step is required.

SUMMARY

The genetics of cardiomyopathies in veterinary patients is an area of great research need. Identifying optimal care for a unique patient profile rather than that of the average population is the basis of precision medicine. To maximize efficacy in veterinary cardiology, collaborations across veterinary and human research disciplines are necessary for the development of constantly changing data sets overarching standard clinical, laboratory testing, next-generation sequencing (NGS), metabolomics, proteomics, and health record data. The development of such a system will require network analytical and systems biology methods for identifying new relationships between disease traits that relies on the harnessing of artificial intelligence. Revolutionizing the prevention and treatment of cardiovascular diseases in veterinary patients will also require for this system to learn and evolve rapidly as the knowledge of cardiovascular diseases improves. Having such a system in place will allow for uncovering and understanding individual differences in genotypes and exposures that account for specific cardiac phenotypes of each individual veterinary patient, thereby, allowing early treatment and preventative recommendations for a single patient and/or a small population of individuals sharing similar molecular profiles. Identifying novel target pathways that mediate complex cardiovascular phenotypes will unlock new strategies for mitigating disease with minimal patient risk.

CLINICS CARE POINTS

- Genetic mutation status (homozygous vs heterozygous genotypes) can influence disease severity, onset, and outcomes particularly in HCM and ARVC.
- All currently cataloged pathogenic mutations for cardiovascular diseases in dogs and cats are referenced in **Table 1** for clinician use; however, genetic status alone is not indicative disease development and/or expression.
- Variability in response to common cardiovascular medications such as ACE inhibitors, antithrombotics, β-blockers, and phosphodiesterase inhibitors are at least partially explained by genetic variants can be tested for to guide therapy.

FUNDING SUPPORT

Support for V.N. Rivas was provided by NIH, United States T32 HL086350 and TL1 TR001861.

DISCLOSURE

The authors declare no disclosures or conflicts of interest.

REFERENCES

1. Hänselmann A, Veltmann C, Bauersachs J, et al. Dilated cardiomyopathies and non-compaction cardiomyopathy. Herz 2020;45(3):212–20. Dilatative Kardiomyopathien und Non-compaction-Kardiomyopathie.

2. Tuohy CV, Kaul S, Song HK, et al. Hypertrophic cardiomyopathy: the future of treatment. Eur J Heart Fail 2020;22(2):228–40.

3. Freeman LM, Rush JE, Stern JA, et al. Feline Hypertrophic Cardiomyopathy: A Spontaneous Large Animal Model of Human HCM. Cardiol Res 2017;8(4): 139–42.

4. Czepluch FS, Wollnik B, Hasenfuß G. Genetic determinants of heart failure: facts and numbers. ESC Heart Fail 2018;5(3):211–7.

5. Ingles J, Burns C, Bagnall RD, et al. Nonfamilial Hypertrophic Cardiomyopathy: Prevalence, Natural History, and Clinical Implications. Circ Cardiovasc Genet 2017;10(2). https://doi.org/10.1161/circgenetics.116.001620.

6. Ramaraj R. Hypertrophic cardiomyopathy: etiology, diagnosis, and treatment. Cardiol Rev 2008;16(4):172–80.

7. Kanzi AM, San JE, Chimukangara B, et al. Next Generation Sequencing and Bioinformatics Analysis of Family Genetic Inheritance. Front Genet 2020;11: 544162.

8. McCarthy MI, Abecasis GR, Cardon LR, et al. Genome-wide association studies for complex traits: consensus, uncertainty and challenges. Nat Rev Genet 2008; 9(5):356–69.

9. Schwarze K, Buchanan J, Fermont JM, et al. The complete costs of genome sequencing: a microcosting study in cancer and rare diseases from a single center in the United Kingdom. Genet Med 2020;22(1):85–94.

10. Zou Y, Song L, Wang Z, et al. Prevalence of idiopathic hypertrophic cardiomyopathy in China: a population-based echocardiographic analysis of 8080 adults. Am J Med 2004;116(1):14–8.

11. Maron BJ, Gardin JM, Flack JM, et al. Prevalence of hypertrophic cardiomyopathy in a general population of young adults. Echocardiographic analysis of 4111 subjects in the CARDIA Study. Coronary Artery Risk Development in (Young) Adults. Circulation 1995;92(4):785–9.

12. Maron BJ, Mathenge R, Casey SA, et al. Clinical profile of hypertrophic cardiomyopathy identified de novo in rural communities. J Am Coll Cardiol 1999;33(6): 1590–5.

13. Pang D, Rondenay Y, Helie P, et al. Sudden cardiac death associated with occult hypertrophic cardiomyopathy in a dog under anesthesia. Can Vet J 2005;46(12):1122–5.

14. Washizu M, Takemura N, Machida N, et al. Hypertrophic cardiomyopathy in an aged dog. J Vet Med Sci 2003;65(6):753–6.

15. Meurs KM, Sanchez X, David RM, et al. A cardiac myosin binding protein C mutation in the Maine Coon cat with familial hypertrophic cardiomyopathy. Hum Mol Genet 2005;14(23):3587–93.

16. Squire JM, Luther PK, Knupp C. Structural evidence for the interaction of C-protein (MyBP-C) with actin and sequence identification of a possible actin-binding domain. J Mol Biol 2003;331(3):713–24.

17. Oakley CE, Hambly BD, Curmi PM, et al. Myosin binding protein C: structural abnormalities in familial hypertrophic cardiomyopathy. Cell Res 2004;14(2): 95–110.

18. Witt CC, Gerull B, Davies MJ, et al. Hypercontractile properties of cardiac muscle fibers in a knock-in mouse model of cardiac myosin-binding protein-C. J Biol Chem 2001;276(7):5353–9.

19. Flavigny J, Souchet M, Sebillon P, et al. COOH-terminal truncated cardiac myosin-binding protein C mutants resulting from familial hypertrophic

cardiomyopathy mutations exhibit altered expression and/or incorporation in fetal rat cardiomyocytes. J Mol Biol 1999;294(2):443–56.

20. Meurs KM, Norgard MM, Ederer MM, et al. A substitution mutation in the myosin binding protein C gene in ragdoll hypertrophic cardiomyopathy. Genomics 2007;90(2):261–4.

21. Ripoll Vera T, Monserrat Iglesias L, Hermida Prieto M, et al. The R820W mutation in the MYBPC3 gene, associated with hypertrophic cardiomyopathy in cats, causes hypertrophic cardiomyopathy and left ventricular non-compaction in humans. Int J Cardiol 2010;145(2):405–7.

22. Meurs KM, Williams BG, DeProspero D, et al. A deleterious mutation in the ALMS1 gene in a naturally occurring model of hypertrophic cardiomyopathy in the Sphynx cat. Orphanet J Rare Dis 2021;16(1):108.

23. Rush JE, Freeman LM, Fenollosa NK, et al. Population and survival characteristics of cats with hypertrophic cardiomyopathy: 260 cases (1990-1999). J Am Vet Med Assoc 2002;220(2):202–7.

24. Schober KE, Fox PR, Abbott J, et al. Retrospective evaluation of hypertrophic cardiomyopathy in 68 dogs. J Vet Intern Med 2022;36(3):865–76.

25. Kittleson MD, Cote E. The Feline Cardiomyopathies: 2. Hypertrophic cardiomyopathy. J Feline Med Surg 2021;23(11):1028–51.

26. Longeri M, Ferrari P, Knafelz P, et al. Myosin-binding protein C DNA variants in domestic cats (A31P, A74T, R820W) and their association with hypertrophic cardiomyopathy. J Vet Intern Med 2013;27(2):275–85.

27. Kittleson MD, Meurs KM, Harris SP. The genetic basis of hypertrophic cardiomyopathy in cats and humans. J Vet Cardiol 2015;17(Suppl 1):S53–73.

28. Marian AJ. Modifier genes for hypertrophic cardiomyopathy. Curr Opin Cardiol 2002;17(3):242–52.

29. Brugada R, Kelsey W, Lechin M, et al. Role of candidate modifier genes on the phenotypic expression of hypertrophy in patients with hypertrophic cardiomyopathy. J Investig Med 1997;45(9):542–51.

30. Stern JA, Ueda Y. Inherited cardiomyopathies in veterinary medicine. Pflugers Arch 2019;471(5):745–53.

31. Meurs KM, Norgard MM, Kuan M, et al. Analysis of 8 sarcomeric candidate genes for feline hypertrophic cardiomyopathy mutations in cats with hypertrophic cardiomyopathy. J Vet Intern Med 2009;23(4):840–3.

32. Tidholm A, Jonsson L. A retrospective study of canine dilated cardiomyopathy (189 cases). J Am Anim Hosp Assoc 1997;33(6):544–50.

33. Dutton E, Lopez-Alvarez J. An update on canine cardiomyopathies - is it all in the genes? J Small Anim Pract 2018. https://doi.org/10.1111/jsap.12841.

34. Petric AD, Stabej P, Zemva A. Dilated cardiomyopathy in Doberman Pinschers: Survival, Causes of Death and a Pedigree Review in a Related Line. J Vet Cardiol 2002;4(1):17–24.

35. Meurs KM, Miller MW, Wright NA. Clinical features of dilated cardiomyopathy in Great Danes and results of a pedigree analysis: 17 cases (1990-2000). J Am Vet Med Assoc 2001;218(5):729–32.

36. Vollmar AC. The prevalence of cardiomyopathy in the Irish wolfhound: a clinical study of 500 dogs. J Am Anim Hosp Assoc 2000;36(2):125–32.

37. Legge CH, Lopez A, Hanna P, et al. Histological characterization of dilated cardiomyopathy in the juvenile toy Manchester terrier. Vet Pathol 2013;50(6):1043–52.

38. Yost O, Friedenberg SG, Jesty SA, et al. The R9H phospholamban mutation is associated with highly penetrant dilated cardiomyopathy and sudden death in a spontaneous canine model. Gene 2019;697:118–22.

39. Harmon MW, Leach SB, Lamb KE. Dilated Cardiomyopathy in Standard Schnauzers: Retrospective Study of 15 Cases. J Am Anim Hosp Assoc 2017; 53(1):38–44.

40. Kittleson MD, Cote E. The Feline Cardiomyopathies: 3. Cardiomyopathies other than HCM. J Feline Med Surg 2021;23(11):1053–67.

41. Grunig E, Tasman JA, Kucherer H, et al. Frequency and phenotypes of familial dilated cardiomyopathy. J Am Coll Cardiol 1998;31(1):186–94.

42. Bozkurt B, Colvin M, Cook J, et al. Current Diagnostic and Treatment Strategies for Specific Dilated Cardiomyopathies: A Scientific Statement From the American Heart Association. Circulation 2016;134(23):e579–646.

43. Tidholm A, Jonsson L. Histologic characterization of canine dilated cardiomyopathy. Vet Pathol 2005;42(1):1–8.

44. Jordan E, Peterson L, Ai T, et al. Evidence-Based Assessment of Genes in Dilated Cardiomyopathy. Circulation 2021;144(1):7–19.

45. Simpson S, Edwards J, Ferguson-Mignan TF, et al. Genetics of Human and Canine Dilated Cardiomyopathy. Int J Genomics 2015;2015:204823.

46. Meurs KM, Friedenberg SG, Kolb J, et al. A missense variant in the titin gene in Doberman pinscher dogs with familial dilated cardiomyopathy and sudden cardiac death. Hum Genet 2019;138(5):515–24.

47. Meurs KM, Lahmers S, Keene BW, et al. A splice site mutation in a gene encoding for PDK4, a mitochondrial protein, is associated with the development of dilated cardiomyopathy in the Doberman pinscher. Hum Genet 2012;131(8): 1319–25.

48. Leach SB, Johnson GS, Gilliam D, et al. Dilated cardiomyopathy in standard schnauzers with a homozygous 22 bp deletion in RBM20. In: Proceedings of the 32nd ACVIM Forum. 2014. Nashville, TN, USA.

49. Meurs KM, Friedenberg SG, Olby NJ, et al. A QIL1 Variant Associated with Ventricular Arrhythmias and Sudden Cardiac Death in the Juvenile Rhodesian Ridgeback Dog. Genes 2019;10(2). https://doi.org/10.3390/genes10020168.

50. Oertle DT, Batcher KL, Stern JA, et al. Sudden death and cardiomyopathy associated with LMNA in the Nova Scotia Duck Tolling Retriever. In: Proceedings of the UC Davis Student Training in Advanced Research (STAR) Symposium. 2022.

51. Philipp U, Vollmar A, Haggstrom J, et al. Multiple Loci are associated with dilated cardiomyopathy in Irish wolfhounds. PLoS One 2012;7(6):e36691.

52. Meurs KM, Stern JA, Sisson DD, et al. Association of dilated cardiomyopathy with the striatin mutation genotype in boxer dogs. J Vet Intern Med 2013;27(6): 1437–40.

53. Schatzberg SJ, Olby NJ, Breen M, et al. Molecular analysis of a spontaneous dystrophin 'knockout' dog. Neuromuscul Disord 1999;9(5):289–95.

54. Fuentes VL, Corcoran B, French A, et al. A double-blind, randomized, placebo-controlled study of pimobendan in dogs with dilated cardiomyopathy. J Vet Intern Med 2002;16(3):255–61.

55. Hambrook LE, Bennett PF. Effect of pimobendan on the clinical outcome and survival of cats with non-taurine responsive dilated cardiomyopathy. J Feline Med Surg 2012;14(4):233–9.

56. Ganesh SK, Arnett DK, Assimes TL, et al. Genetics and genomics for the prevention and treatment of cardiovascular disease: update: a scientific statement from the American Heart Association. Circulation 2013;128(25):2813–51.

57. Meurs KM, Stern JA, Adin D, et al. Assessment of PDK4 and TTN gene variants in 48 Doberman Pinschers with dilated cardiomyopathy. J Am Vet Med Assoc 2020;257(10):1041–4.

58. Jacoby D, McKenna WJ. Genetics of inherited cardiomyopathy. Eur Heart J 2012;33(3):296–304.

59. Cunningham SM, Dos Santos L. Arrhythmogenic right ventricular cardiomyopathy in dogs. J Vet Cardiol 2022;40:156–69.

60. Basso C, Fox PR, Meurs KM, et al. Arrhythmogenic right ventricular cardiomyopathy causing sudden cardiac death in boxer dogs: a new animal model of human disease. Circulation 2004;109(9):1180–5.

61. Nakao S, Hirakawa A, Yamamoto S, et al. Pathological features of arrhythmogenic right ventricular cardiomyopathy in middle-aged dogs. J Vet Med Sci 2011;73(8):1031–6.

62. Meurs KM, Stern JA, Reina-Doreste Y, et al. Natural history of arrhythmogenic right ventricular cardiomyopathy in the boxer dog: a prospective study. J Vet Intern Med 2014;28(4):1214–20.

63. Cunningham SM, Sweeney JT, MacGregor J, et al. Clinical Features of English Bulldogs with Presumed Arrhythmogenic Right Ventricular Cardiomyopathy: 31 Cases (2001-2013). J Am Anim Hosp Assoc 2018;54(2):95–102.

64. Fox PR, Maron BJ, Basso C, et al. Spontaneously occurring arrhythmogenic right ventricular cardiomyopathy in the domestic cat: A new animal model similar to the human disease. Circulation 2000;102(15):1863–70.

65. Ware WA, Reina-Doreste Y, Stern JA, et al. Sudden death associated with QT interval prolongation and KCNQ1 gene mutation in a family of English Springer Spaniels. J Vet Intern Med 2015;29(2):561–8.

66. Mealey KL, Martinez SE, Villarino NF, et al. Personalized medicine: going to the dogs? Hum Genet 2019;138(5):467–81.

67. Duarte JD, Cavallari LH. Pharmacogenetics to guide cardiovascular drug therapy. Nat Rev Cardiol 2021;18(9):649–65.

68. Ueda Y, Li RHL, Nguyen N, et al. A genetic polymorphism in P2RY(1) impacts response to clopidogrel in cats with hypertrophic cardiomyopathy. Sci Rep 2021;11(1):12522.

69. Sabatine MS, Cannon CP, Gibson CM, et al. Effect of clopidogrel pretreatment before percutaneous coronary intervention in patients with ST-elevation myocardial infarction treated with fibrinolytics: the PCI-CLARITY study. JAMA 2005; 294(10):1224–32.

70. Chen ZM, Jiang LX, Chen YP, et al. Addition of clopidogrel to aspirin in 45,852 patients with acute myocardial infarction: randomised placebo-controlled trial. Lancet 2005;366(9497):1607–21.

71. Yusuf S, Zhao F, Mehta SR, et al. Effects of clopidogrel in addition to aspirin in patients with acute coronary syndromes without ST-segment elevation. N Engl J Med 2001;345(7):494–502.

72. Hogan DF, Fox PR, Jacob K, et al. Secondary prevention of cardiogenic arterial thromboembolism in the cat: The double-blind, randomized, positive-controlled feline arterial thromboembolism; clopidogrel vs. aspirin trial (FAT CAT). J Vet Cardiol 2015;17(Suppl 1):S306–17.

73. Li RH, Stern JA, Ho V, et al. Platelet Activation and Clopidogrel Effects on ADP-Induced Platelet Activation in Cats with or without the A31P Mutation in MYBPC3. J Vet Intern Med 2016;30(5):1619–29.

74. Mallouk N, Labruyere C, Reny JL, et al. Prevalence of poor biological response to clopidogrel: a systematic review. Thromb Haemost 2012;107(3):494–506.

75. So DY, Wells GA, McPherson R, et al. A prospective randomized evaluation of a pharmacogenomic approach to antiplatelet therapy among patients with ST-elevation myocardial infarction: the RAPID STEMI study. Pharmacogenomics J 2016;16(1):71–8.

76. Yi X, Zhou Q, Wang C, et al. Platelet receptor Gene (P2Y12, P2Y1) and platelet glycoprotein Gene (GPIIIa) polymorphisms are associated with antiplatelet drug responsiveness and clinical outcomes after acute minor ischemic stroke. Eur J Clin Pharmacol 2017;73(4):437–43.

77. Ueda Y, Li RHL, Tablin F, et al. Nonsynonymous single nucleotide polymorphisms in candidate genes P2RY1, P2RY12 and CYP2C19 for clopidogrel efficacy in cats. Anim Genet 2018;49(4):356–7.

78. Diaz-Villamarin X, Davila-Fajardo CL, Martinez-Gonzalez LJ, et al. Genetic polymorphisms influence on the response to clopidogrel in peripheral artery disease patients following percutaneous transluminal angioplasty. Pharmacogenomics 2016;17(12):1327–38.

79. Lee CR, Luzum JA, Sangkuhl K, et al. Clinical Pharmacogenetics Implementation Consortium Guideline for CYP2C19 Genotype and Clopidogrel Therapy: 2022 Update. Clin Pharmacol Ther 2022;112(5):959–67.

80. Mega JL, Close SL, Wiviott SD, et al. Cytochrome P450 genetic polymorphisms and the response to prasugrel: relationship to pharmacokinetic, pharmacodynamic, and clinical outcomes. Circulation 2009;119(19):2553–60.

81. Mega JL, Simon T, Collet JP, et al. Reduced-function CYP2C19 genotype and risk of adverse clinical outcomes among patients treated with clopidogrel predominantly for PCI: a meta-analysis. JAMA 2010;304(16):1821–30.

82. Lee PM, Faus MCL, Court MH. High interindividual variability in plasma clopidogrel active metabolite concentrations in healthy cats is associated with sex and cytochrome P450 2C genetic polymorphism. J Vet Pharmacol Ther. Jan 2019;42(1):16–25.

83. Hetherington SL, Singh RK, Lodwick D, et al. Dimorphism in the P2Y1 ADP receptor gene is associated with increased platelet activation response to ADP. Arterioscler Thromb Vasc Biol 2005;25(1):252–7.

84. Lev EI, Patel RT, Guthikonda S, et al. Genetic polymorphisms of the platelet receptors P2Y(12), P2Y(1) and GP IIIa and response to aspirin and clopidogrel. Thromb Res 2007;119(3):355–60.

85. Borghi C, Force ST, Rossi F, et al. Role of the Renin-Angiotensin-Aldosterone System and Its Pharmacological Inhibitors in Cardiovascular Diseases: Complex and Critical Issues. High Blood Press Cardiovasc Prev 2015;22(4):429–44.

86. Pfeffer MA, Frohlich ED. Improvements in clinical outcomes with the use of angiotensin-converting enzyme inhibitors: cross-fertilization between clinical and basic investigation. Am J Physiol Heart Circ Physiol 2006;291(5):H2021–5.

87. Danilov SM, Tovsky SI, Schwartz DE, et al. ACE Phenotyping as a Guide Toward Personalized Therapy With ACE Inhibitors. J Cardiovasc Pharmacol Ther 2017; 22(4):374–86.

88. Ames MK, Vaden SL, Atkins CE, et al. Prevalence of aldosterone breakthrough in dogs receiving renin-angiotensin system inhibitors for proteinuric chronic kidney disease. J Vet Intern Med 2022;36(6):2088–97.

89. Mogi M. Aldosterone breakthrough from a pharmacological perspective. Hypertens Res 2022;45(6):967–75.

90. Schilders JE, Wu H, Boomsma F, et al. Renin-angiotensin system phenotyping as a guidance toward personalized medicine for ACE inhibitors: can the

response to ACE inhibition be predicted on the basis of plasma renin or ACE? Cardiovasc Drugs Ther 2014;28(4):335–45.

91. Mayer G. ACE genotype and ACE inhibitor response in kidney disease: a perspective. Am J Kidney Dis 2002;40(2):227–35.

92. Tiret L, Rigat B, Visvikis S, et al. Evidence, from combined segregation and linkage analysis, that a variant of the angiotensin I-converting enzyme (ACE) gene controls plasma ACE levels. Am J Hum Genet 1992;51(1):197–205.

93. Meurs KM, Chdid L, Reina-Doreste Y, et al. Polymorphisms in the canine and feline renin-angiotensin-aldosterone system genes. Anim Genet 2015;46(2):226.

94. Meurs KM, Stern JA, Atkins CE, et al. Angiotensin-converting enzyme activity and inhibition in dogs with cardiac disease and an angiotensin-converting enzyme polymorphism. J Renin Angiotensin Aldosterone Syst 2017;18(4). 1470320317737184.

95. Adin DB, Atkins CE, Friedenberg SG, et al. Prevalence of an angiotensin-converting enzyme gene variant in dogs. Canine Med Genet 2021;8(1):6.

96. Adin D, Atkins C, Domenig O, et al. Renin-angiotensin aldosterone profile before and after angiotensin-converting enzyme-inhibitor administration in dogs with angiotensin-converting enzyme gene polymorphism. J Vet Intern Med 2020; 34(2):600–6.

97. Darbar D. Genomics, heart failure and sudden cardiac death. Heart Fail Rev 2010;15(3):229–38.

98. Shin J, Johnson JA. Beta-blocker pharmacogenetics in heart failure. Heart Fail Rev 2010;15(3):187–96.

99. Oyama MA, Sisson DD, Prosek R, et al. Carvedilol in dogs with dilated cardiomyopathy. J Vet Intern Med 2007;21(6):1272–9.

100. Kveiborg B, Major-Petersen A, Christiansen B, et al. Carvedilol in the treatment of chronic heart failure: lessons from the Carvedilol Or Metoprolol European Trial. Vasc Health Risk Manag 2007;3(1):31–7.

101. Podlowski S, Wenzel K, Luther HP, et al. Beta1-adrenoceptor gene variations: a role in idiopathic dilated cardiomyopathy? J Mol Med (Berl) 2000;78(2):87–93.

102. Parry HM, Doney AS, Palmer CN, et al. State of play of pharmacogenetics and personalized medicine in heart failure. Cardiovasc Ther 2013;31(6):315–22.

103. Maran BA, Mealey KL, Lahmers SM, et al. Identification of DNA variants in the canine beta-1 adrenergic receptor gene. Res Vet Sci 2013;95(1):238–40.

104. Meurs KM, Stern JA, Reina-Doreste Y, et al. Impact of the canine double-deletion beta1 adrenoreceptor polymorphisms on protein structure and heart rate response to atenolol, a beta1-selective beta-blocker. Pharmacogenet Genomics 2015;25(9):427–31.

105. Maran BA, Meurs KM, Lahmers SM, et al. Identification of beta-1 adrenergic receptor polymorphisms in cats. Res Vet Sci 2012;93(1):210–2.

106. Michelakis ED, Tymchak W, Noga M, et al. Long-term treatment with oral sildenafil is safe and improves functional capacity and hemodynamics in patients with pulmonary arterial hypertension. Circulation 2003;108(17):2066–9.

107. Galie N, Ghofrani HA, Torbicki A, et al. Sildenafil citrate therapy for pulmonary arterial hypertension. N Engl J Med 2005;353(20):2148–57.

108. Corbin JD, Francis SH. Cyclic GMP phosphodiesterase-5: target of sildenafil. J Biol Chem 1999;274(20):13729–32.

109. Shekerdemian LS, Ravn HB, Penny DJ. Intravenous sildenafil lowers pulmonary vascular resistance in a model of neonatal pulmonary hypertension. Am J Respir Crit Care Med 2002;165(8):1098–102.

110. Tantini B, Manes A, Fiumana E, et al. Antiproliferative effect of sildenafil on human pulmonary artery smooth muscle cells. Basic Res Cardiol 2005;100(2): 131–8.

111. Kellum HB, Stepien RL. Sildenafil citrate therapy in 22 dogs with pulmonary hypertension. J Vet Intern Med 2007;21(6):1258–64.

112. Brown AJ, Davison E, Sleeper MM. Clinical efficacy of sildenafil in treatment of pulmonary arterial hypertension in dogs. J Vet Intern Med 2010;24(4):850–4.

113. Kellihan HB, Waller KR, Pinkos A, et al. Acute resolution of pulmonary alveolar infiltrates in 10 dogs with pulmonary hypertension treated with sildenafil citrate: 2005-2014. J Vet Cardiol 2015;17(3):182–91.

114. Mondritzki T, Boehme P, Schramm L, et al. New pulmonary hypertension model in conscious dogs to investigate pulmonary-selectivity of acute pharmacological interventions. Eur J Appl Physiol 2018;118(1):195–203.

115. Murphy LA, Russell N, Bianco D, et al. Retrospective evaluation of pimobendan and sildenafil therapy for severe pulmonary hypertension due to lung disease and hypoxia in 28 dogs (2007-2013). Vet Med Sci 2017;3(2):99–106.

116. Johnson LR, Stern JA. Clinical features and outcome in 25 dogs with respiratory-associated pulmonary hypertension treated with sildenafil. J Vet Intern Med 2020;34(1):65–73.

117. Kanjanawart S, Gaysonsiri D, Tangsucharit P, et al. Comparative bioavailability of two sildenafil tablet formulations after single-dose administration in healthy Thai male volunteers. Int J Clin Pharmacol Ther 2011;49(8):525–30.

118. Shon JH, Ku HY, Bae SY, et al. The disposition of three phosphodiesterase type 5 inhibitors, vardenafil, sildenafil, and udenafil, is differently influenced by the CYP3A5 genotype. Pharmacogenet Genomics 2011;21(12):820–8.

119. Jetter A, Lazar A, Schomig E, et al. The CYP2C9 genotype does not influence sildenafil pharmacokinetics in healthy volunteers. Clin Pharmacol Ther 2005; 78(4):441–3.

120. de Denus S, Rouleau JL, Mann DL, et al. CYP3A4 genotype is associated with sildenafil concentrations in patients with heart failure with preserved ejection fraction. Pharmacogenomics J 2018;18(2):232–7.

121. Lin CS, Chow S, Lau A, et al. Human PDE5A gene encodes three PDE5 isoforms from two alternate promoters. Int J Impot Res 2002;14(1):15–24.

122. Cahill KB, Quade JH, Carleton KL, et al. Identification of amino acid residues responsible for the selectivity of tadalafil binding to two closely related phosphodiesterases, PDE5 and PDE6. J Biol Chem 2012;287(49):41406–16.

123. Stern JA, Reina-Doreste Y, Chdid L, et al. Identification of PDE5A:E90K: a polymorphism in the canine phosphodiesterase 5A gene affecting basal cGMP concentrations of healthy dogs. J Vet Intern Med 2014;28(1):78–83.

124. Ueda Y, Johnson LR, Ontiveros ES, et al. Effect of a phosphodiesterase-5A (PDE5A) gene polymorphism on response to sildenafil therapy in canine pulmonary hypertension. Sci Rep 2019;9(1):6899.

125. Campion DP, Dowell FJ. Translating Pharmacogenetics and Pharmacogenomics to the Clinic: Progress in Human and Veterinary Medicine. Front Vet Sci 2019; 6:22.

126. Cooke KL, Snyder PS. Calcium channel blockers in veterinary medicine. J Vet Intern Med 1998;12(3):123–31.

127. Lo ST, Walker AL, Georges CJ, et al. Dual therapy with clopidogrel and rivaroxaban in cats with thromboembolic disease. J Feline Med Surg 2022;24(4): 277–83.

128. de Lima GV, Ferreira FDS. N-terminal-pro brain natriuretic peptides in dogs and cats: A technical and clinical review. Vet World 2017;10(9):1072–82.
129. Li H, Yang Y, Hong W, et al. Applications of genome editing technology in the targeted therapy of human diseases: mechanisms, advances and prospects. Signal Transduct Target Ther 2020;5(1):1.
130. Chery J. RNA therapeutics: RNAi and antisense mechanisms and clinical applications. Postdoc J 2016;4(7):35–50.
131. Ishikawa K, Tilemann L, Fish K, et al. Gene delivery methods in cardiac gene therapy. J Gene Med 2011;13(10):566–72.
132. Shah AS, Lilly RE, Kypson AP, et al. Intracoronary adenovirus-mediated delivery and overexpression of the beta(2)-adrenergic receptor in the heart : prospects for molecular ventricular assistance. Circulation 2000;101(4):408–14.

Predicting Development of Hypertrophic Cardiomyopathy and Disease Outcomes in Cats

Jose Novo Matos, DVM, PhD[a],*,
Jessie Rose Payne, BVetMed, MvetMed, PhD[b]

KEYWORDS

- Arterial thromboembolism • Cardiac death • Congestive heart failure
- Echocardiography • Elongated mitral valve • Left atrial systolic function
- Genotype positive/phenotype negative • Pre-phenotypic

KEY POINTS

- Hypertrophic cardiomyopathy (HCM) is associated with echocardiographic structural and functional changes before left ventricular hypertrophy (overt HCM) is observed (pre-phenotypic changes).
- Echocardiographic features that have been shown to predict the development of HCM in cats include decreased left atrial fractional shortening and an elongated anterior mitral valve leaflet.
- Prognosis for cats with HCM is very variable, with some cats dying of congestive heart failure, arterial thromboembolism, or sudden death, whereas in other cats, death is unrelated to the cardiac disease.
- Independent predictors of outcome include measures of left atrial size and function.
- Novel treatments aiming to modulate HCM and delay its progression should ideally target patients at risk of developing HCM and patients with high-risk HCM; therefore, detecting these subpopulations in clinical practice is paramount.

INTRODUCTION

Hypertrophic cardiomyopathy (HCM) is a myocardial disease in humans and cats characterized by a hypertrophied and non-dilated left ventricle in the absence of abnormal loading conditions, such as other cardiac or systemic disease capable of

[a] Department of Veterinary Medicine, University of Cambridge, Madingley Road, Cambridge CB3 0ES, UK; [b] Langford Vets Small Animal Referral Hospital, University of Bristol, Langford House, Langford BS40 5DU, UK
* Corresponding author.
E-mail address: jms330@cam.ac.uk

Vet Clin Small Anim 53 (2023) 1277–1292
https://doi.org/10.1016/j.cvsm.2023.05.012
0195-5616/23/© 2023 Elsevier Inc. All rights reserved.

producing left ventricular hypertrophy (LVH).[1–3] HCM is the most common heart disease in cats affecting up to 15% of the general feline population, that is, approximately one in seven cats.[4,5]

Echocardiography is the clinical gold standard for HCM diagnosis in cats, and the primary and most commonly used diagnostic modality in humans.[2,3,6] Echocardiography is also used for prognostication and follow-up of HCM patients.[7] The morphologic hallmark of HCM is LVH, and thus, the diagnosis is based on the measurement of maximal diastolic left ventricular (LV) wall thickness on echocardiography. Besides LVH, other important pathologic features in HCM include myocardial fibrosis (interstitial and replacement), small vessel disease (intramural arteriosclerosis), and myocyte disarray, which cannot be quantified on echocardiography but also affect LV myocardial function and outcomes.[1,8–11] All these morphologic changes contribute to HCM functional hallmark of LV diastolic dysfunction.[8] Systolic function is classically hyperdynamic; however, in some cases, LV systolic impairment occurs associated with marked myocardial fibrosis.[12,13] Occasionally, thin and hypokinetic myocardial LV segments are observed on echocardiography and seem to be caused by regional transmural myocardial scars.[14]

Diastolic function can be assessed on echocardiography by standard Doppler, tissue Doppler, and speckle-tracking imaging,[15,16] but left atrial (LA) size and function also reflect LV diastolic function in HCM. LA size has been considered a morphophysiologic expression of LV diastolic function[17]; thus, LA dilation reflects severity and chronicity of diastolic dysfunction.[18] LA remodeling (dilation) and dysfunction are associated with worsening diastolic function and disease progression.[15–17]

Another important and common feature of human and feline HCM is the presence of systolic anterior motion of the mitral valve (SAM) causing dynamic LV outflow tract obstruction.[2,19,20] Echocardiography also plays a major role at identifying SAM and grading LV outflow tract obstruction severity.[20]

Prognosis for cats with HCM is very variable, with median survival times from diagnosis in large, heterogenous populations being reported as 596 to 1276 days.[21–26] Cardiac-related deaths include sudden cardiac death, death due to congestive heart failure (CHF) and death due to arterial thromboembolism (ATE).[22,26–29] However, 18.6% to 25.7% of cats with HCM die due to noncardiac causes[22,24] and numerous studies have identified cats being diagnosed with HCM at ≥16 years of age,[21–25] suggesting that HCM may have a relatively benign course in some individuals.

Predicting which cats are at an increased risk of developing HCM and which cats with HCM are more likely to develop cardiovascular events or die of HCM are highly desirable goals in clinical cardiology, as these will impact patient's prognosis and management. Predicting HCM and adverse outcomes (high-risk HCM phenotypes) will help identifying and targeting which patients might profit from treatment and early interventions. These will become increasingly relevant as treatments that can modify disease progression are identified.

PREDICTING DEVELOPMENT OF HYPERTROPHIC CARDIOMYOPATHY

In people, changes in LV function and geometry precede LVH, suggesting that LVH is not the first manifestation of HCM[30]; thus, it is likely that HCM has a spectrum of phenotypic changes which start even before an increase in LV wall thickness is apparent.

Several recent studies in humans have looked for HCM pre-phenotypic changes, that is, clinical and echocardiographic characteristics that precede LVH (overt HCM). These studies have focused on genotype positive/phenotype (LVH) negative (G+/LVH-) individuals, that is, HCM mutation carriers that have not yet fully developed the disease phenotype (LVH), which are a subgroup of people revealed by the exponential growth in clinical genetics.[31,32] Certain clinical characteristics have been suggested to precede the development of LVH (overt HCM), including increased LV ejection fraction,[30,33,34] impaired LA function,[35] systolic and diastolic myocardial dysfunction on tissue Doppler imaging and strain,[33,36–39] smaller LV diameters and volumes,[30] ECG changes,[34,40–42] elongated mitral valve leaflets,[34,43,44] myocardial crypts,[43,45] higher N-terminal pro-B-type natriuretic peptide,[34] impaired myocardial energetics,[46] and profibrotic state.[47,48]

So far, only a few mutations causing HCM have been described in cats,[49–52] so the genotype in most cats is unknown. Nevertheless, some of the echocardiographic features identified in humans as pre-phenotypic HCM might also help predicting which cats are at an increased risk of developing HCM.

A recent prospective longitudinal study in cats from rehoming centers (CatScan II study)[28] followed a cohort of cats that were normal at baseline and developed HCM during the study period, and assessed for baseline echocardiographic variables that were associated with an increased risk of developing HCM. Most cats in the CatScan population were non-pedigree and thus were not genotyped, so it is not known whether they had sarcomere gene mutations and included individuals that were G+/LVH−. Nevertheless, multivariable analysis showed that decreased LA systolic function (measured by LA fractional shortening [LA%FS]) and increased LV systolic function (measured by LV fractional shortening [LV%FS]) were independent predictors of an increased hazard for developing HCM.

Another study has also recently shown that normal cats with elongated anterior mitral valve leaflet had an increased risk of developing HCM.[53] It has also been speculated that Maine Coon cats carrying MYBPC3 A31P mutation have diastolic dysfunction before developing LVH.[54–56]

Decreased Left Atrial Fractional Shortening

The CatScan II study suggested that decreased LA%FS is an HCM pre-phenotypic change in cats, as cats that developed HCM had a decreased LA%FS at baseline (**Fig. 1**), even though they had a normal LA size. Likewise, in people, LA dysfunction

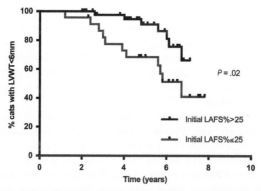

Fig. 1. The CatScan II study followed normal cats over time and showed that cats with lower left atrial fractional shortening (LA%FS) had an increased risk of developing hypertrophic cardiomyopathy later in life. This Kaplan–Meier curve shows the percentage of cats developing HCM over time according to their initial LA%FS. (*Data from* Novo Matos J, Payne JR, Seo J, et al. Natural history of hypertrophic cardiomyopathy in cats from rehoming centers: The CatScan II study. *J Vet Intern Med* 2022;36:1900–1912.)

with normal LA size has been suggested as an HCM early phenotypic change.[35] In people, there is a profibrotic state and interstitial myocardial fibrosis before development of LVH, which might cause abnormal myocardial tissue properties.[48] Therefore, it has been speculated that LA dysfunction reflects early changes in myocardial tissue composition.[35] A recent study showed that LA%FS in cats with subclinical HCM (cats with no history of clinical signs, stage B) was correlated with LV extracellular volume, a measure of interstitial fibrosis, but not with LV wall thickness.[57] Abnormal collagen metabolism has been also suggested in G+/LVH− Ragdoll cats (ie, MYBPC3 R820W mutation carriers),[58] and interstitial fibrosis has been described on histopathology in cats diagnosed antemortem with mild subclinical HCM.[59] Thus, LA dysfunction in cats might, as in humans, reflect abnormal myocardial properties that precede overt HCM.

Increased Left Ventricular Fractional Shortening

The CatScan II study also documented an increased LV%FS in the cats that later developed HCM (LVH). In people, LV ejection fraction is also reported to be higher in pre-phenotypic HCM (pre-LVH).[30,33,34,60] It has been suggested that a hyperdynamic contraction might reflect intrinsic myocardial changes caused by sarcomere mutations.[33] Sarcomere mutations cause increased sarcomere power output (hypercontractility),[61] which is believed to be the main trigger for LVH in HCM.[33,61] Recent pharmacologic trials have targeted sarcomere hypercontractility by using cardiac myosin inhibitors.[61–65] A myosin inhibitor in a mouse model of HCM halted the development and progression of HCM,[61] and recent randomized clinical trials in people showed that cardiac myosin inhibitors reduced hypercontractility and LV outflow tract obstruction improving symptoms and exercise performance.[63,64] These groundbreaking results support the hypothesis that enhanced sarcomere function is the driving mechanism of HCM (LVH). In cats with HCM from a research colony, cardiac myosin inhibitors have also been shown to decrease myocardial hypercontractility and relieve LV outflow tract obstruction.[62,65]

It is unclear why pre-phenotypic HCM is associated with LV hypercontractility but decreased LA systolic function. The LA dysfunction might reflect an increased LA afterload (pressure overload) associated with early LV myocardial changes.

Elongated Mitral Valve Leaflets

An abnormal mitral valve apparatus with elongated mitral valve leaflets and/or abnormal papillary muscle morphology and attachments has been described as part of the HCM phenotype in humans and cats[20,44,66] and might play a critical role in SAM and LV outflow tract obstruction.[20,44] Moreover, an elongated anterior mitral valve leaflet was present in G+/LVH− people and has been suggested as an early morphologic marker of HCM.[34,43,44]

A recent study in cats measured the length of the anterior mitral leaflet on echocardiography (**Fig. 2**) and showed an association between mitral valve length and later development of HCM (LVH). The study showed that an elongated anterior mitral valve preceded the development of HCM and thus can be used as a predictor of HCM.[53]

A cohort of cats with SAM and normal LV wall thickness has been described,[28,67] and when a small number of these cats were followed over time they showed increased LV wall thickness and LA enlargement, that is, developed an HCM phenotype.[28] It is unresolved if SAM represents an early phenotypic (pre-LVH/HCM) change in this subpopulation of cats. However, as increased mitral valve leaflet length is associated with SAM and has been suggested as an early morphologic marker of HCM,[20,43,44,53] it sounds plausible that cats with SAM and normal LV wall thickness

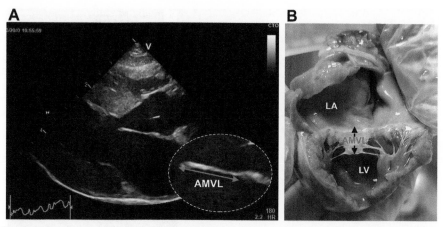

Fig. 2. The anterior mitral valve leaflet (AMVL) can be measured on echocardiography from the aortic valve cusp to the tip of the leaflet using a right parasternal five-chamber view in late diastole (*A*, zoomed image of the AMVL). (*B*) Gross postmortem image of the mitral valve apparatus of a cat heart showing the location of the echocardiographic AMVL measurement. AMVL, anterior mitral valve leaflet; LA, left atrium; LV, left ventricle. (*From* Seo J, Novo Matos J, Payne JR, et al. Anterior mitral valve leaflet length in cats with hypertrophic cardiomyopathy. J Vet Cardiol 2021;37:62–70; with permission.)

represent pre-phenotypic HCM. However, larger longitudinal studies in this cohort of cats will be needed to prove this hypothesis.

Diastolic Dysfunction

Tissue Doppler imaging and speckle tracking have been shown to be more sensitive than conventional echocardiography for detection of early/subtle myocardial changes. In people, these imaging modalities detected the presence of diastolic dysfunction in G+/LVH− individuals, suggesting that sarcomere mutations affect myocardial function before overt HCM (LVH) is present.[33,36–38]

Similarly, diastolic dysfunction detected on tissue Doppler imaging and speckle tracking was described in two cats before LVH was detected.[55,68] Also, studies in Maine coon cats carrying MYBPC3 A31P mutation without LVH (G+/LVH−) documented diastolic dysfunction on tissue Doppler imaging.[54,56] Although this was observed in a limited number of cats without long-term follow-up, thus it is unknown if these changes are just a marker of underlying disease or can predict the development of HCM. Nevertheless, tissue Doppler imaging and strain might also be useful at detecting pre-phenotypic HCM in cats.

As our understanding of pre-phenotypic changes and HCM natural history increase, these and other echocardiographic features can become useful in HCM screening, especially in cases with equivocal LVH (**Fig. 3**) and for targeting early HCM in clinical trials aiming to modulate disease development and progression.

PREDICTING CARDIOVASCULAR EVENTS AND MORTALITY IN CATS WITH HYPERTROPHIC CARDIOMYOPATHY

Several studies have set out to evaluate prognostic indicators in cats with HCM.[21,22,24–27,69–72] Factors that influence outcome can be identified within the signalment, history, physical examination findings, echocardiographic findings, and

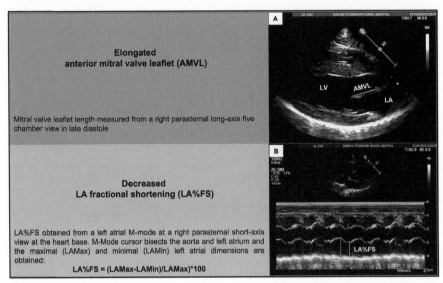

Fig. 3. Echocardiographic predictors of HCM. Two-year-old Maine coon cat negative for MYBPC3 A31P mutation with equivocal/borderline left ventricular wall thickness (interventricular septum 5.5 mm, left ventricular free wall 5.1 mm). Left ventricular diastolic function was normal (E/A 1.4, E′/A′ 2.0; E′ 9 cm/s), but left atrial fractional shortening was reduced (LA%FS 17%) and the anterior mitral valve leaflet was long (AMVL 13 mm). A decreased LA%FS and elongated AMVL have been suggested as HCM pre-phenotypic changes and predictors of later development of HCM (overt left ventricular hypertrophy). (*A*) Right parasternal long-axis five-chamber view; (*B*) left atrial M-Mode from a right parasternal short-axis view at the heart base. LA, left atrium; LA%FS, left atrial fractional shortening; LV, left ventricle; LV%FS, left ventricular fractional shortening.

results of cardiac biomarker testing. A small number of factors have been found to be independently predictive of outcome, and some factors are associated with a specific cardiac end point.

Signalment, History, and Physical Examination

Cats that are older at diagnosis of HCM are generally reported to have shorter survival times compared with younger cats[22,24,71] and the risk of cardiac morbidity and mortality increased progressively at 1, 5, and 10 years post-diagnosis in one study.[19] Interestingly, one study demonstrated that a young age at diagnosis (<3.5 years) was also associated with a poor outcome.[73] Conversely, survival time has not been found to be influenced by sex in HCM.[21,24,71]

Overall, being a pedigree cat does not seem to confer a prognostic advantage or disadvantage compared with being a non-pedigree cat[21,71]; however, individual pedigree breeds may have a worse clinical course. Studies have suggested that Ragdolls[24] and Maine Coons[25] may have shorter survival times following diagnosis of HCM than other cat breeds. Genetic mutations might influence outcome, although we still have limited information about the genetic mutations associated with HCM in cats. Ragdolls that are homozygous for the myosin binding protein C3 mutation (MYBPC3 R820W) are more likely to die a cardiac death and have a shorter time to cardiac death than Ragdolls that are either heterozygous for MYBPC3 R820W mutation or have the wildtype.[74]

The presence of clinical signs at initial diagnosis is associated with a negative prognosis for the cat.[21,22,24,25,71–73] Cats without clinical signs at diagnosis (subclinical HCM, stage B) are significantly more likely to die of noncardiac disease than cats that present showing clinical signs.[22] Indeed, only 27.9% of cats with subclinical HCM die due to their cardiac disease, although this is obviously a much higher rate of cardiovascular mortality than occurs in cats without apparent cardiac disease at initial assessment.[19] Median survival times from initial diagnosis in cats with subclinical HCM have been reported as varying between 1129 and greater than 3617 days, whereas cats with CHF had average survival times between 92 and 563 days and cats with ATE between 61 and 184 days.[21,22,24] The influence of presenting with a history of syncope on average survival times is less clear. One study showed no difference in survival between cats presenting with syncope and CHF,[22] whereas another study showed that cats with syncope had a longer survival time than cats with either CHF or ATE and with no difference in survival times between cats without clinical signs and cats with syncope.[71] These discordant results are likely due to the small proportion of cats with HCM that present with a history of syncope. With only 3.8% to 5.7%[22,71] cats presenting with syncope, clinically relevant differences in outcome compared with other presentations are difficult to achieve.

Although cats that are diagnosed with HCM have a greater body weight than those without HCM,[5] body weight does not carry prognostic value in cats with HCM.[21,71] Auscultation findings do carry prognostic value, with the absence of a heart murmur, the presence of a gallop sound, and the presence of an auscultable arrhythmia all being associated with a reduced survival time.[71] One study demonstrated that ventricular arrhythmias were common in cats with HCM; however, the study failed to identify any prognostic importance for number of ventricular premature complexes or number of runs of ventricular tachycardia, potentially due to low numbers of cats enrolled.[75] Conversely, the presence of atrial fibrillation has been found to indicate a poor prognosis in a group of cats with a number of different underlying diagnoses, including HCM.[76] A heart rate of ≥200 bpm at initial diagnosis was found to be negatively associated with survival in an early study[21] but has not been demonstrated in more recent studies.[22,24,71] Sleeping respiratory rate is routinely used to assess how well controlled the signs of CHF have been,[77] but the cats respiratory rate in the clinic is not associated with prognosis,[72] perhaps being confounded by some cats being tachypnoeic due to anxiety.

Echocardiography

One study demonstrated that the presence of extreme LV hypertrophy (≥9.0 mm) is associated with a poor outcome (**Fig. 4**).[71] This is in concordance with a small retrospective study which showed that non-survivors had a greater wall thickness than survivors.[70] The impact of the morphologic distribution of LVH is unclear, with one study demonstrating that cats with asymmetric LV free wall hypertrophy were associated with a worse outcome,[72] whereas morphologic distribution of LVH had no prognostic value in another study.[69]

Measures of LV diastolic function are associated with outcome, with cats with restrictive diastolic physiology having a poor prognosis compared with those with normal, delayed, or pseudonormal diastolic physiology.[71,73] Measures of systolic function are also prognostically important. A LV%FS of less than 30% (see **Fig. 4**) was associated with a worse outcome in one study,[71] and another study demonstrated that non-survivors had lower LV%FS values than survivors.[69] Reduced mitral and tricuspid annular plane systolic excursion, both measures of longitudinal ventricular

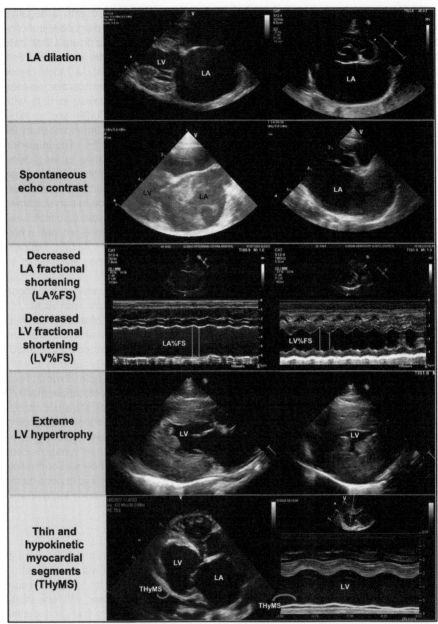

Fig. 4. Echocardiographic features associated with an increased risk of cardiovascular events and cardiac death in cats with hypertrophic cardiomyopathy (HCM). Left atrial (LA) dilation and reduced atrial function have been repeatedly shown to be associated with an increased risk of cardiac death. Spontaneous echo contrast ("smoke") has been associated with an increased risk of arterial thromboembolism (ATE), but in fact this is most likely a surrogate marker of severe LA dysfunction. Decreased left ventricular fractional shortening (LV%FS) is an independent predictor of death due to congestive heart failure (CHF) and decreased LA fractional shortening (LA%FS) is an independent predictor of death due to ATE. Extreme left ventricular hypertrophy (wall thickness ≥9 mm) is a predictor of cardiac mortality. Finally,

systolic function, was associated with a poor outcome, although did not persist to multivariable modeling.[78] In addition, the presence of thin and hypokinetic myocardial segments, presumed to represent myocardial infarction (see **Fig. 4**), is associated with a decreased survival time.[14,71,73]

Cats with SAM have longer survival times than those without SAM in numerous heterogenous populations,[22,24,70,71] but the effect does not persist when the influence of clinical signs is taken into account.[22,24,71] SAM is not a predictor of outcome in populations of cats without clinical signs (HCM stage B) or in populations of cats with CHF (HCM stage C).[19,24,79]

LA enlargement is the most commonly reported negative prognostic indicator in cats.[22,24,26,69–73] More recently, measures of LA function, including LA%FS, have been shown to have important prognostic information and might be more important than LA size[71,73] and the rate of change of LA size over time might also be prognostically useful.[26] The presence of spontaneous echo contrast or a thrombus within the left atrium has also been shown to carry a negative prognosis (see **Fig. 4**).[71,72]

Cardiac Biomarkers

Cardiac troponins, markers of myocardial cell damage, have been demonstrated to have prognostic value in cats with HCM. Troponin T and troponin I are both predictive of outcome in cats with HCM,[80] although only troponin T was predictive at the multivariable level. Troponin I was predictive of outcome in another study.[73] Studies have also demonstrated that N-terminal pro-B-type natriuretic peptide was predictive of outcome,[26,73] although the effect seems to be negated by the impact of LA size.

Independent Predictors of Outcome

Several studies have created multivariable models to look at independent predictors of outcome,[22,24,71–73] and a measure of LA size or LA function was a consistent independent predictor in all studies. Models of independent predictors of outcome have included LA size and age[22]; LA enlargement, age greater than 6 years and being a Ragdoll[24]; LA%FS, extreme LVH ($\geq$9.0 mm) and LV%FS less than 30%[71]; LA to aortic root ratio greater than 1.76, presence of CHF and troponin I greater than 0.7 ng/mL[73]; and LA enlargement and the presence of spontaneous echo contrast and/or LA thrombus (see **Fig. 4**; **Table 1**).[72]

The presence of CHF at initial diagnosis and decreasing LV%FS independently predicted a CHF death. The presence of an ATE at initial diagnosis and decreasing LA%FS independently predicted an ATE death. No multivariable models could be generated to predict sudden death due to low numbers of patients that experienced sudden death.[27] Given how frequently cats with ATE do not survive the episode,[81] treatments aiming to reduce the chances of this occurring have been investigated. Knowing that cats that have already had an ATE are at an increased risk of dying of another ATE, this patient population was investigated and demonstrated that treatment with clopidogrel increased survival time after the first ATE compared with treatment with aspirin.[82] Therefore, treatment with clopidogrel is considered the first-line therapy for cats following an ATE, and cardiologists will often start treatment with clopidogrel in cats

---

thin and hypokinetic myocardial segments are seen in cats with advanced HCM and are associated with a poor outcome. LA, left atrium; LA%FS, left atrial fractional shortening; LV, left ventricle; LV%FS, left ventricular fractional shortening; THyMS, thin and hypokinetic myocardial segments.

Table 1
Independent predictors of poor outcome in cats with hypertrophic cardiomyopathy

Predictor	Comments
Echocardiographic features	
LA dilation[a]	-
Decreased LA%FS[a]	-
Extreme LV hypertrophy	LVWT ≥9.0 mm
Decreased LV%FS	LV%FS <30%;
Spontaneous echo contrast ± LA thrombus	-
Signalment, presentation, biomarkers	
Older cats	>6 years old
Breed	Ragdoll
Clinical signs	CHF and/or ATE
Increased cardiac troponin I	>0.7 ng/mL

Abbreviations: ATE, arterial thromboembolism; CHF, congestive heart failure; LA, left atrial; LA% FS, left atrial fractional shortening; LV, left ventricular; LV%FS, left ventricular fractional shortening; LVWT, left ventricular wall thickness.
[a] Measures of left atrial size or function were consistent independent predictors of outcome across several studies.

considered at risk of ATE, including cats with LA enlargement and spontaneous echo contrast.

CONCLUSION

Recent studies have suggested that decreased LA%FS and an elongated anterior mitral valve leaflet precede overt HCM (precede LVH) and thus are pre-phenotypic changes that can help predict cats at an increased risk of developing HCM. These echocardiographic features might be especially useful in cats with equivocal LVH to help clinicians assessing the probability of HCM in individual cats.

Several studies have identified independent predictors of adverse outcome in cats with HCM, namely older age, LA dilation, decreased LA and LV systolic function, extreme LVH, increased cardiac troponin I, and CHF or ATE at presentation. These can help clinicians identifying cats at high risk of developing cardiovascular events or suffer cardiac death.

SUMMARY

HCM is the most common cardiac disease in cats, but the prognosis is very variable with many cats having a normal life expectancy while approximately 30% develop severe complications, such as CHF or ATE and die of their heart disease. Predicting which cats are at an increased risk of developing HCM and which cats with HCM are more likely to develop cardiovascular events or suffer a cardiac-related death are highly desirable goals in clinical cardiology, as these will impact patient's prognosis and management. Recent studies suggested that decreased LA%FS and an elongated mitral valve leaflet precede overt HCM (precede LVH) and thus are pre-phenotypic changes that can help predict cats at an increased risk of developing HCM. Several studies have looked for predictors of outcome in cats with HCM, and independent predictors of cardiovascular events or cardiac death have included left atrial dilation, decreased left atrial and ventricular systolic function, extreme LVH, increased cardiac troponin I, and CHF or ATE at presentation. Left atrial dysfunction is an important feature of HCM, as it seems to be both a predictor of HCM in normal cats and a predictor of outcome in cats with overt HCM.

CLINICS CARE POINTS

- Standard of care echocardiography variables can help identifying cats at risk of hypertrophic cardiomyopathy (HCM) and cats with HCM at risk of adverse cardiovascular events.

- Decreased left atrial fractional shortening and elongated anterior mitral valve leaflet are early phenotypic changes in feline HCM that can help identifying normal cats with an increased risk of developing HCM. These might be especially useful in cats with equivocal left ventricular hypertrophy.

- Measures of left atrial size and function are consistently identified as prognostic indicators in HCM.

- Thin and hypokinetic left ventricular myocardial segments are associated with advanced HCM and a very poor outcome.

- Up to 70% of cats with subclinical HCM do not die due to their cardiac disease. Cats that die due to their heart disease can die due to congestive heart failure, arterial thromboembolism, or sudden death. Cats that initially present with congestive heart failure are most likely to eventually die due to congestive heart failure, whereas cats that initially present with arterial thromboembolism are most likely to eventually die due to arterial thromboembolism.

CONFLICT OF INTEREST DECLARATION

Authors disclose no conflict of interest.

FUNDING

The authors are grateful to the Petplan Charitable Trust, Everts Luff Feline Endowment and IDEXX Laboratories for funding several of the studies here reported.

REFERENCES

1. Fox PR. Hypertrophic cardiomyopathy. Clinical and pathologic correlates. J Vet Cardiol 2003;5:39–45.
2. Elliott P, Anastasakis A, Borger M, et al. 2014 ESC guidelines on diagnosis and management of hypertrophic cardiomyopathy: the task force for the diagnosis and management of hypertrophic cardiomyopathy of the european society of cardiology (ESC). Eur Heart J 2014;35:2733–79.
3. Luis Fuentes V, Abbott J, Chetboul V, et al. ACVIM consensus statement guidelines for the classification, diagnosis, and management of cardiomyopathies in cats. J Vet Intern Med 2020;34:1062–77.
4. Paige CE, Abbott JA, Elvinger F, et al. Prevalence of cardiomyopathy in apparently healthy cats. J Am Vet Med Assoc 2009;234:1398–403.
5. Payne JR, Brodbelt DC, Luis Fuentes V. Cardiomyopathy prevalence in 780 apparently healthy cats in rehoming centres (the CatScan study). J Vet Cardiol 2015;17:S244–57.
6. Nagueh SF, Bierig SM, Budoff MJ, et al. American society of echocardiography clinical recommendations for multimodality cardiovascular imaging of patients with hypertrophic cardiomyopathy: endorsed by the American society of nuclear

cardiology, society for cardiovascular magnetic resonance, and society of cardio-vascular computed tomography. J Am Soc Echocardiogr 2011;24(5):473–98.

7. Kitai T, Xanthopoulos A, Nakagawa S, et al. Contemporary diagnosis and management of hypertrophic cardiomyopathy: The role of echocardiography and multimodality imaging. J Cardiovasc Dev Dis 2022;9:169.

8. Kwon DH, Smedira NG, Rodriguez ER, et al. Cardiac magnetic resonance detection of myocardial scarring in hypertrophic cardiomyopathy. Correlation with histopathology and prevalence of ventricular aachycardia. J Am Coll Cardiol 2009; 54:242–9.

9. Varnava AM, Elliott PM, Mahon N, et al. Relation between myocyte disarray and outcome in hypertrophic cardiomyopathy. Am J Cardiol 2001;88:275–9.

10. Hughes SE. The pathology of hypertrophic cardiomyopathy. Histopathology 2004;44:412–27.

11. Maragiannis D, Alvarez PA, Ghosn MG, et al. Left ventricular function in patients with hypertrophic cardiomyopathy and its relation to myocardial fibrosis and exercise tolerance. Int J Cardiovasc Imaging 2018;34:121–9.

12. Olivotto I, Maron BJ, Appelbaum E, et al. Spectrum and clinical significance of systolic function and myocardial fibrosis assessed by cardiovascular magnetic resonance in hypertrophic cardiomyopathy. Am J Cardiol 2010;106:261–7.

13. Olivotto I, Cecchi F, Poggesi C, et al. Patterns of disease progression in hypertrophic cardiomyopathy an individualized approach to clinical staging. Circ Hear Fail 2012;5:535–46.

14. Novo Matos J, Sargent J, Silva J, et al. Thin and hypokinetic myocardial segments in cats with cardiomyopathy. J Vet Cardiol 2023;46:5–17.

15. Schober KE, Chetboul V. Echocardiographic evaluation of left ventricular diastolic function in cats: Hemodynamic determinants and pattern recognition. J Vet Cardiol 2015;17:S102–33.

16. Rohrbaugh MN, Schober KE, Rhinehart JD, et al. Detection of congestive heart failure by Doppler echocardiography in cats with hypertrophic cardiomyopathy. J Vet Intern Med 2020;34:1091–101.

17. Tsang TSM, Barnes ME, Gersh BJ, et al. Left atrial volume as a morphophysiologic expression of left ventricular diastolic dysfunction and relation to cardiovascular risk burden. Am J Cardiol 2002;90:1284–9.

18. Abhayaratna WP, Seward JB, Appleton CP, et al. Left atrial size. Physiologic determinants and clinical applications. J Am Coll Cardiol 2006;47:2357–63.

19. Fox PR, Keene BW, Lamb K, et al. International collaborative study to assess cardiovascular risk and evaluate long-term health in cats with preclinical hypertrophic cardiomyopathy and apparently healthy cats: the REVEAL Study. J Vet Intern Med 2018;32:930–43.

20. Schober K, Todd A. Echocardiographic assessment of left ventricular geometry and the mitral valve apparatus in cats with hypertrophic cardiomyopathy. J Vet Cardiol 2010;12:1–16.

21. Atkins CE, Gallo AM, Kurzman ID, et al. Risk factors, clinical signs, and survival in cats with a clinical diagnosis of idiopathic hypertrophic cardiomyopathy: 74 cases (1985-1989). J Am Vet Med Assoc 1992;201:613–8.

22. Rush JE, Freeman LM, Fenollosa NK, et al. Population and survival characteristics of cats with hypertrophic cardiomyopathy: 260 cases (1990-1999). J Am Vet Med Assoc 2002;220:202–7.

23. Ferasin L, Sturgess CP, Cannon MJ, et al. Feline idiopathic cardiomyopathy: a retrospective study of 106 cats (1994-2001). J Feline Med Surg 2003;5:151–9.

24. Payne J, Luis Fuentes V, Boswood A, et al. Population characteristics and survival in 127 referred cats with hypertrophic cardiomyopathy (1997 to 2005). J Small Anim Pract 2010;51:540–7.

25. Trehiou-Sechi E, Tissier R, Gouni V, et al. Comparative echocardiographic and clinical features of hypertrophic cardiomyopathy in 5 breeds of cats: a retrospective analysis of 344 cases (2001-2011). J Vet Intern Med 2012;26:532–41.

26. Ironside VA, Tricklebank PR, Boswood A. Risk indictors in cats with preclinical hypertrophic cardiomyopathy: a prospective cohort study. J Feline Med Surg 2021; 23:149–59.

27. Payne JR, Borgeat K, Brodbelt DC, et al. Risk factors associated with sudden death vs. congestive heart failure or arterial thromboembolism in cats with hypertrophic cardiomyopathy. J Vet Cardiol 2015;17:S318–28.

28. Novo Matos J, Payne JR, Seo J, et al. Natural history of hypertrophic cardiomyopathy in cats from rehoming centers: the CatScan II study. J Vet Intern Med 2022;36:1900–12.

29. Spalla I, Payne JR, Borgeat K, et al. Prognostic value of mitral annular systolic plane excursion and tricuspid annular plane systolic excursion in cats with hypertrophic cardiomyopathy. J Vet Cardiol 2018;20:154–64.

30. Ho CY, Day SM, Colan SD, et al. The burden of early phenotypes and the influence of wall thickness in hypertrophic cardiomyopathy mutation carriers: findings from the HCMNet study. JAMA Cardiol 2017;2:419–28.

31. Semsarian C, Ingles J, Maron MS, et al. New perspectives on the prevalence of hypertrophic cardiomyopathy. J Am Coll Cardiol 2015;65:1249–54.

32. Maron BJ, Semsarian C. Editorial: Emergence of gene mutation carriers and the expanding disease spectrum of hypertrophic cardiomyopathy. Eur Heart J 2010; 31(13):1551–3.

33. Ho CY, Sweitzer NK, McDonough B, et al. Assessment of diastolic function with Doppler tissue imaging to predict genotype in preclinical hypertrophic cardiomyopathy. Circulation 2002;105:2992–7.

34. Ho CY, Cirino AL, Lakdawala NK, et al. Evolution of hypertrophic cardiomyopathy in sarcomere mutation carriers. Heart 2016;102:1805–12.

35. Farhad H, Seidelmann SB, Vigneault D, et al. Left Atrial structure and function in hypertrophic cardiomyopathy sarcomere mutation carriers with and without left ventricular hypertrophy. J Cardiovasc Magn Reson 2017;19:107.

36. Ho CY, Carlsen C, Thune JJ, et al. Echocardiographic strain imaging to assess early and late consequences of sarcomere mutations in hypertrophic cardiomyopathy. Circ Cardiovasc Genet 2009;2:314–21.

37. Cardim N, Perrot A, Ferreira T, et al. Usefulness of Doppler myocardial imaging for identification of mutation carriers of familial hypertrophic cardiomyopathy. Am J Cardiol 2002;90:128–32.

38. Nagueh SF, McFalls J, Meyer D, et al. Tissue Doppler imaging predicts the development of hypertrophic cardiomyopathy in subjects with subclinical disease. Circulation 2003;108:395–8.

39. Captur G, Ho CY, Schlossarek S, et al. The embryological basis of subclinical hypertrophic cardiomyopathy. Sci Rep 2016;6:27714.

40. Lakdawala NK, Thune JJ, Maron BJ, et al. Electrocardiographic features of sarcomere mutation carriers with and without clinically overt hypertrophic cardiomyopathy. Am J Cardiol 2011;108:1606–13.

41. Gray B, Ingles J, Semsarian C. Natural history of genotype positive-phenotype negative patients with hypertrophic cardiomyopathy. Int J Cardiol 2011;152: 258–9.

42. Maurizi N, Michels M, Rowin EJ, et al. Clinical course and significance of hypertrophic cardiomyopathy without left ventricular hypertrophy. Circulation 2019;139: 830–3.

43. Captur G, Lopes LR, Mohun TJ, et al. Prediction of sarcomere mutations in subclinical hypertrophic cardiomyopathy. Circ Cardiovasc Imaging 2014;7:863–71.

44. Maron MS, Olivotto I, Harrigan C, et al. Mitral valve abnormalities identified by cardiovascular magnetic resonance represent a primary phenotypic expression of hypertrophic cardiomyopathy. Circulation 2011;124:40–7.

45. Brouwer WP, Germans T, Head MC, et al. Multiple myocardial crypts on modified long-axis view are a specific finding in pre-hypertrophic HCM mutation carriers. Eur Heart J Cardiovasc Imaging 2012;13:292–7.

46. Crilley JG, Boehm EA, Blair E, et al. Hypertrophic cardiomyopathy due to sarcomeric gene mutations is characterized by impaired energy metabolism irrespective of the degree of hypertrophy. J Am Coll Cardiol 2003;41:1776–82.

47. Ho CY, López B, Coelho-Filho OR, et al. Myocardial fibrosis as an early manifestation of hypertrophic cardiomyopathy. N Engl J Med 2010;363:552–63.

48. Ho CY, Abbasi SA, Neilan TG, et al. T1 Measurements Identify Extracellular Volume Expansion in Hypertrophic Cardiomyopathy Sarcomere Mutation Carriers With and Without Left Ventricular Hypertrophy. Circ Cardiovasc Imaging 2013;6:415–22.

49. Meurs KM, Sanchez X, David RM, et al. A cardiac myosin binding protein C mutation in the Maine Coon cat with familial hypertrophic cardiomyopathy. Hum Mol Genet 2005;14:3587–93.

50. Meurs KM, Norgard MM, Ederer MM, et al. A substitution mutation in the myosin binding protein C gene in Ragdoll hypertrophic cardiomyopathy. Genomics 2007; 90:261–4.

51. Schipper T, Van Poucke M, Sonck L, et al. A feline orthologue of the human MYH7 c.5647G>A (p.(Glu1883Lys)) variant causes hypertrophic cardiomyopathy in a Domestic Shorthair cat. Eur J Hum Genet 2019;27:1724–30.

52. Meurs KM, Williams BG, DeProspero D, et al. A deleterious mutation in the ALMS1 gene in a naturally occurring model of hypertrophic cardiomyopathy in the Sphynx cat. Orphanet J Rare Dis 2021;16(1):108.

53. Seo J, Matos JN, Payne JR, et al. Anterior mitral valve leaflet length in cats with hypertrophic cardiomyopathy. J Vet Cardiol 2021;37:62–70.

54. Sampedrano CC, Chetboul V, Mary J, et al. Prospective echocardiography and tissue Doppler imaging screening of a population of maine coon cats tested for the A31P mutation in the myosin-binding protein c gene: A specific analysis of the heterozygous status. J Vet Intern Med 2009;23:91–9.

55. Chetboul V, Carlos Sampedrano C, Gouni V, et al. Two-dimensional color tissue doppler imaging detects myocardial dysfunction before occurrence of hypertrophy in a young maine coon cat. Vet Radiol Ultrasound 2006;47:295–300.

56. MacDonald KA, Kittleson MD, Kass PH, et al. Tissue Doppler imaging in maine coon cats with a mutation of myosin binding protein C with or without hypertrophy. J Vet Intern Med 2007;21:232–7.

57. Fries RC, Kadotani S, Keating SCJ, et al. Cardiac extracellular volume fraction in cats with preclinical hypertrophic cardiomyopathy. J Vet Intern Med 2021;35: 812–22.

58. Borgeat K, Stern J, Meurs KM, et al. The influence of clinical and genetic factors on left ventricular wall thickness in Ragdoll cats. J Vet Cardiol 2015;17:S258–67.

59. Khor KH, Campbell FE, Owen H, et al. Myocardial collagen deposition and inflammatory cell infiltration in cats with pre-clinical hypertrophic cardiomyopathy. Vet J 2015;203:161–8.

60. De S, Borowski AG, Wang H, et al. Subclinical echocardiographic abnormalities in phenotype-negative carriers of myosin-binding protein C3 gene mutation for hypertrophic cardiomyopathy. Am Heart J 2011;162:262–7.
61. Green EM, Wakimoto H, Anderson RL, et al. Heart disease: A small-molecule inhibitor of sarcomere contractility suppresses hypertrophic cardiomyopathy in mice. Science 2016;351:617–21.
62. Stern JA, Markova S, Ueda Y, et al. A small molecule inhibitor of sarcomere contractility acutely relieves left ventricular outflow tract obstruction in feline hypertrophic cardiomyopathy. PLoS One 2016;11:e0168407.
63. Olivotto I, Oreziak A, Barriales-Villa R, et al. Mavacamten for treatment of symptomatic obstructive hypertrophic cardiomyopathy (EXPLORER-HCM): a randomised, double-blind, placebo-controlled, phase 3 trial. Lancet 2020;396:759–69.
64. Maron MS, Masri A, Choudhury L, et al. Phase 2 Study of aficamten in patients with obstructive hypertrophic cardiomyopathy. J Am Coll Cardiol 2023;81:34–45.
65. Sharpe AN, Oldach MS, Rivas VN, et al. Effects of aficamten on cardiac contractility in a feline translational model of hypertrophic cardiomyopathy. Sci Reports 2023;13:32.
66. Klues HG, Maron BJ, Dollar AL, et al. Diversity of structural mitral valve alterations in hypertrophic cardiomyopathy. Circulation 1992;85:1651–60.
67. Ferasin L, Kilkenny E, Ferasin H. Evaluation of N-terminal prohormone of brain natriuretic peptide and cardiac troponin-I levels in cats with systolic anterior motion of the mitral valve in the absence of left ventricular hypertrophy. J Vet Cardiol 2020;30:23–31.
68. Suzuki R, Mochizuki Y, Yoshimatsu H, et al. Early detection of myocardial dysfunction using two-dimensional speckle tracking echocardiography in a young cat with hypertrophic cardiomyopathy. J Feline Med Surg Open Rep 2018;4. 2055116918 756219.
69. Peterson EN, Moise NS, Brown CA, et al. Heterogeneity of hypertrophy in feline hypertrophic heart disease. J Vet Intern Med 1993;7:183–9.
70. Fox PR, Liu SK, Maron BJ. Echocardiographic assessment of spontaneously occurring feline hypertrophic cardiomyopathy: an animal model of human disease. Circulation 1995;92(9):2645–51.
71. Payne JR, Borgeat K, Connolly DJ, et al. Prognostic indicators in cats with hypertrophic cardiomyopathy. J Vet Intern Med 2013;27:1427–36.
72. Spalla I, Locatelli C, Riscazzi G, et al. Survival in cats with primary and secondary cardiomyopathies. J Feline Med Surg 2016;18:501–9.
73. Borgeat K, Sherwood K, Payne JR, et al. Plasma cardiac troponin I concentration and cardiac death in cats with hypertrophic cardiomyopathy. J Vet Intern Med 2014;28:1731–7.
74. Borgeat K, Casamian-Sorrosal D, Helps C, et al. Association of the myosin binding protein C3 mutation (MYBPC3 R820W) with cardiac death in a survey of 236 Ragdoll cats. J Vet Cardiol 2014;16:73–80.
75. Bartoszuk U, Keene BW, Baron Toaldo M, et al. Holter monitoring demonstrates that ventricular arrhythmias are common in cats with decompensated and compensated hypertrophic cardiomyopathy. Vet J 2019;243:21–5.
76. Côté E, Harpster NK, Laste NJ, et al. Atrial fibrillation in cats: 50 Cases (1979-2002). J Am Vet Med Assoc 2004;225:256–60.
77. Porciello F, Rishniw M, Ljungvall I, et al. Sleeping and resting respiratory rates in dogs and cats with medically-controlled left-sided congestive heart failure. Vet J 2016;207:164–8.

78. Spalla I, Payne JR, Borgeat K, et al. Mitral annular plane systolic excursion and tricuspid annular plane systolic excursion in cats with hypertrophic cardiomyopathy. J Vet Intern Med 2017;31:691–9.

79. Schober KE, Zientek J, Li X, et al. Effect of treatment with atenolol on 5-year survival in cats with preclinical (asymptomatic) hypertrophic cardiomyopathy. J Vet Cardiol 2013;15:93–104.

80. Langhorn R, Tarnow I, Willesen JL, et al. Cardiac troponin I and T as prognostic markers in cats with hypertrophic cardiomyopathy. J Vet Intern Med 2014;28: 1485–91.

81. Borgeat K, Wright J, Garrod O, et al. Arterial thromboembolism in 250 Cats in general practice: 2004-2012. J Vet Intern Med 2014;28:102–8.

82. Hogan DF, Fox PR, Jacob K, et al. Secondary Prevention of Cardiogenic Arterial Thromboembolism in the Cat: The Double-Blind, Randomized, Positive-Controlled Feline Arterial Thromboembolism; Clopidogrel vs. Aspirin Trial (FAT CAT). J Vet Cardiol 2015;S306–17.

Advancing Treatments for Feline Hypertrophic Cardiomyopathy

The Role of Animal Models and Targeted Therapeutics

Joanna L. Kaplan, DVM, DACVIM (Cardiology)[a],*, Victor N. Rivas, MS[a],
David J. Connolly, BSc, BVetMed, PhD, CertVC, Cert SAM, DipECVIM (Cardiology),
MRCVS[b]

KEYWORDS

- Novel • Mavacamten • Aficamten • Rapamycin • Induced pluripotent stem cells
- Inter-cellular communication

KEY POINTS

- Therapeutic intervention of feline HCM is challenging in large part due to the vast heterogeneity in genotype and clinical disease presentation.
- Exploration of key molecular and cellular pathways that drive HCM pathophysiology facilitates the discovery of novel therapeutics.
- Development of innovative in vitro multicellular culture systems enables understanding of these aberrant pathways.
- Further characterization and development of animal models are vital to further explore novel therapeutics that advance treatment of feline cardiomyopathy and hold translational potential for human medicine.

INTRODUCTION

Despite being well-described as the most common cardiovascular disease in the cat, hypertrophic cardiomyopathy (HCM) continues to challenge currently available treatment strategies due to its vast heterogeneity in clinical presentation and disease progression.[1,2] Although some cats may remain subclinical throughout life, many develop severe consequences of disease including left-sided congestive heart failure (CHF),

[a] Department of Medicine and Epidemiology, School of Veterinary Medicine, University of California, Davis, CA, USA; [b] Department of Clinical Science and Services, Royal Veterinary College, Hatfield, Hertfordshire, UK
* Corresponding author. 2108 Tupper Hall, One Shields Avenue, Davis, CA 95616.
E-mail address: jlkkaplan@ucdavis.edu

Vet Clin Small Anim 53 (2023) 1293–1308
https://doi.org/10.1016/j.cvsm.2023.05.011
0195-5616/23/© 2023 Elsevier Inc. All rights reserved.

arterial thromboembolism (ATE), ventricular arrhythmias, or sudden death. Unfortunately, for many cats, the first indication of HCM is one of these devastating outcomes, and detailed risk stratification to aid clinicians in understanding which cats progress to more severe disease is lacking. Despite numerous efforts, there still remains no effective medical or surgical options for this disease in the subclinical phase to prolong lifespan or reduce the risk of developing one of these severe outcomes.[1–12] Previously investigated drug therapies, including calcium channel blockers (ie, diltiazem), beta blockers (ie, atenolol), ace-inhibitors (enalapril, benazepril, ramipril), spironolactone, or disopyramide, often target clinical signs and nonspecific hemodynamic consequences of disease rather than the initiating underlying pathophysiologic mechanism of hypercontractility, hypertrophy, and diastolic dysfunction.[3–14] This has led numerous investigators to explore novel drug therapies that more precisely target specific molecular pathways involved in the development of HCM. These challenges and opportunities demand better understanding of the complex disease mechanisms involved in HCM. This article will describe crucial work in animal and cellular models that has led to and will continue to propel the development of new therapies.

ANIMAL MODELS OF HYPERTROPHIC CARDIOMYOPATHY

Several animal species including cats, genetically engineered rabbits, pigs, rodents, and more recently a colony of rhesus macaques have been used to model HCM.[15–20] Hypertrophic cardiomyopathy in cats provide a unique opportunity to investigate a naturally occurring disease model that exhibits considerable similarities at the subcellular, cellular, and whole organ levels with humans.[15] Shared phenotypic features include ventricular wall thickening, atrial enlargement, and histologically cardiomyocyte hypertrophy and disarray, interstitial and replacement fibrosis, interstitial inflammatory cell infiltration and intramural vascular wall dysplasia.[21,22] Similarities in clinical presentation range from no clinical signs to life-threatening ventricular arrhythmias, heart failure, sudden death, and thromboembolism.[23] Importantly, compared to other animal models of HCM, only cats show left ventricular outflow tract obstruction (one of the clinical hallmarks of the human disease). A study that demonstrated the efficacy of a new class of myosin inhibitors in reducing dynamic outflow tract obstruction in Maine coon cats with obstructive HCM highlights this important aspect of the feline model, as this drug has now achieved FDA approval for use in humans.[24] Likewise, from a veterinary perspective, humans can be considered an excellent model for feline HCM given the analogous nature of the disease in both species.[25]

However, animal models also possess inherent limitations, particularly when considering engineered mice which have been used extensively in cardiac research. For instance, cardiac size, heart rate and action potential duration, cardiac output, and metabolism differ between species. Furthermore, in mice the α-myosin heavy chain isoforms predominate compared to the slower β-isoforms in humans which impacts on sarcomeric function and is particularly relevant for research in myocardial disease.[26] With reference to the feline model, a major limitation remains the restricted knowledge of the genetic architecture of HCM in this species with only a small number of causative mutations identified to date.[27]

In vitro Models of Hypertrophic Cardiomyopathy: in vitro Motility Assays

Studies on septal myectomy tissue from human patients with HCM and from engineered rodent models indicate that many but not all sarcomeric mutations enhance myofilament Ca^{2+} sensitivity leading to a hypercontractile phenotype with subsequent energy deficiency, mitochondrial dysfunction, disrupted autophagy, and eventually cell death, which act as the major common pathway promoting HCM.[28,29] Much of the detailed exploration of Ca^{2+} kinetics was performed using the *in vitro* motility assay, a standardized test system enabling the investigation of the interaction between actin and myosin, the 2 main proteins responsible for cardiomyocyte contraction. Our laboratory used the same assay to investigate contractile and regulatory proteins in left ventricular tissue from a range of outbred and pedigree cats with and without HCM. We included Ragdoll cats with and without the homozygous *MYBPC3* R820W mutation and feline samples were compared with myectomy samples from human patients. We found that fundamental Ca^{2+} regulatory abnormalities exemplified by increased Ca^{2+} sensitivity in cats with HCM are virtually the same as in the human samples. Furthermore, we were able to restore modulation of Ca^{2+} sensitivity by adding the calcium desensitizer Epigallocatechin 3-gallate.[30] Similar findings using a wider range of small molecules have been shown for human-derived samples expressing a variety of HCM-causing mutations.[31]

In vitro Models of Hypertrophic Cardiomyopathy: Induced Pluripotent Stem Cells

The induction of pluripotency is a process where fully differentiated cells are reprogrammed into a pluripotent state by introducing specific transcription factors initially identified in embryonic stem cells into the target cell.[32] In the initial development of iPSC technology reprogramming efficiencies were very low (0.05%–0.08%) and relied on integrating retroviruses which raised the possibility of insertional mutagenesis and reactivation of silenced retroviral genes.[33] Further refinement utilized non-integrating viruses such as adenoviruses and separately using plasmid delivery, however reprogramming efficiencies remained very low (0.001%–0.0001%).[34] The use of the Sendai virus system represented a significant breakthrough since this single stranded RNA non-integrating virus replicates in the cytoplasm and achieves reprogramming efficiencies in fully optimised conditions of up to 3%.[35] Other non-viral methods including mRNA transfection, protein transfection, PiggyBac vectors and cocktails of small molecules have been employed but are either technically challenging, labor intensive or have low efficiency.[36]

Induced pluripotent stem cells (iPSCs) have the potential to differentiate into derivatives of all 3 germ layers, engendering great promise for their use in regenerative medicine and disease modeling.[33,37] iPSCs can be derived from patients with disease-causing genetic mutations, allowing patient-specific iPSC lines to be developed for basic research and potentially in the long-term personalized medicine. For example, cardiomyocytes derived from iPSC lines (iPSC-CM) harboring HCM-causing mutations effectively recapitulate the disease by displaying cellular hypertrophy, altered contraction kinetics, and abnormal calcium handling, facilitating the exploration of novel therapeutic modalities including gene therapy.[38,39] Furthermore, the ability to control for other factors, such as genetic, epigenetic, and environmental effects, in a consistent manner makes iPSC disease models excellent platforms for rapid drug discovery.[26] This has been made possible by the development of gene editing techniques which means that iPSC lines can be precisely edited to insert or repair a specific mutation, facilitating generation of isogenic clones where the mutation of interest is the only modified variable. This controls for background genetic variation and epigenetic status in the starting somatic cell population which may hinder the interpretation of results and represents a significant advantage over patient-specific versus wild type cell lines[40] (**Fig. 1**). This is particularly relevant for disorders with incomplete penetrance such as HCM and provides a powerful tool for analyzing disease-causing mutations whilst controlling for genetic background.[40,41] Another advantage of iPSC-CM lines is that they can be cultured for extended periods of time unlike isolated adult

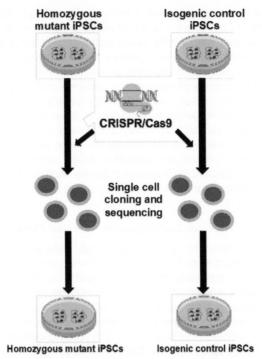

Homozygous mutant iPSCs

Isogenic control iPSCs

CRISPR/Cas9

Single cell cloning and sequencing

Homozygous mutant iPSCs

Isogenic control iPSCs

Fig. 1. Generation of mutant iPSCs and wild-type isogenic controls using CRISPR/Cas9 gene editing. Gene editing techniques enable the generation of isogenic clones where the mutation of interest is the only modified variable. iPSCs, induced pluripotent stem cells.

cardiomyocytes. These advantages have resulted in iPSC-CM being increasingly utilized in HCM research.[40,42–45]

The initial goal of our group was to explore the influence of the *MYBPC3* R820W mutation in Ragdoll cats by developing iPSC-CM lines from homozygous and genotype-negative (wild type) individuals. We chose this genetic variant since it is one of the few known HCM-causing mutations in cats and the phenotype had been well characterised.[46–48] Our initial approach employed the Sendai virus system but despite several attempts and successful reprogramming of a human fibroblast line as a control, we were unable to generate iPSCs from feline dermal or adipose-tissue fibroblasts using this method. Based on these results, we employed a less elegant retrovirus system to introduce the transcription factors Oct4, Sox2, Klf4, cMyc, and Nanog that had successfully reprogrammed dermal fibroblasts from a snow leopard and were able to generate and fully characterize a feline iPSC line.[49–51] However, despite culturing our iPSCs to beyond passage 20, we found that the inserted reprogramming transcription factors remained upregulated which maintained the cells in a highly pluripotent state and may explain why we were unable to fully differentiate the cells toward a cardiomyocyte lineage.

Because of the difficulties we encountered with our feline iPSCs and given the similarities between human and feline HCM, we opted to investigate the effect of the R820W mutation using a human cell system. To achieve this, we used gene editing techniques (CRISPR/Cas9) to introduce the R820W mutation into a well-characterized human iPSC line (that had been derived using the non-integrating

Sendai virus system). This approach had the further advantage of standardizing culture techniques without the use of undefined animal-derived media. We successfully engineered multiple iPSC lines that were homozygous or heterozygous for the MYBPC3/R820W mutation as well as isogenic controls and then differentiated these lines into beating cardiomyocyte populations of high purity containing greater than 99% Troponin T positive cells.[52] We chose to focus further experiments on iPSC-CM lines carrying the R820W homozygous mutation since homozygous cats present at a young age with a severe HCM phenotype, whereas heterozygous cats can have a relatively benign clinical course with normal life expectancy.[47]

We showed that homozygous iPSC-CMs had a larger cell area compared to wild-type (WT) cells, consistent with cell hypertrophy. Using a combination of immunocytochemistry and ELISA analysis we demonstrated that cells in both groups expressed an equal quantity of cMyBPC protein similar to a previous report and this was incorporated into the A-band of sarcomeres as expected. This suggest that the MYPBC3 R820W mutation does not cause haploinsufficiency.[30] Our functional analysis of contracting cardiomyocytes indicated that mutant cells had a longer relaxation phase, longer contraction duration, and lower contraction amplitude compared to WT cells.[52] This preliminary data shows that CRISPR mediated knockin of the R820W mutation in iPSC-CMs effectively recapitulates morphologic and functional features characteristic of HCM and creates a platform for further research.

Maturation of Induced Pluripotent Stem Cell-CMs

Although genetically edited iPSC-CMs provide enormous potential for elucidating HCM-associated aberrant cellular pathways as well as a platform for rapid drug screening, several obstacles remain. The main limitation is their immature cellular features which more closely resemble fetal cardiomyocytes due to their expression of fetal genes.[53] Their immaturity embodies a wide range of features including smaller size, reduced electrical and contractile function, disorganized sarcomeres, and characteristically an absence of T-tubules and an inadequate sarcoplasmic reticulum organization.[54,55] Numerous techniques have been employed to foster the maturation of iPSC-CMs including culturing cells in a 3-dimensional (3D) environment on hydrogel-based micropatterned substrates mimicking the extracellular matrix, switching metabolic substrate use from glucose to fatty acids to promote oxidative phosphorylation, applying auxotonic mechanical loading and electrical pacing to the cells in 3D culture and introducing other cardiac cell types such as cardiac fibroblasts and endothelial cells to the 3D culture.[26,54,56–65] The goal of such techniques particularly when employed in combination is to recapitulate as closely as possible the cellular environment of the adult heart in a 3D format.

FUTURE DIRECTIONS – FOCUS ON FIBROSIS

A particular focus of our group is the development of interstitial fibrosis in HCM and in agreement with findings in human HCM we have shown upregulation of key mediators of fibrosis including lumican and members of the lysyl oxidase and TGF-β families in the myocardium of HCM cats.[66–69] We hypothesize that myocardial fibrosis is not directly caused by sarcomeric mutations per se but rather is contingent on and secondary to cardiac muscle dysfunction at the molecular, cellular or whole organ level. Consequently, the development of fibrosis is a universal feature of HCM irrespective of the specific HCM mutation. Although mechanisms responsible for myocardial fibrosis remain elusive, they likely involve the interactions between dysfunctional cardiomyocytes and the cardiac non-myocyte population including cardiac fibroblasts, endothelial and inflammatory cells.[70,71] This reciprocal cellular crosstalk may occur through primary secretion of cytokines such as TGF-β by dysfunctional myocytes, paracrine stimulation of non-myocytes which then secrete TGF-β, or some combination thereof. Furthermore, once myofibroblast transformation has occurred, the process of myocardial fibrosis becomes self-perpetuating and is independent of myocyte dysfunction, possibly driving further cardiac pathology through a myriad of pleiotropic consequences. These include effects on matrix remodeling, cytokine elaboration, inflammation, and cardiomyocyte hypertrophy.[72,73]

To explore processes driving fibrosis in HCM we are developing a standardized electrically paced 3D Engineered Heart Tissue (EHT) model to which varying loading conditions can be applied. The EHT model will comprise Ragdoll *MYBPC3* R820W wild-type (R820W−/−) or homozygous (R820W+/+) isogenic iPSC-CM lines, cardiac fibroblast ± endothelial cells. This model will facilitate quantification of the crosstalk (via direct cell to cell contact, paracrine or secretory signaling) between constituent cell types, enabling detailed investigation of mechanisms of fibrosis and hypertrophy in HCM and may inform novel therapeutic approaches. Using specific blocking experiments will enable us to identify the most important signaling pathways and determine those most amenable to therapeutic intervention. For instance, inhibitors of the TGF-β1/ Smad and JNK/c-Jun signaling pathways show profound antifibrotic effects in part by reducing the expression of the lysyl oxidase family. Their efficacy has recently been documented in a variety of disease processes including pulmonary fibrosis, sarcopenia and atrial fibrosis.[74–77] More direct inhibitors of the lysyl oxidase family have also proven effective in the management of hepatic fibrosis and systemic sclerosis.[78,79]

NOVEL DRUG THERAPIES FOR TREATMENT OF HYPERTROPHIC CARDIOMYOPATHY
Small Molecular Inhibitors

In health, the sarcomere of the cardiomyocyte is made up of 2 motor proteins, actin, and myosin.[80] In the resting heart, myosin is separated from actin by the troponin-tropomyosin complex. However, once calcium enters the cell, this complex is altered, allowing for actin and myosin to interact. In order for myosin to bind to actin, and therefore cause contraction of the cardiomyocyte, a four-step process must take place, involving a myosin adenosine triphosphatase (ATPase). In diastole, ATP bound to myosin undergoes hydrolysis, forming ADP and inorganic phosphate (P_i), which remain bound to myosin. Once P_i is released, actin and myosin can form a cross-bridge with one another, leading to contraction. The remaining ADP is then released, leading to a rigor complex, followed by replacement with a new ATP molecule that dissociates actin from myosin, and returns the cardiac myosin to its resting state.

Genetic variants associated with HCM often disrupt the proper assembly of proteins within the sarcomere, can lead to destabilization of the cardiac myosin in the relaxed state, and formation of excessive cross-bridges between actin and myosin.[13,81] This is thought to result in hypercontractility, compensatory hypertrophy, and diastolic dysfunction, ultimately leading to the development of left ventricular outflow tract obstruction (LVOTO), reduced coronary artery perfusion to the myocardium, increased myocardial oxygen consumption, replacement fibrosis, and arrhythmias. Thus far, 2 small molecule inhibitors, mavacamten, and aficamten, have been developed to specifically target the myosin ATPase of the beta cardiac myosin heavy chain to normalize cross-bridge formation and therefore, normalize contractility, relieve LVOTO, and improve relaxation and myocardial energetics (**Fig. 2**).[13,14,24,81–88]

Mavacamten (trade name: Camzyos) is the first of its class of cardiac myosin inhibitors to achieve FDA approval for the treatment of obstructive HCM in human

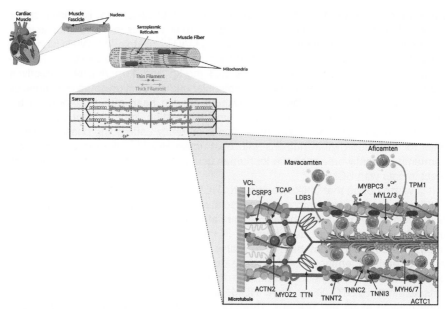

Fig. 2. Targets of mavacamten and aficamten. Cardiac myosin inhibitors target the myosin ATPase within the sarcomere to reduce the force of contraction. ACTC1, actin alpha cardiac muscle-1; ACTN2, actinin alpha-2; Ca2+, calcium; CSRP3, cysteine and glycine-rich protein-3; LDB3, LIM domain binding-3; MYBPC3, myosin binding protein-C3; MYH6/7, myosin heavy chain-6/-7; MYL2/3, myosin light chain-2/-3; MYOZ2, myozenin-2; TCAP, telethonin; TNNC2, troponin-C2; TNNI3, cardiac troponin-I; TNNT2, cardiac troponin-T; TPM1, tropomyosin alpha-1 chain; TTN, titin; VCL, vinculin.

medicine.[86] Although this drug is currently unavailable in veterinary medicine, it shows excellent translational potential to treat clinical feline HCM.[2,24] In a study utilizing a transgenic HCM mouse model, *in vitro* and *in vivo* experiments demonstrated that mavacamten successfully reduced cardiac myosin heavy chain ATPase activity and therefore, contractility in a dose-dependent fashion.[88] Furthermore, when given to genetically engineered mice harboring a pathogenic HCM mutation, mavacamten prevented the development of ventricular hypertrophy, cardiomyocyte disarray, and myocardial fibrosis, and attenuated hypertrophic and profibrotic gene expression. In mice expressing the HCM phenotype, mavacamten reduced left ventricular wall thickness and fractional shortening.

Finally, a small prospective study involving five A31P MYPBC3 genotype-positive cats with naturally-occurring HCM and LVOTO demonstrated that mavacamten successfully reduced contractility and alleviated LVOTO.[24] Interestingly, unlike beta blockers and calcium channel blockers which have both negative inotropic and chronotropic effects, mavacamten reduced percent fractional shortening without impacting heart rate. This study was pivotal in leading to clinical trials in human HCM, which ultimately led to its FDA approval.[82,83] Once available in veterinary medicine, future long-term studies would serve useful to determine if mavacamten benefits cats with occult HCM with or without LVOTO.

Aficamten is another promising cardiac myosin inhibitor that showed dose-dependent reductions in cardiac fractional shortening in healthy rats, dogs, and more recently HCM affected cats.[14,84,85] In 2 prospective, randomized, cross-over studies in purpose-bred HCM affected cats with LVOTO, aficamten, like mavacamten reduced left ventricular fractional shortening due to an increased left ventricular internal dimension (LVID) in systole, while preserving LVID in diastole.[14,85] While high-dose aficamten (2 mg/kg) led to an increased heart rate (suspected to be due to a reflex tachycardia), aficamten at lower doses (0.3 mg/kg and 1 mg/kg) still effectively reduced systolic function and peak left ventricular outflow tract pressure gradients, ultimately resolving LVOTO obstruction without altering heart rate. Furthermore, aficamten reduced isovolumic relaxation time suggesting improvement in diastolic function following administration. Aficamten is currently undergoing phase III clinical trials for FDA approval in humans with obstructive HCM.[87] Like mavacamten, aficamten is currently only available for human use, but shows great potential for treatment in cats with HCM.[14,85]

It is worth noting that unlike people with HCM in which LVOTO is an independent risk factor for sudden death and is associated with increased morbidity and mortality, this finding has not been recapitulated in the cat.[1] It is unknown if this dissimilarity is due to a true difference in the affected feline population. Alternatively, this difference may be due to a bias in veterinary studies, in which LVOTO leads to earlier identification of disease due to the higher likelihood of a murmur being detected on physical exam, and therefore closer monitoring. In contrast, cats without LVOTO likely have HCM identified later in the disease process once clinical signs are present. Therefore, many cats with more mild cases of non-obstructive HCM are less likely to be identified than cases of the mild obstructive form of disease, leading to a false perception that the presence of LVOTO is associated with a better prognosis. Finally, LVOTO is still a component of HCM that contributes to increased wall stress, myocardial oxygen consumption, and consequently myocardial ischemia and fibrosis.[89,90] This emphasizes the utility to understanding novel drug therapies that have the potential to alleviate LVOTO, especially in cats with severe LVOTO (>4.5–5.0 m/s) and cats that are symptomatic for this sequelae.[2]

Rapamycin

Rapamycin, also known as sirolimus, is currently under investigation for the treatment of HCM in cats (**Fig. 3**). Rapamycin is a macrolide that is produced by the bacterium *Streptomyces hygroscopicus* and was originally discovered to target and inhibit genes that encode a protein called TOR in yeast.[91,92] A mammalian homolog called mammalian or mechanistic target of rapamycin (mTOR) was later discovered. mTOR is an atypical serine/threonine protein kinase that interacts with numerous proteins to form 2 types of multiprotein complexes, called mTOR complex 1 (mTORC1) and mTOR complex 2 (mTORC2).[91–93] These complexes have different upstream inputs and downstream effects, as well as different sensitivities to rapamycin. Generally, mTORC1 upregulates protein and lipid synthesis and down regulates autophagy, playing an important role in promoting adaptive cardiac remodeling in response to pressure overload. mTORC2 regulates glucose and lipid metabolism, helps maintain normal cardiac physiology, and promotes cardiomyocyte survival when confronted with pressure overload. Both mTORC1 and mTORC2 play essential roles in cardiac health and complete disruption of mTORC1 and mTORC2 functions lead to metabolic derangements and cardiovascular disease.[93] However, studies have demonstrated that partial inhibition of mTORC1 may in fact have advantageous outcomes in the aging heart, as it may lead to reduced energy expenditure and abnormal protein accumulation, as well upregulation of autophagy (**Fig. 3**).

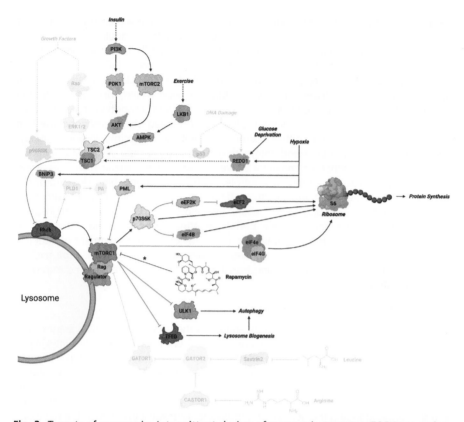

Fig. 3. Targets of rapamycin. Intermittent dosing of rapamycin targets mTORC1 to reduce protein synthesis and upregulate lysosome biogenesis and autophagy. AKT, protein kinase-B; AMPK, AMP-activated protein kinase; BNIP3, Bcl-2 interacting protein-3; CASTOR1, cytosolic arginine sensor for MTORC1 subunit-1; eEF2, eukaryotic translation elongation factor-2; eEF2K, eukaryotic translation elongation factor-2 kinase; eIF4B, eukaryotic translation initiation factor-4B; eIF4e, eukaryotic translation initiation factor-4e; eIF4G, eukaryotic translation initiation factor-4G; ERK1/2, extracellular signal-regulated kinase-1/-2; GATOR1, GTPase-activating protein activity toward Rags-1; GATOR2, GTPase-activating protein activity toward Rags-2; LB1, nuclear lamin-B1; mTORC1, mammalian target of rapamycin complex-1; mTORC2, mammalian target of rapamycin complex-2; p53, tumor protein; p70S6K, ribosomal protein S6 kinase beta-1; PA, polymerase acidic protein; PDK1, pyruvate dehydrogenase kinase-1; PI3K, phosphoinositide 3-kinase; PLD1, phospholipase-D1; PML, promyelocytic leukemia; Rag, recombination activating gene; Ras, rat sarcoma virus; REDD1, regulated in DNA damage and development-1; Rheb, Ras homolog enriched in brain; S6, ribosomal protein S6; sp90RSK, serine/threonine kinase; TFEB, transcription factor-EB; TSC1, tuberous sclerosis complex-1; TSC2, tuberous sclerosis complex-2; ULK1, Unc-51-like kinase-1.

A challenge when treating with rapamycin is determining a dosing strategy that partially and selectively inhibits mTORC1 while minimizing the inhibition of mTORC2. While mTORC1 is sensitive to acute or intermittent doses of rapamycin, mTORC2 is less sensitive to rapamycin, and typically becomes activated with chronic continuous exposure.[91] Thus, intermittent dosing strategies may be employed to partially inhibit mTORC1 effects while minimizing inhibition of mTORC2, thereby maximizing therapeutic benefit while minimizing adverse side effects. More recently, intermittent dosing of rapamycin has shown to reverse pathologic left ventricular hypertrophy in mouse models and humans receiving renal transplants.[94–97] Therefore, intermittent dosing of rapamycin is an intriguing novel therapy to treat feline HCM.

This has led to the development of a new formulation of delayed-released (DR) rapamycin which was utilized in a clinical trial via once weekly oral administration in cats with subclinical HCM and no LVOTO.[98] Data collection for this two-centered, randomized, double-blinded, placebo-controlled study has concluded, in which cats were dosed with either low-dose or high-dose rapamycin once weekly, or placebo over a 6-month period. Interestingly, preliminary data demonstrate statistically significant reductions in maximal left ventricular wall thickness in cats receiving low-dose rapamycin compared to controls or those receiving high-dose formulations. It is postulated that the positive effect observed in cats treated with low-dose rapamycin may be due to successful inhibition of mTORC1, where high-dose rapamycin may offset some of the beneficial effects observed via activation of mTORC2. This drug is currently undergoing FDA review for the treatment of subclinical feline HCM. Further long-term studies are needed to determine if rapamycin's positive effects on cardiac remodeling translate into a survival benefit and improvement in quality of life.

Discovery of Future Novel Drug Therapies

Arguably the largest challenges to discovering new therapies to treat HCM are the vast heterogeneity in disease genotype and phenotype.[15] With recent advancements in genetic techniques, extensive research efforts are currently underway to further identify causative and disease modifying genetic variants in feline HCM (unpublished data). A large-scale study is currently in the process of utilizing whole-genome sequencing and RNA sequencing in HCM-affected cats of all breeds and healthy controls with the goal of further understanding the genetic and molecular pathways involved in the development of HCM and modification of disease severity. A better understanding of the genotype-phenotype relationship will help propel future novel treatment discoveries. The ultimate goal would be to use personalized medicine to develop therapies that better target specific characteristics of an individual's expression of disease.

SUMMARY

Feline HCM remains a challenging disease to effectively treat, particularly in the subclinical phase.[1,2] This is largely due to our lack of understanding of how to predict disease progression within the individual patient. Advancements in our understanding of the genetic and molecular mechanisms associated with HCM in small and large animal models have led to exciting discoveries of novel drug therapies and treatment strategies that ultimately benefit both people and animals with HCM.[15] Further investigations using this comparative and translational medicine approach will continue to drive future discovery of novel ways to manage HCM in our feline population. Additional preclinical and clinical trials exploring new drug therapies are already underway.

CLINICS CARE POINTS

- Utilization of translational animal models is vital to explore and develop novel therapies for treatment of HCM in both veterinary species and people.

- Small molecule inhibitors have great potential for treatment in cats with HCM, although clinical trials are currently lacking.
- Results of a current clinical trial demonstrate that domestic cats receiving a new formulation of delayed-release rapamycin at low doses have significantly less echocardiographic cardiac remodeling compared to their control counterparts.
- Identifying and characterising aberrant molecular pathways using precise and unambiguous in vitro models can facilitate development of novel therapies.

DISCLOSURES

The authors have no disclosures or conflicts of interest.

REFERENCES

1. Fuentes VL, Abbott J, Chetboul V, et al. ACVIM consensus statement guidelines for the classification, diagnosis, and management of cardiomyopathies in cats. J Vet Intern Med 2020;34(3):1062–77.
2. Kittleson MD, Côté E. The feline Cardiomyopathies: 2. Hypertrophic cardiomyopathy. J Feline Med Surg 2021;23(11):1028–51.
3. Bright JM, Golden AL, Gompf RE, et al. Evaluation of the calcium channel-blocking agents diltiazem and verapamil for treatment of feline hypertrophic cardiomyopathy. J Vet Intern Med 1991;5(5):272–82.
4. Bright JM, Golden AL. Evidence for or against the efficacy of calcium channel blockers for management of hypertrophic cardiomyopathy in cats. Vet Clin North Am Small Anim Pract 1991;21(5):1023–34.
5. Schober KE, Zientek J, Li X, et al. Effect of treatment with atenolol on 5-year survival in cats with preclinical (asymptomatic) hypertrophic cardiomyopathy. J Vet Cardiol 2013;15(2):93–104.
6. Coleman AE, DeFrancesco TC, Griffiths EH, et al. Atenolol in cats with subclinical hypertrophic cardiomyopathy: a double-blind, placebo-controlled, randomized clinical trial of effect on quality of life, activity, and cardiac biomarkers. J Vet Cardiol 2020;30:77–91.
7. MacDonald KA, Kittleson MD, Larson RF, et al. The effect of ramipril on left ventricular mass, myocardial fibrosis, diastolic function, and plasma neurohormones in Maine Coon cats with familial hypertrophic cardiomyopathy without heart failure. J Vet Intern Med 2006;20(5):1093–105.
8. MacDonald KA, Kittleson MD, Kass PH, et al. Effect of spironolactone on diastolic function and left ventricular mass in Maine Coon cats with familial hypertrophic cardiomyopathy. J Vet Intern Med 2008;22(2):335–41.
9. Rush JE, Freeman LM, Brown DJ, et al. The use of enalapril in the treatment of feline hypertrophic cardiomyopathy. J Am Anim Hosp Assoc 1998;34(1):38–41.
10. King JN, Martin M, Chetboul V, et al. Evaluation of benazepril in cats with heart disease in a prospective, randomized, blinded, placebo-controlled clinical trial. J Vet Intern Med 2019;33(6):2559–71.
11. Wall M, Calvert CA, Sanderson SL, et al. Evaluation of extended-release diltiazem once daily for cats with hypertrophic cardiomyopathy. J Am Anim Hosp Assoc 2005;41(2):98–103.
12. Amberger CN, Glardon O, Glaus T, et al. Effects of benazepril in the treatment of feline hypertrophic cardiomyopathy results of a prospective, open-label, multicenter clinical trial. J Vet Cardiol 1999;1(1):19–26.

13. Masri A, Olivotto I. Cardiac myosin inhibitors as a novel treatment option for obstructive hypertrophic cardiomyopathy: addressing the core of the matter. J Am Heart Assoc 2022;11(9):e024656.
14. Sharpe AN, Oldach MS, Kaplan JL, et al. Pharmacokinetics of a single dose of aficamten (CK-274) on cardiac contractility in a A31P MYBPC3 hypertrophic cardiomyopathy cat model. J Vet Pharmacol Therap 2023;46(1):52–61.
15. Ueda Y, Stern JA. A one health approach to hypertrophic cardiomyopathy. Yale J Biol Med 2017;90(3):433–48.
16. Fox PR, Liu SK, Maron BJ. Echocardiographic assessment of spontaneously occurring feline hypertrophic cardiomyopathy. An animal model of human disease. Circulation 1995;92(9):2645–51.
17. Hornyik T, Rieder M, Castiglione A, et al. Transgenic rabbit models for cardiac disease research. Br J Pharmacol 2022;179(5):938–57.
18. Montag J, Petersen B, Flögel AK, et al. Successful knock-in of hypertrophic cardiomyopathy-mutation R723G into the MYH7 gene mimics HCM pathology in pigs. Sci Rep 2018;8(1):4786.
19. Lin CS, Sun YL, Liu CY. Structural and biochemical evidence of mitochondrial depletion in pigs with hypertrophic cardiomyopathy. Res Vet Sci 2003;74(3): 219–26.
20. Flenner F, Jungen C, Küpker N, et al. Translational investigation of electrophysiology in hypertrophic cardiomyopathy. J Mol Cell Cardiol 2021;157:77–89.
21. Aupperle H, Baldauf K, März I. An immunohistochemical study of feline myocardial fibrosis. J Comp Pathol 2011;145(2–3):158–73.
22. Kitz S, Fonfara S, Hahn S, et al. Feline hypertrophic cardiomyopathy: che Consequence of cardiomyocyte-initiated and macrophage-driven remodeling processes? Vet Pathol 2019;56(4):565–75.
23. Freeman LM, Rush JE, Stern JA, et al. Feline hypertrophic cardiomyopathy: a spontaneous large animal model of human HCM. Cardiol Res 2017;8(4):139–42.
24. Stern JA, Markova S, Ueda Y, et al. A small molecule inhibitor of sarcomere contractility acutely relieves left ventricular outflow tract obstruction in feline hypertrophic cardiomyopathy. PLoS One 2016;11(12):e0168407.
25. Maron BJ, Fox PR. Hypertrophic cardiomyopathy in man and cats. J Vet Cardiol 2015;17(Suppl 1):S6–9.
26. Santini L, Palandri C, Nediani C, et al. Modelling genetic diseases for drug development: Hypertrophic cardiomyopathy. Pharmacol Res 2020;160:105176.
27. Kittleson MD, Meurs KM, Harris SP. The genetic basis of hypertrophic cardiomyopathy in cats and humans. J Vet Cardiol 2015;17(Suppl 1):S53–73.
28. Marston SB. How do mutations in contractile proteins cause the primary familial cardiomyopathies? J Cardiovasc Transl Res 2011;4(3):245–55. Review.
29. Ušaj M, Moretto L, Månsson A. Critical evaluation of current hypotheses for the pathogenesis of hypertrophic cardiomyopathy. Int J Mol Sci 2022;23(4):2195.
30. Messer AE, Chan J, Daley A, et al. Investigations into the sarcomeric protein and $Ca2+$-regulation abnormalities underlying hypertrophic cardiomyopathy in cats (Felix catus). Front Physiol 2017;8:348.
31. Sheehan A, Messer AE, Papadaki M, et al. Molecular defects in cardiac myofilament $Ca2+$-regulation due to cardiomyopathy-linked mutations can be reversed by small molecules binding to troponin. Front Physiol 2018;9:243.
32. Stadtfeld M, Hochedlinger K. Induced pluripotency: history, mechanisms, and applications. Genes Dev 2010;24(20):2239–63.
33. Takahashi K, Yamanaka S. Induction of pluripotent stem cells from mouse embryonic and adult fibroblast cultures by defined factors. Cell 2006;126(4):663–76.

34. Okita K, Nakagawa H, Ichisaka T, et al. Generation of mouse induced pluripotent cells without viral vectors. Science 2008;322(5903):949–53.

35. Fusaki N, Ban H, Nishiyama A, et al. Efficient induction of transgene-free human pluripotent stem cells using a vector based on Sendai virus, an RNA virus that does not integrate into the host genome. Proc Jpn Acad Ser B Phys Biol Sci 2009;85(8):348–62.

36. Lyra-Leite DM, Gutiérrez-Gutiérrez Ó, Wang M, et al. A review of protocols for human iPSC culture, cardiac differentiation, subtype-specification, maturation, and direct reprogramming. STAR Protoc 2022;3(3):101560.

37. Takahashi K, Tanabe K, Ohnuki M, et al. Induction of pluripotent stem cells from adult human fibroblasts by defined factors. Cell 2007;131(5):861–72.

38. Prondzynski M, Krämer E, Laufer SD, et al. Evaluation of MYBPC3 trans-Splicing and gene replacement as therapeutic options in human iPSC-derived cardiomyocytes. Mol Ther Nucleic Acids 2017;7:475–86.

39. Prondzynski M, Mearini G, Carrier L. Gene therapy strategies in the treatment of hypertrophic cardiomyopathy. Eur J Physiol 2019;471(5):807–15.

40. Bhagwan JR, Mosqueira D, Chairez-Cantu K, et al. Isogenic models of hypertrophic cardiomyopathy unveil differential phenotypes and mechanism-driven therapeutics. J Mol Cell Cardiol 2020;145:43–53.

41. Gähwiler EKN, Motta SE, Martin M, et al. Human iPSCs and genome editing technologies for precision cardiovascular tissue engineering. Front Cell Dev Biol 2021;9:639699.

42. Kondo T, Higo S, Shiba M, et al. Human-induced pluripotent stem cell-derived cardiomyocyte model for TNNT2 Δ160E-induced cardiomyopathy. Circ Genom Precis Med 2022;15(5):e003522.

43. Dainis A, Zaleta-Rivera K, Ribeiro A, et al. Silencing of MYH7 ameliorates disease phenotypes in human iPSC-cardiomyocytes. Physiol Genomics 2020;52(7):293–303.

44. Smith JGW, Owen T, Bhagwan JR, et al. Isogenic pairs of hiPSC-CMs with hypertrophic cardiomyopathy/LVNC-associated ACTC1 E99K mutation unveil differential functional deficits. Stem Cell Rep 2018;11(5):1226–43.

45. Birket MJ, Ribeiro MC, Kosmidis G, et al. Contractile defect caused by mutation in MYBPC3 revealed under conditions optimized for human PSC-cardiomyocyte function. Cell Rep 2015;13(4):733–45.

46. Meurs KM, Norgard MM, Ederer MM, et al. A substitution mutation in the myosin binding protein C gene in ragdoll hypertrophic cardiomyopathy. Genomics 2007;90(2):261–4.

47. Borgeat K, Casamian-Sorrosal D, Helps C, et al. Association of the myosin binding protein C3 mutation (MYBPC3 R820W) with cardiac death in a survey of 236 Ragdoll cats. J Vet Cardiol 2014;16(2):73–80.

48. Borgeat K, Stern J, Meurs KM, et al. The influence of clinical and genetic factors on left ventricular wall thickness in Ragdoll cats. J Vet Cardiol 2015;17(Suppl 1):S258–67.

49. Verma R, Holland MK, Temple-Smith P, et al. Inducing pluripotency in somatic cells from the snow leopard (Panthera uncia), an endangered felid. Theriogenology 2012;77(1):220–8.e2.

50. Verma R, Liu J, Holland MK, et al. Nanog Is an essential factor for induction of pluripotency in somatic cells from endangered felids. Biores Open Access 2013;2(1):72–6.

51. Dutton LC, Dudhia J, Guest DJ, et al. Inducing pluripotency in the domestic cat (Felis catus). Stem Cells Dev 2019;28(19):1299–309.

52. Dutton LC, Dudhia J, Guest DJ. Connolly D.J., CRISPR/Cas9 genome engineering to model the R820W mutation effects in iPSC-derived cardiomyocytes. Research communications of the 30th ecvim-ca online congress 2-5 September 2020. J Vet Intern Med, 34 (6), 2020, 3058-3166.

53. van den Berg CW, Okawa S, Chuva de Sousa Lopes SM, et al. Transcriptome of human foetal heart compared with cardiomyocytes from pluripotent stem cells. Development 2015;142(18):3231–8.

54. Ribeiro MC, Tertoolen LG, Guadix JA, et al. Functional maturation of human pluripotent stem cell derived cardiomyocytes in vitro–correlation between contraction force and electrophysiology. Biomaterials 2015;51:138–50.

55. Pioneer JM, Racca AW, Klaiman JM, et al. Isolation and mechanical measurements of myofibrils from human induced pluripotent stem cell-derived cardiomyocytes. Stem Cell Rep 2016;6(6):885–96.

56. Pioner JM, Santini L, Palandri C, et al. Optical investigation of action potential and calcium handling maturation of hiPSC-Cardiomyocytes on biomimetic substrates. Int J Mol Sci 2019;20(15):3799.

57. Mannhardt I, Breckwoldt K, Letuffe-Brenière D, et al. Human engineered heart tissue: analysis of contractile force. Stem Cell Rep 2016;7(1):29–42.

58. Tiburcy M, Hudson JE, Balfanz P, et al. Defined engineered human myocardium with advanced maturation for applications in heart failure modeling and repair. Circulation 2017;135(19):1832–47.

59. Ronaldson-Bouchard K, Ma SP, Yeager K, et al. Advanced maturation of human cardiac tissue grown from pluripotent stem cells. Nature 2018;556(7700):239–43.

60. Leonard A, Bertero A, Powers JD, et al. Afterload promotes maturation of human induced pluripotent stem cell derived cardiomyocytes in engineered heart tissues. J Mol Cell Cardiol 2018;118:147–58.

61. Hirt MN, Boeddinghaus J, Mitchell A, et al. Functional improvement and maturation of rat and human engineered heart tissue by chronic electrical stimulation. J Mol Cell Cardiol 2014;74:151–61.

62. Jackman CP, Carlson AL, Bursac N. Dynamic culture yields engineered myocardium with near-adult functional output. Biomaterials 2016;111:66–79.

63. Ramachandra CJA, Mehta A, Wong P, et al. Fatty acid metabolism driven mitochondrial bioenergetics promotes advanced developmental phenotypes in human induced pluripotent stem cell derived cardiomyocytes. Int J Cardiol 2018; 272:288–97.

64. Shadrin IY, Allen BW, Qian Y, et al. Cardiopatch platform enables maturation and scaleup of human pluripotent stem cell-derived engineered heart tissues. Nat Commun 2017;8(1):1825.

65. Ruan JL, Tulloch NL, Razumova MV, et al. Mechanical stress conditioning and electrical stimulation promote contractility and force maturation of induced pluripotent stem cell-derived human cardiac tissue. Circulation 2016;134(20):1557–67.

66. Coats CJ, Heywood WE, Virasami A, et al. Proteomic analysis of the myocardium in hypertrophic obstructive cardiomyopathy. Circ Genom Precis Med 2018; 11(12):e001974. PMID: 30562113.

67. Al-U'datt D, Allen BG, Nattel S. Role of the lysyl oxidase enzyme family in cardiac function and disease. Cardiovasc Res 2019 Nov 1;115(13):1820–37.

68. Yang J, Savvatis K, Kang JS, et al. Targeting LOXL2 for cardiac interstitial fibrosis and heart failure treatment. Nat Commun 2016;7:13710.

69. Cheng WC, Wilkie L, Dobromylsky M, et al. Cellular localization of key proteins controlling pro-fibrotic pathways in cats with hypertrophic cardiomyopathy

2020 ACVIM Forum On Demand Research Abstract Program. J Vet Intern Med, 34 (6), 2020, 2830-2989. https://doi.org/10.1111/jvim.15904.

70. Wang BX, Kit-Anan W, Terracciano CMN. Many cells make life work-multicellularity in stem cell-based cardiac disease modelling. Int J Mol Sci 2018;19(11):3361.

71. Perbellini F, Watson SA, Bardi I, et al. Heterocellularity and cellular cross-talk in the cardiovascular system. Front Cardiovasc Med 2018;5:143.

72. Meng Q, Bhandary B, Bhuiyan MS, et al. Myofibroblast-specific TGFβ receptor II signaling in the fibrotic response to cardiac myosin binding protein c-induced cardiomyopathy. Circ Res 2018;123(12):1285–97.

73. Heras-Bautista CO, Mikhael N, Lam J, et al. Cardiomyocytes facing fibrotic conditions re-express extracellular matrix transcripts. Acta Biomater 2019;89: 180–92.

74. Chapman HA, Wei Y, Montas G, et al. Reversal of TGFβ1- driven profibrotic state in patients with pulmonary fibrosis. N Engl J Med 2020;382(11):1068–70.

75. Tong X, Zhang S, Wang D, et al. Azithromycin attenuates bleomycin-induced pulmonary fibrosis partly by inhibiting the expression of LOX and LOXL-2. Front Pharmacol 2021;12:709819.

76. Wu Y, Wu Y, Yang Y, et al. Lysyl oxidase-like 2 inhibitor rescues D-galactose-induced skeletal muscle fibrosis. Aging Cell 2022;21(7):e13659.

77. Wu Y, Can J, Hao S, et al. LOXL2 inhibitor attenuates angiotensin II-induced atrial fibrosis and vulnerability to atrial fibrillation through inhibition of transforming growth factor beta-1 Smad2/3 pathway. Cerebrovasc Dis 2022;51(2):188–98.

78. Yao Y, Findlay A, Stolp J, et al. Pan-lysyl oxidase inhibitor PXS-5505 ameliorates multiple-organ fibrosis by inhibiting collagen crosslinks in rodent models of systemic sclerosis. Int J Mol Sci 2022;23(10):5533.

79. Chen W, Yang A, Jia J, et al. Lysyl Oxidase (LOX) Family Members: Rationale and Their Potential as Therapeutic Targets for Liver Fibrosis. Hepatology 2020;72(2): 729–41.

80. Katz AM. Physiology of the heart. In: DeStefano F, editor. Ch 4 the contractile proteins. 5th edition. Philadelphia, PA: Wolters Kluwer Health/Lippincott Williams & Wilkins Health; 2010. p. 88–106.

81. Ho CY, Mealiffe ME, Bach RG, et al. Evaluation of mavacamten in symptomatic patients with nonobstructive hypertrophic cardiomyopathy. J Am Coll Cardiol 2020;75:2649–60.

82. Heitner SB, Jacoby D, Lester SJ, et al. Mavacamten treatment for obstructive hypertrophic cardiomyopathy: a clinical trial. Ann Intern Med 2019;170(11):741–8.

83. Olivotto I, Oreziak A, Barriales-Villa R, et al. Mavacamten for treatment of symptomatic obstructive hypertrophic cardiomyopathy (EXPLORER-HCM): a randomized, double-blind, placebo-controlled, phase 3 trial. Lancet 2020;396(10253): 759–69.

84. Chuang C, Collibee S, Ashcraft L, et al. Discovery of aficamten (CK-274), a next generation cardiac myosin inhibitor for the treatment of hypertrophic cardiomyopathy. J Med Chem 2021;64(19):14142–52.

85. Sharpe AN, Oldach MS, Rivas VN, et al. Effects of aficamten on cardiac contractility in a feline translational model of hypertrophic cardiomyopathy. Sci Rep 2023; 13(1):32.

86. FDA. FDA approves new drug to improve heart function in adults with rare heart condition. Available at: https://www.fda.gov/drugs/news-events-human-drugs/fda-approves-new-drug-improve-heart-function-adults-rare-heart-condition. Accessed February 15, 2023.

87. Cytokinetics. Cytokinetics announces start of SEQUOIA-HCM, a phase 3 clinical trial of aficamten in patients with symptomatic obstructive hypertrophic cardiomyopathy. Available at: https://ir.cytokinetics.com/news-releases/news-release-details/cytokinetics-announces-start-sequoia-hcm-phase-3-clinical-trial. Accessed February 15, 2023.

88. Green EM, Wakimoto K, Anderson RL, et al. A small-molecule inhibitor of sarcomere contractility suppresses hypertrophic cardiomyopathy in mice. Science 2016;351(6273):617–21.

89. Abbott JA. Feline hypertrophic cardiomyopathy: an update. Vet Clin North Am Small Anim Pract 2010;40(4):685–700.

90. Maron MS, Olivotto I, Betocchi S, et al. Effect of left ventricular outflow tract obstruction on clinical outcome in hypertrophic cardiomyopathy. N Engl J Med 2003;348:295–303.

91. Apelo SIA, Lamming DW. Rapamycin: an inhibitor of aging emerges from the soil of easter island. J Gerontol A Biol Sci Med Sci 2016;71(7):841–9.

92. Laplante M, Sabatini DM. mTOR signaling in growth control and disease. Cell 2012;149(2):274–93.

93. Sciarretta S, Forte M, Frati G, et al. New insights into the role of mTOR signaling in the cardiovascular system. Circ Res 2018;122(3):489–505.

94. Shioi T, McMullen JR, Tarnavski O, et al. Rapamycin attenuates load-induced cardiac hypertrophy in mice. Circulation 2003;107(12):1664–70.

95. Marin TM, Keith K, Davies B, et al. Rapamycin reverses hypertrophic cardiomyopathy in a mouse model of LEOPARD syndrome-associated PTPN11 mutation. J Clin Invest 2011;121(3):1026–43.

96. McMullen JR, Sherwood MC, Tarnavski O, et al. Inhibition of mTOR signaling with rapamycin regresses established cardiac hypertrophy induced by pressure overload. Circulation 2004;109:3050–5.

97. Paoletti E, Amidone M, Cassottana P. Effect of sirolimus on left ventricular hypertrophy in kidney transplant recipients: a 1-year nonrandomized controlled trial. Am J Kidney Dis 2008;52:324–30.

98. Stern JA et al. Oral Rapamycin Therapy in Feline Subclinical Hypertrophic Cardiomyopathy: Results of the RAPACAT Clinical Trial. Proceedings of the International Cardio-renal Veterinary Symposium (ICVS) Americas 2022. Presented October 16, 2022. Fort Lauderdale, FL.

Preventing Cardiogenic Thromboembolism in Cats

Literature Gaps, Rational Recommendations, and Future Therapies

Meg Shaverdian, BS[a], Ronald H.L. Li, DVM, MVetMed, PhD, DACVECC[b],*

KEYWORDS

- Immunothrombosis • Hypertrophic cardiomyopathy • Platelet priming
- Neutrophil extracellular traps • Thromboprophylaxis

KEY POINTS

- Underlying causes of cardiogenic arterial thromboembolism (CATE) in cats are complex and not well understood.
- Immunothrombosis involving platelets, inflammation, and neutrophils likely plays a crucial role in CATE pathogenesis and presents a novel therapeutic target.
- Primary prevention should be optimized using precision medicine or dual-agent therapy to prevent CATE.

INTRODUCTION

Cardiogenic arterial thromboembolism (CATE) is one of the leading causes of morbidity and mortality in cats with cardiomyopathies. CATE occurs when a thrombus, originated from the left atrium (LA) or left atrial appendage (LAA), dislodges and embolizes to the distal aorta and/or arteries causing tissue ischemia, necrosis, and subsequent ischemic reperfusion injury.[1] Hypertrophic cardiomyopathy (HCM) is the main underlying cause of CATE with a reported prevalence of 11.3% among cats affected by HCM.[2,3] Severe inflammation, burn injuries, and smoke inhalation may also result in transient myocardial thickening and CATE. Because cats with CATE often present acutely with congestive heart failure (CHF) and extreme pain without any prior clinical signs, it is a distressing emergency for pet owners with a high rate of euthanasia at the time of diagnosis.[4] Owing to a high mortality rate of up to 54.1% and a high recurrence

[a] Department of Surgical and Radiological Sciences, School of Veterinary Medicine, University of California, Davis, 2108 Tupper Hall, One Shields Avenue, Davis, CA 95616, USA;
[b] Department of Clinical Sciences, College of Veterinary Medicine, North Carolina State University, Raleigh, NC, USA
* Corresponding author.
E-mail address: rhli@ucdavis.edu

Vet Clin Small Anim 53 (2023) 1309–1323
https://doi.org/10.1016/j.cvsm.2023.06.002
0195-5616/23/© 2023 Elsevier Inc. All rights reserved.

rate of up to 49%, long-term thromboprophylaxis is the most important prevention strategy in cats with HCM and CATE.[3,5–7] However, optimal strategies for preventing CATE have not been established. The development of novel therapeutics in the treatment of CATE also is a challenge because little is known regarding the underlying pathophysiology of this disease. This review aims to summarize our understanding of CATE pathophysiology, recommendations for thromboprophylaxis, and the knowledge gaps in the literature and clinical practice.

CURRENT UNDERSTANDING OF CARDIOGENIC ARTERIAL THROMBOEMBOLISM PATHOPHYSIOLOGY

According to Virchow's triad, thrombosis occurs in the setting of an overall hypercoagulable state, abnormal blood flow, and endothelial injury. Although the pathophysiology of CATE in cats is not well understood, alterations of all three components of Virchow's triad are considered the main contributing factors (**Fig. 1**).[1]

Hypercoagulability

A delicate balance between antithrombotic and prothrombotic properties of the hemostatic system must be maintained to prevent life-threatening hemorrhage and thrombosis. It involves an intricate network of platelets, circulating blood cells, humoral proteins, and many feedback mechanisms that regulate the system. HCM has been shown to disrupt this dynamic balance of hemostasis causing hypercoagulability, clinically manifesting as intracardiac thrombosis and CATE (see **Fig. 1**).

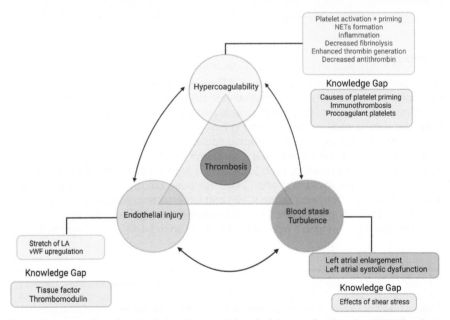

Fig. 1. Summary of Virchow's triad and potential underlying mechanisms in CATE. Blood stasis occurs due to left atrial enlargement and dysfunction resulting in intracardiac thrombosis and damage of the endocardium. Endothelial injury may initiate coagulation, by upregulating von Willebrand factor (vWF), tissue factor (TF), or downregulating thrombomodulin (TM), further exacerbating a hypercoagulable state, by facilitating platelet–neutrophil interactions and immunothrombosis.

Platelets

Platelets are the primary effectors in coagulation and hemostasis. In response to vascular injuries, platelets adhere to exposed subendothelial matrixes and, in a multi-step process, undergo activation and recruitment of nearby platelets. This initial step is crucial to the formation of the platelet plug and fibrin network.[8] Findings in several *ex vivo* studies in HCM cats indicate that platelet activation and priming have an important role in the pathogenesis of CATE. A study by Tablin and colleagues showed that platelets from a colony of Maine Coon cats with occult HCM had increased platelet-derived microparticles and surface P-selectin expression, a marker for platelet activation.[9] In addition, the severity of HCM, characterized by LA enlargement, left ventricular (LV) wall thickness, and LV end-systolic cavity obliteration, correlated with the degree of platelet activation. These findings were further confirmed by Helenski and Ross, who demonstrated that some cats with cardiomyopathies display irreversible platelet aggregation in response to adenosine diphosphate (ADP), indicating that their platelets may be hyperresponsive.[10] Such a process, known as platelet priming, can be caused by exposure to molecules that either modulate intracellular inhibitory pathways or potentiate activating pathways in platelets. This, in turn, causes unrestrained and amplified response to physiologic agonists.[11,12] Platelet priming was confirmed by Tan and colleagues, who showed that client-owned cats with occult HCM had elevated response to thrombin compared with healthy cats without HCM.[12] Another study conducted in a separate colony of Maine Coon/outbred mixed cats showed that cats homozygous for the mutation in the myosin-binding protein C (*MYBPC3*) gene had increased platelet activation in response to ADP compared with wild-type cats.[11] Interestingly, none of the cats at the time of study had echocardiographic evidence of HCM, which suggests that platelet priming may occur before the diagnosis of occult HCM.[11] Collectively, these studies support the notion that platelet priming causing increased platelet activation plays a role in conjuring an overall hypercoagulable state in cats with HCM.

Secondary hemostasis and fibrinolysis

Secondary hemostasis consists of a series of enzymatic reactions that activate thrombin, a proteolytic enzyme that cleaves fibrinogen to fibrin monomers. Polymerization and stabilization of fibrin give rise to fibrin clot, which is crucial to stabilizing the platelet plug. Fibrin formation is dampened when thrombin binds to antithrombin (AT) to inhibit coagulation factors via glycosaminoglycans, heparins, and heparin sulfates. Fibrinolysis controls clot remodeling by cleaving fibrin clots allowing blood flow to be reestablished after thrombus formation. Fibrinolysis is activated by plasmin, which is, in turn, activated by tissue plasminogen activator (TPA) or urinary-type plasminogen activator, producing fibrin degradation products (FDPs) like D-dimer.[13]

Evidence suggests that overactivation of secondary hemostasis may contribute to hypercoagulability in HCM cats. Elevated thrombin–AT (TAT) complexes and FDPs, which are used to measure the activation of secondary hemostasis and fibrinolysis, have been documented in cats with cardiomyopathies.[14–16] Although one study found increased AT concentrations in cats with cardiomyopathies, another showed that HCM cats had reduced AT suggesting that AT may be consumed more readily in a hypercoagulable state.[14,15] A study by Stokol and colleagues further confirmed these findings by demonstrating increased TAT complexes and D-dimer in cats with cardiomyopathies.[16] The clinical use of TAT and D-dimer as biomarkers for identifying cats at risk of CATE has not been evaluated and requires further investigation.

Immunothrombosis

Immunothrombosis describes the complex interactions between innate immunity and the coagulation system. Under normal conditions, immunothrombosis facilitates microvascular thrombosis to prevent pathogen dissemination during vascular injuries and infection. Dysregulation of immunothrombosis caused by many cardiovascular diseases has been linked to systemic hypercoagulability and thrombosis. Neutrophils, which are the most abundant granulocytes, is a main player of immunothrombosis.[17] In addition to degranulation and phagocytosis, neutrophils release neutrophil extracellular traps (NETs) in response to various stimuli. NETs, which are composed of cell-free DNA (cfDNA), citrullinated histones (citH), and antimicrobial proteins not only contribute to host defense by ensnaring and eliminating pathogens but they also possess prothrombotic properties.[18] Research in various species identifies five major pathways in which NETs may contribute to thrombosis (**Fig. 2**).[17–23]

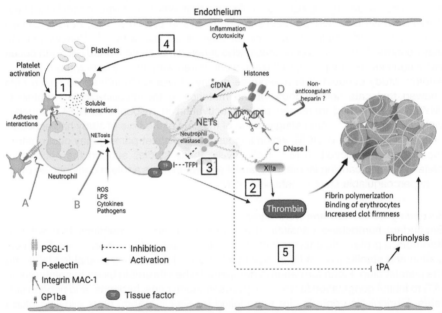

Fig. 2. Potential pathways of immunothrombosis during CATE and therapeutic targets. (1) Activated platelets interact with neutrophils via adhesive or soluble interactions forming neutrophil extracellular traps (NETs). NETs formation may also be initiated in response to reactive oxygen species (ROS), lipopolysaccharides (LPS), cytokines, and pathogens, (2) NETs may amplify thrombin and fibrin polymerization by activating Factor XII via the negatively charged surfaces of cfDNA and by amplifying tissue factor-dependent thrombin generation, (3) granular proteins, such as neutrophil elastase, found on NETs may augment thrombin generation by degrading natural anticoagulants like tissue factor pathway inhibitor (TFPI), (4) extracellular histones on NETs may activate platelets and promote inflammation, (5) NETs may impair fibrinolysis by inhibiting activity of tissue plasminogen activator (TPA). Potential therapeutic targets: (A) Inhibiting adhesive interactions between platelets and neutrophils using peptides or monoclonal antibodies to dampen neutrophil activation and NETs formation, (B) pharmacologic inhibition of NETs formation, (C) dismantling of NET structures by DNase I, (D) scavenging of free histones using peptides like non-anticoagulant heparins to prevent cytotoxicity and platelet activation.

Plasma cfDNA, as a marker of NETs, was found to be elevated in cats with HCM and CATE but did not correlate with LA function or neutrophil count. Further analysis of cfDNA fragment size discovered that prothrombotic cfDNA fragments around 100 to 500 base pairs were found only in cats with HCM and CATE.[24] Using immunofluorescence microscopy to characterize and quantify NETs in thrombi within the aortic bifurcations and external iliac arteries in cats, NETs were found to be dynamic structural elements of arterial thrombi with altering distributions in relations to their proximity to the distal aorta.[25] These differences in thrombus composition could be due to neutrophil entrapment at the site of vascular occlusion or neutrophil activation as they are exposed to extreme variations in shear stress. The role of pathologic shear stress and NETs in cats with HCM is unclear.

Extracellular histones can be released extracellularly via NETs formation or necrosis. Once released, they act as danger-associated molecular patterns by inducing inflammation and apoptosis. Free histones also have been shown to increase platelet activation and promote NETs formation in mice and human beings.[18,21] Free citH are considered by some investigators a specific marker of systemic NETs formation. Histone citrullination is a posttranslational modification process that converts arginine to citrulline residues, which alters the electrostatic interactions between DNA and histones causing nucleosome decondensation and cfDNA release.[18] High concentrations of citH have been identified in arterial thrombi retrieved from cats and human stroke patients indicative of active NETs formation during cardiovascular diseases.[24,26] Li and colleagues demonstrated that plasma citH concentration was significantly increased in HCM cats and approximately 50% of cats with subclinical HCM had increased citH3 concentrations. Interestingly, none of the healthy cats in the control group had any detectable levels of citH. Plasma citH3 also correlated with predisposing factors for CATE, such as LA enlargement and LA systolic dysfunction. These findings suggest that citH may serve as a future therapeutic target or biomarker for HCM cats at risk of CATE.[24]

Systemic inflammation is one of the driving forces of global hypercoagulability. Although systemic inflammation has previously been characterized in some human patients with HCM, its role in the pathogenesis of feline CATE is not well understood. Neutrophil-to-lymphocyte ratio (NLR) is a well-established biomarker indicating the balance between innate and adaptive immunity. In human medicine, elevated NLR signals systemic inflammation and stress, which can be used as a prognostic marker in short- and long-term outcomes in patients with ischemic stroke and HCM.[27,28] Similarly elevated NLR was observed in cats with severe HCM and was shown to be an independent predictor of cardiac-related deaths.[29]

Blood Stasis

Cats with HCM that develop CATE or CHF have moderate to severe LA enlargement and LA systolic dysfunction. Decreased LA function results in blood flow stasis, which is associated with the formation of spontaneous echocardiographic contrast (SEC), and/or intracardiac thrombus within the LA appendage (see **Fig. 1**).[1,30] Schober and Maerz found that LAA blood flow velocity of less than 0.2 m/s was an independent predictor for spontaneous echocardiographic contrast (SEC) and may be used to identify cats at an increased risk of CATE.[30] SEC was postulated to be caused by low blood low, which facilitates the formation of red blood cell fibrinogen aggregates giving rise to a swirling pattern of blood flow "smoke" on echocardiogram.[31] However, another study found that human patients with SEC had more activated platelets, leukocytes, and platelet-leukocyte aggregates within the LA suggesting that platelet leukocytes may be involved in the formation of intracardiac thrombus and may be at least in part responsible for the origin of SEC.[32]

Endothelial Injury

Under normal physiologic conditions, endothelium releases molecules such as nitric oxide (NO), prostaglandin I2, and thrombomodulin to restrict platelet aggregation and subsequent fibrin deposition. During endothelial injury, these protective mechanisms are likely compromised and prothrombotic molecules such as von Willebrand factor (vWF) and tissue factor are upregulated and released.[33] vWF is a large glycoprotein synthesized and released by endothelial cells, platelets, and megakaryocytes. Once released, it binds to circulating platelets via platelet glycoproteins causing tethering and rolling of platelets on the endothelium. This initial adhesion to the endothelium is short-term and is proportional to shear stress.[33] Elevated vWF levels have been documented in human patients with atrial fibrillation, myocardial infarct, inflammatory vascular disease, and HCM and have been used as an indicator of disease progression.[34–36] In HCM cats, endocardial damage due to LA enlargement and stretching of the endocardium may also lead to upregulation of vWF.[1,37] Stokol and colleagues showed that plasma vWF concentrations were significantly elevated in cats with acute CATE indicating the presence of endothelial damage.[16] A recent study by Cheng and colleagues detected upregulation of endocardial vWF in cats with severe HCM and CATE and found an abundance of vWF within intracardiac thrombi. These findings indicate that vWF is upregulated in HCM, which may likely contribute to thrombosis in cats.[38]

KNOWLEDGE GAP

According to various human and murine studies, activated platelets can be further categorized into aggregatory and procoagulant platelets. Although aggregatory platelets contribute to the growth of the initial platelet plug, procoagulant platelets provide a membrane surface for the assembly of coagulation complexes to propagate thrombin generation and fibrin polymerization. The exact mechanisms underlying the transformation of platelets to their procoagulant phenotypes are unclear but may be mediated by the mitochondrial necrosis pathway (**Fig. 3**). Conventional antiplatelet drugs, which target the aggregatory functions of platelets, may not prevent procoagulant platelet formation and their effects on thrombin generation. In humans, procoagulant platelets are associated with an elevated risk of thrombosis in cardiovascular diseases such as stroke. A better understanding of how they are formed and their contribution in CATE pathophysiology may identify novel therapeutic targets (see **Fig. 3**).[39]

Although NETs have been characterized in plasma and thrombi in cats with HCM and CATE, the underlying mechanisms regulating their formation are unknown. Because the extreme variations in blood shear stress in cats with HCM and CATE may play a role in the pathogenesis of thrombosis, studies are being conducted to investigate the molecular interactions between neutrophils and platelets under hydrodynamic shear stress that may be essential for NETs formation.[25] Also, revealing the mechanisms of immunothrombosis in platelet priming also is essential in optimizing thromboprophylaxis in cats with cardiomyopathies.

RISK ASSESSMENT FOR CATS WITH CARDIOMYOPATHIES AND DIAGNOSIS OF CARDIOGENIC ARTERIAL THROMBOEMBOLISM

Several risk factors are associated with the development and progression of CATE such as reduced LA fractional shortening and severe LA enlargement on echocardiogram (**Box 1**). In addition, cats with preexisting CATE have the highest risk for the recurrence of CATE.[40] Unfortunately, existing methods of identifying risk factors rely solely on echocardiograms. This is complicated by the fact that many cats at risk do not have

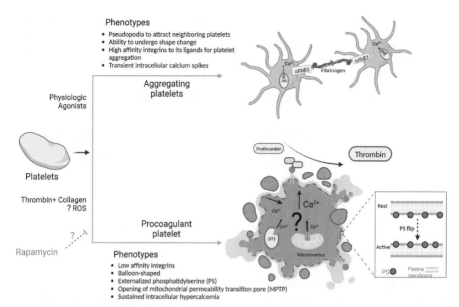

Fig. 3. Summary of phenotypes and functions of aggregatory and procoagulant platelets. Activated platelets commit to become procoagulant platelets on strong physiologic agonists such as thrombin and collagen. Sustained increase in intracellular calcium occurs through a multistep process which involves calcium influx through plasma membrane, calcium release from the dense tubular system (DTS), reactive oxygen species, and mitochondria. A cascade of intracellular events leads to calcium release via mitochondrial permeability transition pores (mPTP), which causes externalization of the negatively charged phospholipid, phosphatidylserine (PS). Exposure of PS provides a membrane surface where coagulation proteins bind to form complexes to amplify thrombin generation. Drugs such as rapamycin might reduce the formation of procoagulant platelet function by stabilization of mitochondrial membrane potential.

Box 1

Summary of risk factors in cats for cardiogenic arterial thromboembolism

Known risk factors for cardiogenic arterial thromboembolism in cats
  History and signalment
    • Male
    • Previous thromboembolic events
    • Gallop sounds
  Echocardiogram findings:
    • LA enlargement
    • LA systolic dysfunction such as low LAA flow velocity
    • SEC/intracardiac thrombus

Potential risk factors for future research
  Biomarkers
    • Citrullinated histones
    • vWF
    • Cell-free DNA fragments (500–1000 base pairs)
    • Increased platelet activation/procoagulant platelets
    • Platelet–neutrophil aggregates

auscultatory abnormalities, hence are unlikely to undergo echocardiographic screening. No biomarkers or validated risk model analyses are available to evaluate thrombotic risk in HCM cats. **Box 1** summarizes known risk factors and potential biomarkers for identifying cats at risk for CATE.

RECOMMENDATIONS FOR PREVENTING CARDIOGENIC ARTERIAL THROMBOEMBOLISM

Primary prevention aims to prevent the first incidence of a thromboembolic event, whereas secondary prevention aims to prevent or limit the recurrence of CATE. Given the high morbidity and mortality rates of CATE, cats at risk of CATE should be treated with thromboprophylaxis that is cost-effective, safe, and efficacious.[1]

Primary Prevention in Cats with Stage B2 Cardiomyopathy

Primary prevention should be implemented in cats diagnosed with stage B2 cardiomyopathy with LA enlargement and/or observed LA systolic dysfunction. **Fig. 3** outlines the risk assessments and primary prevention strategies in cats with Stage B2 cardiomyopathy. The efficacy of antiplatelet drugs for the primary prevention of CATE is lacking. However, a multicenter, randomized, double-blinded clinical trial feline arterial thromboembolism; clopidogrel vs. aspirin trial (FATCAT) comparing clopidogrel with aspirin in CATE recurrence in 75 cats that survived a thromboembolic event revealed that clopidogrel was superior to aspirin in reducing the incidence of CATE recurrence.[7] Both drugs modulate platelet activation and platelet aggregation via different mechanisms of action with high interindividual variability (**Table 1**).[1] However, on-treatment recurrence rate remained high at 36% for clopidogrel and 75% for aspirin indicating that an antiplatelet drug alone does not eliminate the risk of CATE.[7] For that reason, aspirin therapy alone does not seem to be an effective thromboprophylaxis. These findings also support the use of precision medicine to identify genetic polymorphisms that impact the inhibitory effects of clopidogrel in cats. Precision medicine uses genetic testing to identify mutations that influence the pharmacodynamics of drugs in individuals and is an emerging field in human cardiovascular medicine. A prospective observational study in 49 HCM cats found that nonsynonymous single-nucleotide polymorphism in the *P2RY1* gene, which encodes the platelet ADP receptor, P2Y1, was significantly associated with clopidogrel resistance after 10 to 14 days of clopidogrel therapy. Because a high number of HCM cats was shown to have the P2RY1:A236 G variant (51% heterozygous, 16.3% homozygous), genetic testing for this variant is highly recommended, whereas the patient is started on clopidogrel (**Fig. 4**).[41] A multimodal thromboprophylaxis approach also should be considered in cats tested positive for this variant. In human studies, dual-agent therapy (DAT) consisting of an antiplatelet drug and a direct oral anticoagulant (DOAC) such as rivaroxaban is superior to single-agent therapy in preventing and reducing the incidence of acute thrombosis.[42] Although dose escalation of clopidogrel was shown to be beneficial in humans with clopidogrel resistance due to cytochrome P450 2C gene mutations, Yu and colleagues did not find any significant associations between clopidogrel active metabolites and platelet inhibition. This finding indicates that dose escalation would not likely be effective at potentiating the inhibitory effect of clopidogrel in cats with the *P2RY1*:A236 G variant.[41] If DOAC is not a viable option, unfractionated heparin (UFH), low-molecular weight heparin (LMWH), or addition of aspirin can be considered.

A dual-agent approach with an antiplatelet drug such as clopidogrel and DOAC such as rivaroxaban or apixaban should be considered in cats with Stage B2 cardiomyopathy with atrial fibrillation, SEC, or LA intracardiac thrombi. UFH or LMWH may

Table 1
Summary of common drugs used for primary and secondary prevention of cardiogenic arterial thromboembolism in cats

Drug	Recommended Dose	Mechanism of Action
Antiplatelet		
Aspirin	81 mg PO q72 h 5 mg/kg PO q48 h	Irreversible inhibition of platelet cyclooxygenase-1, responsible for converting arachidonic acid to thromboxane A_2, which induces platelet activation and aggregation
Clopidogrel	18.75 mg PO q24 h Single loading dose: 37.5 mg PO q24 h	Metabolized by liver to clopidogrel active metabolite, which binds irreversibly to adenosine diphosphate (ADP) receptor, $P2Y_{12}$, preventing ADP binding to the receptor
Anticoagulant		
Unfractionated heparin	250 U/kg SC q6h	Binds to antithrombin to potentiate its activity to inhibit factors IIa, IXa, Xa, XIa, and XIIa
Enoxaparin Dalteparin	75–100 IU/kg SC q4 to 6h 0.7–1 mg/kg SC q4 to 6h	Forms complex with antithrombin and preferentially inhibits factor Xa
Direct oral anticoagulant		
Rivaroxaban Apixaban	2.5 mg to 5 mg PO q24 h 0.2 mg/kg PO	Binds to and inhibits factor Xa directly
Thrombolytics		
Tissue plasminogen activator	1 mg/kg (maximum 6 mg) IV slow bolus over 30 min OR 1 mg/cat IV bolus then 2.5 mg/cat over 30 min	Catalyzes enzymatic conversion of plasminogen to plasmin which cleaves fibrin polymers

be used in place of DOAC but a few studies have found that multiple subcutaneous administrations of up to every 6 hours are required to obtain effective anticoagulant activity.[43] This could greatly compromise owner and patient compliance. To date, two DOACs (rivaroxaban and apixaban) have been studied in cats and are shown to be safe, well-tolerated, and effective in inhibiting factor Xa.[44,45] A retrospective study describing the use of DAT with clopidogrel and rivaroxaban reported no on-treatment thrombotic events in cats with cardiomyopathy and SEC or intracardiac thrombi. Adverse effects were also low at 15% with clinically insignificant bleeding.[46] This finding suggests that DAT may be an effective thromboprophylaxis for primary prevention. Comparative studies of metabolism and excretion of rivaroxaban in dogs, humans, and rats found that ~66% of the drug was excreted unchanged by the kidneys.[47] Therefore, drug clearance may be inversely proportional to the degree of renal function impairment. In the Rivaroxaban versus Warfarin in Nonvalvular Atrial Fibrillation (ROCKET AF) trial, which evaluated the efficacy of dose reduction of rivaroxaban in human patients with atrial fibrillation and moderate renal impairment, major bleeding events were reported more frequently among patients on rivaroxaban or warfarin.[48] Because apixaban is largely excreted unchanged via the gastrointestinal routes (59%) in dogs, it is reasonable to consider using apixaban in cats with severe renal disease.[49] Further studies are required to study the effects of DOACs in cats with severe renal disease. Given the high interindividual variability in response to clopidogrel therapy in cats, genetic testing for the P2RY1:A236 G variant is highly recommended in

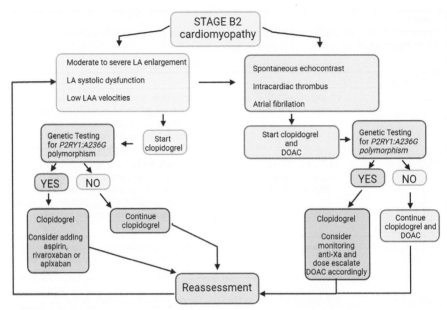

Fig. 4. Recommendations for primary prevention of CATE in cats in Stage B2 cardiomyopathy.

cats at high risk of CATE. If SEC or LA thrombus remains static or worsens after starting DAT, increased dosing frequency or dose escalation of DOACs based on anti-Xa activity may be warranted (see **Fig. 4**).

Secondary Prevention in Cats with Stage C Cardiomyopathy

In addition to stabilizing cardiopulmonary status, commencement of thromboprophylaxis to prevent further thrombus growth and thrombotic events is of utmost importance. In patients that tolerate oral medications, clopidogrel should be started (see **Table 1**). According to the Consensus on the Rational Use of Antithrombotics in Veterinary Critical Care (CURATIVE) guidelines, a single loading dose of 37.5 mg may be effective at increasing therapeutic plasma concentrations more quickly.[50] The FAT-CAT study, which compared aspirin to clopidogrel as sole thromboprophylactic treatment in cats after a CATE event, demonstrated that clopidogrel was superior to aspirin by prolonging the recurrence of arterial thromboembolism (ATE) (median time: 346 days vs 128 days).[7] Despite the lack of high-quality evidence, DAT with a DOAC or anticoagulant should be considered as part of their in-hospital thromboprophylaxis strategy.[50] In a retrospective case series by Lo and colleagues describing the use of DAT with clopidogrel and rivaroxaban in 18 cats following CATE, recurrence rate was 17% with a median survival time of 502 days.[46] This is the longest survival time and lowest recurrence rate ever reported when compared with the FATCAT study, which reported a recurrence rate of 36% in the clopidogrel group.[7] It is important to note that both studies included cats that survived to hospital discharge while previous retrospective studies reported cats that were euthanized at presentation or within 48 hours of hospitalization when mortality rate was the highest. Nonetheless, this further supports the notion that a DAT may be superior to single-agent approach in preventing recurrence of CATE. In an *ex vivo* study, we demonstrated that 7 days of DAT treatment with rivaroxaban and clopidogrel resulted in synergistic platelet inhibition in healthy cats. Compared with treatment with clopidogrel or rivaroxaban alone, DAT was more effective at modulating tissue factor-induced thrombin generation and thrombin-mediated platelet activation.51 The study also found that mono-agent treatment alone with rivaroxaban resulted in potentiation in platelet aggregation and activation.[46]

Cats that are hospitalized for CATE may be in respiratory distress due to concurrent CHF and, hence, may not tolerate oral medications. In these cats, injectable anticoagulants should be administered. Although UFH is inexpensive and widely available, its efficacy has not been investigated in cats with CATE. As mentioned earlier, LMWH requires multiple dosing to maintain anti-Xa activity.[43] For that reason, LMWH or UFH may be more suitable for in-hospital treatment before patients can be transitioned to oral medications. Although the current CURATIVE guidelines recommend individual dose adjustments based on therapeutic monitoring, no studies to date have shown an optimal range of anti-Xa activities that would safely deliver thromboprophylaxis in clinical cats.[50]

Once patients are discharged from hospital, reassessment by echocardiogram and physical examination for worsening of LA function, SEC, intracardiac thrombus, and perfusion to previously thrombosed sites are highly recommended to assess efficacy of thromboprophylaxis. Cats that develop on-treatment return of SEC or intracardiac thrombus should be monitored for DOAC anti-Xa activity for dose escalation or increase in dosing frequency. **Fig. 5** outlines the risk assessments and secondary prevention strategies in cats with Stage C cardiomyopathy.

THROMBOLYTIC THERAPY

The use of streptokinase or TPA to accelerate fibrinolysis in cats with CATE is controversial.[4] Based on human guidelines, TPA should be administered in cats shortly, ideally within 6 hours after thromboembolic events. A recent prospective multicenter

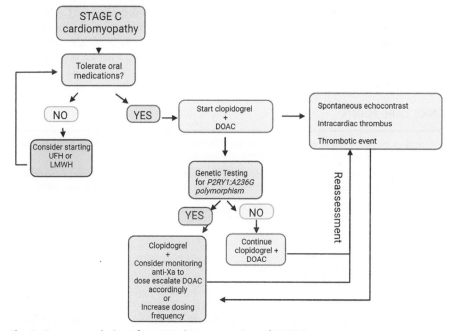

Fig. 5. Recommendations for secondary prevention of CATE in cats.

randomized placebo-controlled trial did not demonstrate any benefit of TPA on short-term survival and limb perfusion compared with conventional therapy despite enrollment within 6 hours of CATE.[52] Although this study did not find gross evidence of hemorrhage in necropsy of cats treated with TPA, it is, nevertheless, a known and potentially life-threatening complication of TPA. Clinicians are advised to weigh the risks and benefits of TPA administration cautiously.

FUTURE THERAPIES

Given the important role of platelets in clot formation, targeting procoagulant platelet formation while sparing the aggregatory function of platelets may be a more effective and safe approach in preventing and treating CATE (see **Fig. 3**). Platelet integrin $\alpha IIb\beta 3$ antagonists such as abciximab and eptifibatide may offer better thromboprophylaxis than conventional antiplatelet drugs. The efficacy of abciximab has been studied in a feline arterial injury model, which showed that the combination of abciximab and aspirin was superior to aspirin in reducing thrombus formation.[53] However, its in vitro inhibitory effect on platelet aggregation could not be determined suggesting that abciximab may not bind to feline platelet integrins. Eptifibatide was shown to cause unpredictable circulatory and sudden death in cats; hence, its use is not recommended in clinical patients.[54] Larger scale clinical trials are required to assess the efficacy and safety of $\alpha IIb\beta 3$ antagonists in clinical HCM cats.

Novel therapies directed at disrupting NETs formation, scavenging NETs proteins, and dismantling NETs structure may have synergistic effects on existing therapies by modulating thrombin generation, platelet activation, and augmenting clot remodeling (see **Fig. 2**).

SUMMARY

Platelet–neutrophil interaction and immunothrombosis likely play an important role in the complex pathophysiology of CATE. Early recognition of risk factors for CATE is the key to prevent thromboembolic events and to implement effective and safe primary prevention strategies. To improve patient outcomes, future research should aim to improve our understanding of the molecular and mechanistic interactions involved in this disease process. Precision medicine could aid in identifying cats at risk of CATE and optimizing antithrombotic treatments.

CLINICS CARE POINTS

- Precision medicine using genetic testing for *P2RY1:A236 G* polymorphism to provide the optimal thromboprophylaxis in cats at risk of developing CATE
- Dual-agent therapy consisting of clopidogrel and direct oral anticoagulant is recommended in cats with P2RY1:A236 G mutation or those at high risk of developing CATE and CATE recurrence.

DISCLOSURE

The authors have nothing to disclose.

REFERENCES

1. Hogan DF. Feline Cardiogenic Arterial Thromboembolism: Prevention and Therapy. Vet Clin North Am Small Anim Pract 2017;47(5):1065–82.

2. Payne JR, Brodbelt DC, Luis Fuentes V. Cardiomyopathy prevalence in 780 apparently healthy cats in rehoming centres (the CatScan study). J Vet Cardiol 2015;17(Suppl 1):S244–57.

3. Fox PR, Keene BW, Lamb K, et al. International collaborative study to assess cardiovascular risk and evaluate long-term health in cats with preclinical hypertrophic cardiomyopathy and apparently healthy cats: The REVEAL Study [published correction appears in J Vet Intern Med. 2018 Nov;32(6):2310]. J Vet Intern Med 2018;32(3):930–43.

4. Luis Fuentes V. Arterial thromboembolism: risks, realities and a rational first-line approach. J Feline Med Surg 2012;14(7):459–70.

5. Smith SA, Tobias AH, Jacob KA, et al. Arterial thromboembolism in cats: acute crisis in 127 cases (1992-2001) and long-term management with low-dose aspirin in 24 cases. J Vet Intern Med 2003;17(1):73–83.

6. Borgeat K, Wright J, Garrod O, et al. Arterial thromboembolism in 250 cats in general practice: 2004-2012. J Vet Intern Med 2014;28(1):102–8.

7. Hogan DF, Fox PR, Jacob K, et al. Secondary prevention of cardiogenic arterial thromboembolism in the cat: The double-blind, randomized, positive-controlled feline arterial thromboembolism; clopidogrel vs. aspirin trial (FAT CAT). J Vet Cardiol 2015;17(Suppl 1):S306–17.

8. Jurk K, Kehrel BE. Platelets: physiology and biochemistry. Semin Thromb Hemost 2005;31(4):381–92.

9. Tablin F, Schumacher T, Pombo M, et al. Platelet activation in cats with hypertrophic cardiomyopathy. J Vet Intern Med 2014;28(2):411–8.

10. Helenski CA, Ross JN Jr. Platelet aggregation in feline cardiomyopathy. J Vet Intern Med 1987;1(1):24–8.

11. Li RH, Stern JA, Ho V, et al. Platelet Activation and Clopidogrel Effects on ADP-Induced Platelet Activation in Cats with or without the A31P Mutation in MYBPC3. J Vet Intern Med 2016;30(5):1619–29.

12. Tan AWK, Li RHL, Ueda Y, et al. Platelet Priming and Activation in Naturally Occurring Thermal Burn Injuries and Wildfire Smoke Exposure Is Associated With Intracardiac Thrombosis and Spontaneous Echocardiographic Contrast in Feline Survivors. Front Vet Sci 2022;9:892377.

13. Chapin JC, Hajjar KA. Fibrinolysis and the control of blood coagulation. Blood Rev 2015;29(1):17–24.

14. Welles EG, Boudreaux MK, Crager CS, et al. Platelet function and antithrombin, plasminogen, and fibrinolytic activities in cats with heart disease. Am J Vet Res 1994;55(5):619–27.

15. Bédard C, Lanevschi-Pietersma A, Dunn M. Evaluation of coagulation markers in the plasma of healthy cats and cats with asymptomatic hypertrophic cardiomyopathy. Vet Clin Pathol 2007;36(2):167–72.

16. Stokol T, Brooks M, Rush JE, et al. Hypercoagulability in cats with cardiomyopathy. J Vet Intern Med 2008;22(3):546–52 [published correction appears in J Vet Intern Med. 2009 Jan-Feb;23(1):224. Gelzer, A L [corrected to Gelzer, A R]].

17. Stark K, Massberg S. Interplay between inflammation and thrombosis in cardiovascular pathology. Nat Rev Cardiol 2021;18(9):666–82.

18. Goggs R, Jeffery U, LeVine DN, et al. Neutrophil-Extracellular Traps, Cell-Free DNA, and Immunothrombosis in Companion Animals: A Review. Vet Pathol 2020;57(1):6–23.

19. von Brühl ML, Stark K, Steinhart A, et al. Monocytes, neutrophils, and platelets cooperate to initiate and propagate venous thrombosis in mice in vivo. J Exp Med 2012;209(4):819–35.

20. Massberg S, Grahl L, von Bruehl ML, et al. Reciprocal coupling of coagulation and innate immunity via neutrophil serine proteases. Nat Med 2010;16(8):887–96.

21. Semeraro F, Ammollo CT, Morrissey JH, et al. Extracellular histones promote thrombin generation through platelet-dependent mechanisms: involvement of platelet TLR2 and TLR4. Blood 2011;118(7):1952–61.

22. Jeffery U, LeVine DN. Canine Neutrophil Extracellular Traps Enhance Clot Formation and Delay Lysis. Vet Pathol 2018;55(1):116–23.

23. Hogwood J, Pitchford S, Mulloy B, et al. Heparin and non-anticoagulant heparin attenuate histone-induced inflammatory responses in whole blood. PLoS One 2020;15(5):e0233644.

24. Li RHL, Fabella A, Nguyen N, et al. Circulating neutrophil extracellular traps in cats with hypertrophic cardiomyopathy and cardiogenic arterial thromboembolism. J Vet Intern Med 2023;37(2):490–502.

25. Li RH, Nguyen N, Stern JA, et al. Neutrophil extracellular traps in feline cardiogenic arterial thrombi: a pilot study. J Feline Med Surg 2022;24(6):580–6.

26. Laridan E, Denorme F, Desender L, et al. Neutrophil extracellular traps in ischemic stroke thrombi. Ann Neurol 2017;82(2):223–32.

27. Xue J, Huang W, Chen X, et al. Neutrophil-to-Lymphocyte Ratio Is a Prognostic Marker in Acute Ischemic Stroke. J Stroke Cerebrovasc Dis 2017;26(3):650–7.

28. Ozyilmaz S, Akgul O, Uyarel H, et al. The importance of the neutrophil-to-lymphocyte ratio in patients with hypertrophic cardiomyopathy. Rev Port Cardiol 2017;36(4):239–46.

29. Fries RC, Kadotani S, Stack JP, et al. Prognostic Value of Neutrophil-to-Lymphocyte Ratio in Cats With Hypertrophic Cardiomyopathy. Front Vet Sci 2022;9:813524.

30. Schober KE, Maerz I. Assessment of left atrial appendage flow velocity and its relation to spontaneous echocardiographic contrast in 89 cats with myocardial disease. J Vet Intern Med 2006;20(1):120–30.

31. Rastegar R, Harnick DJ, Weidemann P, et al. Spontaneous echo contrast videodensity is flow-related and is dependent on the relative concentrations of fibrinogen and red blood cells. J Am Coll Cardiol 2003;41(4):603–10.

32. Zotz RJ, Müller M, Genth-Zotz S, et al. Spontaneous echo contrast caused by platelet and leukocyte aggregates? Stroke 2001;32(5):1127–33.

33. Yau JW, Teoh H, Verma S. Endothelial cell control of thrombosis. BMC Cardiovasc Disord 2015;15:130.

34. Lip GY, Blann A. von Willebrand factor: a marker of endothelial dysfunction in vascular disorders? Cardiovasc Res 1997;34(2):255–65.

35. Spiel AO, Gilbert JC, Jilma B. von Willebrand factor in cardiovascular disease: focus on acute coronary syndromes. Circulation 2008;117(11):1449–59.

36. Cambronero F, Vilchez JA, García-Honrubia A, et al. Plasma levels of von Willebrand factor are increased in patients with hypertrophic cardiomyopathy. Thromb Res 2010;126(1):e46–50.

37. Liu SK, Maron BJ, Tilley LP. Feline hypertrophic cardiomyopathy: Gross anatomic and quantitative histologic features. Am J Pathol 1981;102:388–95.

38. Cheng WC, Wilkie L, Kurosawa TA, et al. Immunohistological Evaluation of Von Willebrand Factor in the Left Atrial Endocardium and Atrial Thrombi from Cats with Cardiomyopathy. Animals (Basel) 2021;11(5):1240.

39. Chu Y, Guo H, Zhang Y, et al. Procoagulant platelets: Generation, characteristics, and therapeutic target. J Clin Lab Anal 2021;35(5):e23750.

40. Payne JR, Borgeat K, Connolly DJ, et al. Prognostic indicators in cats with hypertrophic cardiomyopathy. J Vet Intern Med 2013;27(6):1427–36.

41. Ueda Y, Li RHL, Nguyen N, et al. A genetic polymorphism in P2RY$_1$ impacts response to clopidogrel in cats with hypertrophic cardiomyopathy. Sci Rep 2021;11(1):12522.
42. Yuan J. Efficacy and safety of adding rivaroxaban to the anti-platelet regimen in patients with coronary artery disease: a systematic review and meta-analysis of randomized controlled trials. BMC Pharmacol Toxicol 2018;19(1):19.
43. Alwood AJ, Downend AB, Brooks MB, et al. Anticoagulant effects of low-molecular-weight heparins in healthy cats. J Vet Intern Med 2007;21(3):378–87.
44. Myers JA, Wittenburg LA, Olver CS, et al. Pharmacokinetics and pharmacodynamics of the factor Xa inhibitor apixaban after oral and intravenous administration to cats. Am J Vet Res 2015;76(8):732–8.
45. Dixon-Jimenez AC, Brainard BM, Brooks MB, et al. Pharmacokinetic and pharmacodynamic evaluation of oral rivaroxaban in healthy adult cats. J Vet Emerg Crit Care 2016;26(5):619–29.
46. Lo ST, Walker AL, Georges CJ, et al. Dual therapy with clopidogrel and rivaroxaban in cats with thromboembolic disease. J Feline Med Surg 2022;24(4):277–83.
47. Weinz C, Schwarz T, Kubitza D, et al. Metabolism and excretion of rivaroxaban, an oral, direct factor Xa inhibitor, in rats, dogs, and humans. Drug Metab Dispos 2009;37(5):1056–64.
48. Patel MR, Mahaffey KW, Garg J, et al. Rivaroxaban versus warfarin in nonvalvular atrial fibrillation. N Engl J Med 2011;365(10):883–91.
49. Zhang D, He K, Raghavan N, et al. Comparative metabolism of 14C-labeled apixaban in mice, rats, rabbits, dogs, and humans. Drug Metab Dispos 2009;37(8):1738–48.
50. Blais MC, Bianco D, Goggs R, et al. Consensus on the Rational Use of Antithrombotics in Veterinary Critical Care (CURATIVE): Domain 3-Defining antithrombotic protocols. J Vet Emerg Crit Care 2019;29(1):60–74.
51. Lo ST, Li RHL, Georges CJ, et al. Synergistic inhibitory effects of clopidogrel and rivaroxaban on platelet function and platelet-dependent thrombin generation in cats. J Vet Intern Med 2023;1:11.
52. Guillaumin J, DeFrancesco TC, Scansen BA, et al. Bilateral lysis of aortic saddle thrombus with early tissue plasminogen activator (BLASTT): a prospective, randomized, placebo controlled study in feline acute aortic thromboembolism. J Feline Med Surg 2022;24(12):e535–45.
53. Bright JM, Dowers K, Powers BE. Effects of the glycoprotein IIb/IIIa antagonist abciximab on thrombus formation and platelet function in cats with arterial injury. Vet Ther 2003;4(1):35–46.
54. Bright JM, Dowers K, Hellyer P. In vitro anti-aggregatory effects of the GP IIb/IIIa antagonist eptifibatide on feline platelets. J Vet Intern Med 2002;16(6):v. https://doi.org/10.1111/j.1939-1676.2002.tb01316.x.

Hypertrophic Cardiomyopathy–Advances in Imaging and Diagnostic Strategies

Ryan Fries, DVM

KEYWORDS

- Cat • Echocardiogram • Heart • Biomarker

KEY POINTS

- Timely and accurate diagnosis of HCM is essential in combating this global disease impacting the feline population.
- Cardiac biomarkers have the potential to substantially improve screening practices for at-risk populations.
- Echocardiography is considered the reference standard for diagnosing HCM in cats; however, advanced imaging methods such as tissue strain, contrast-enhanced echocardiography, and cardiac MRI are improving diagnosis, accuracy, and risk-stratification.

 Video content accompanies this article at http://www.vetsmall.theclinics.com.

INTRODUCTION

Hypertrophic cardiomyopathy (HCM) is the most common heart disease in cats and is reported to affect between 15% and 34% of overtly healthy cats.[1,2] HCM is characterized by concentric hypertrophy resulting in a reduction of left ventricular chamber size, impaired ventricular relaxation, and increased wall thickness, all of which impede diastolic filling.[3] HCM is a genetic disease and familial HCM has been reported to be caused by a mutation in myosin binding protein C in Maine coon and Ragdoll cats.[4,5] Hallmark histopathologic myocardial lesions in cats with HCM include myofiber disarray, small coronary arteriosclerosis, and interstitial and replacement fibrosis.[6] In humans with HCM, myocardial interstitial changes can be focal or global with the potential for reversibility with treatment in early stages.[7,8]

Identification of left ventricular hypertrophy cannot be used as the sole means for diagnosing primary HCM. Left ventricular hypertrophy can be primary, the result of

Department of Veterinary Clinical Medicine, University of Illinois at Urbana-Champaign, 1008 West Hazelwood Drive, Urbana, IL 61802, USA
E-mail address: rfries@illinois.edu

Vet Clin Small Anim 53 (2023) 1325–1342
https://doi.org/10.1016/j.cvsm.2023.05.010
0195-5616/23/© 2023 Elsevier Inc. All rights reserved.

genetic HCM, or it can be secondary to other diseases such as systemic hypertension, hyperthyroidism, acromegaly, pseudohypertrophy, left ventricular outflow (LVOT) tract obstructions, or transient myocardial thickening.[9] Therefore, a wholistic patient-specific diagnostic workup and management plan must be undertaken. The ability to distinguishing between primary and secondary HCM is paramount because many of the secondary causes of HCM are reversible and will dramatically alter both treatment and prognosis. Although beyond the scope of this article, prognosis for cats with HCM is highly variable across all stages of the disease. The most common sequalae attributed to HCM are congestive heart failure, arterial thromboembolism, and sudden cardiac death.[10] There is a substantial risk associated with HCM, and a 10-year cardiovascular mortality rate of approximately 30% of cats.[10] Additionally, even in cats with noncardiovascular death, the presence of preclinical HCM is associated with significantly greater mortality and shorter survival times.[11] Collectively, given the high prevalence of HCM and the significant morbidity and mortality associated with its presence, prompt diagnosis and management of this condition is essential.

DISCUSSION
Genetic and Breed Risk Factors

HCM is primarily a disease of middle-aged to older cats but can affect cats of all ages and all breeds, including mixed breeds. There is no sex-lined heritability pattern for HCM, although male cats typically account for greater than 70% of cats diagnosed with HCM in most reports. Breeds considered or suspected to have a higher incidence of HCM than the general feline population are Maine Coon, American short-haired, Ragdoll, Persian, Sphynx, British short-haired, Norwegian forest cat, Siberian, Scottish fold, Birman, Himalayan, Chartreux, and Bengal. Testing for HCM-related genetic markers is available for Maine Coon and Ragdoll breeds and recently Sphynx cats. Genetic testing should always be interpreted in the context of an individual patient. Although causative mutations have been identified in some breeds, these mutations are of variable penetrance, and they do not represent the totality of all possible genetic causes of HCM.[12,13] This has the combined effect of both false positives and false negatives associated with presence of a genetic mutation. At best, a genetically affected cat should always have definitive testing, such as an echocardiogram to determine if HCM is present. Although some cardiologists may not consider breed alone to be reason enough to pursue additional diagnostics, the author often recommends screening evaluations for high-risk pure-bred cats especially if they are part of a breeding colony.

Physical Examination

The most commonly identified abnormality on physical examination in cats with HCM remains auscultatory abnormalities including a systolic heart murmur, a gallop heart sound, or an irregular heart rhythm. Although these abnormalities may indicate the presence of heart disease, none is specific for HCM. Of these, gallop or irregular heart rhythms are most predictive of a cardiac abnormality, whereas functional heart murmurs are heard in many cats without identifiable cardiac disease or occur secondary to a systemic problem (eg, anemia). Importantly, the absence of auscultatory abnormalities does not preclude the presence of HCM. In asymptomatic cats, the presence of a murmur in the general population can be as high as 72% in cats aged older than 9 years; however, the positive predictive value of a murmur identifying HCM never exceeds 50%.[10] Although this may be somewhat disheartening, evidence also indicates that the lack of a murmur does carry relatively high-negative predictive values (75%–

100%) depending on the age of the cat.[14] Despite these inconsistencies, auscultation remains the primary method by which cats that may benefit from further testing can be identified.

Echocardiography

In veterinary medicine, echocardiography is the gold standard test for diagnosing HCM. It is widely accepted that for HCM to be confirmed, there must be symmetric or asymmetric left ventricular concentric hypertrophy in the absence of other causes such as aortic stenosis, systemic hypertension, acromegaly, or hyperthyroidism. Concentric hypertrophy is defined as end-diastolic left ventricular free wall or interventricular septal thickness of 6 mm or greater, with an equivocal zone from 5.5 to 5.9 mm (**Fig. 1**). There is no validation of which cutoff values (>5.5 or > 6 mm) is the most appropriate for diagnosing the presence of left ventricular hypertrophy and HCM, although standard practice typically uses a maximal thickness of 6 mm or greater in any part of the wall segment.[15] Importantly, these values must be interpreted on a patient-specific basis and include the use of breed and weight-based references values whenever possible.[16–18]

Currently, the author recommends echocardiography to establish the location of left ventricular hypertrophy, the presence of systolic anterior motion (SAM) and LVOT obstruction, diastolic dysfunction, and left atrial size and function including the presence of spontaneous echo-contrast or a thrombus (Video 1). In veterinary medicine, 2 forms of HCM are routinely described: obstructive and nonobstructive HCM. Although in humans, there are multiple anatomic variants of HCM, based on the location and extent of the hypertrophied myocardium. For example, HCM may be described as reverse curvature septum, the most common form, describes a septum with the convexity to left ventricle (LV) cavity because the cavity has a crescent shape. Neutral HCM refers to a straight septum. The sigmoid form of HCM involves a basal septum bulge, with the concavity to the LV cavity; it usually produces SAM. Apical HCM involves the hypertrophy of the apex.[19] Each of these phenotypes carries a different prognosis and treatment regimen, highlighting both the heterogeneity of the HCM phenotype and more importantly, the need for patient-specific treatment recommendations rather than a one-size-fits-all approach.

Echocardiography provides meaningful information regarding left ventricular systolic function, which has been shown to be impaired in some cats with HCM. Although global systolic function assessed by fractional shortening or ejection fraction is mostly

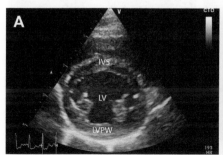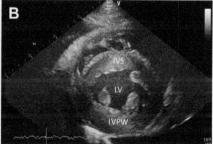

Fig. 1. Right parasternal, short-axis view of the left ventricle using 2D transthoracic imaging at the level of the papillary muscles. (*A*) Image from a normal cat and (*B*) image from a cat with symmetrical left ventricular concentric hypertrophy. IVS; interventricular septum, LV; left ventricle, LVPW; left ventricular posterior wall.

preserved, indices of systolic function measured by strain support an overall decreased systolic function in cats with HCM.[20-22] Impairment of contractile function in HCM assessed by strain is associated with left ventricular mass but not markers of extracellular fibrosis.[22] This suggests that impairment of contractility in feline HCM is mediated by mechanisms other than extracellular expansion and is consistent with results of regional strain imaging in people with HCM.[23] Therefore, left ventricular function should be evaluated by tissue Doppler and strain echocardiography whenever possible. In humans with HCM, decreased longitudinal strain values are associated with a more severe form of the disease, as well as an increased risk of major cardiovascular events, independent of other echocardiographic criteria while this relationship has not been evaluated in cats with HCM.

HCM and progressive myocardial fibrosis lead to worsening diastolic function in HCM. Echocardiography and, specifically, spectral and tissue Doppler imaging techniques, involving transmitral flow and mitral annular tissue velocities, are indispensable in assessing diastolic function. For an accurate evaluation of diastolic function, multiple parameters should be assessed, including Doppler of mitral valve inflow, left atrial size and function, and mitral annular tissue Doppler imaging. Although transmitral flow is highly influenced by loading conditions, heart rate, and other disease states, tissue Doppler imaging is less sensitive to loading conditions and heart rates. For these reasons, tissue Doppler imaging is the preferred method for evaluating diastolic function in cats.

Echocardiography provides information about LVOT obstructions and the presence of SAM. For optimal results, SAM is typically visualized using high temporal resolution two-dimensional (2D) imaging from the right parasternal inflow outflow or 5-chamber view (**Fig. 2**). As a consequence of SAM, mitral valve coaptation is reduced in systole causing secondary mitral regurgitation proportional with the degree of obstruction. Spectral Doppler examination of the LVOT can be used to detect hemodynamically significant obstructions, which the author classifies as greater than 80 mm Hg at heart rates less than 180 bpm (**Fig. 3**).

Despite what may seem to be a straightforward approach to diagnosing HCM, echocardiography is often inadequate due to poor visualization of all wall segments (apex, midventricle, base), inadequate delineation of the endocardial surface (especially with endocardial thickening), leading to overestimation of wall thickness, isolated or segmental hypertrophy of one region of the myocardium, papillary muscle hypertrophy,

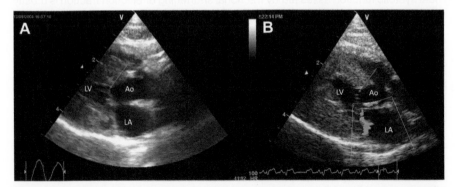

Fig. 2. Right parasternal, long-axis 5-chamber view using 2D transthoracic imaging. (A) Image demonstrating SAM of mitral valve (*red arrow*) and (B) SAM of mitral valve (*red arrow*) and color Doppler imaging demonstrating turbulent flow in the LVOT tract as well as mitral regurgitation. Ao; aorta, LA; left atrium, LV; left ventricle.

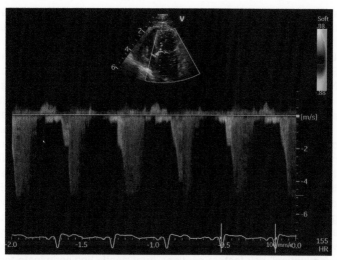

Fig. 3. Spectral Doppler interrogation of LVOT tract velocities obtained from the left-apical, 5-chamber view. The spectral profiles are dynamic and the average maximum velocity obtained was 4.79 m/s, estimating a severe obstructive gradient of 92 mm Hg at a heart rate of 155 bpm.

and a limited number of acoustic windows. As a result of these limitations, hypertrophied ventricular segments can be missed, underestimated, or overestimated by echocardiography (Video 2). In humans, CMR has become the gold standard evaluation in patients with HCM because it provides a complete evaluation of both ventricles, wall thicknesses, characterization of the myocardium, and cardiac volumes with high spatial and temporal resolution in all planes.[24] (Video 3) A recent study in humans demonstrated the effectiveness of CMR in detecting cardiac hypertrophy over other imaging methods, with a 1.4% detection of LVH among the supposed healthy general population, a significantly higher percentage than by echocardiography.[25]

Biomarkers

The gold standard for the diagnosis of HCM remains echocardiography; however, its widespread use is limited in many areas, and it is a technically challenging modality. Advances in cardiac biomarker assays have alternatively allowed for the routine use in clinical practice for the screening of cardiac disease in cats and diagnosis of respiratory distress secondary to cardiac disease.[26–31] Cardiac biomarkers are appealing in general and specialty practice due to their ease of use, minimally invasive approach, and increase the availability with national laboratories and point-of-care assays available.

Biomarkers are defined as a characteristic that is objectively measured and evaluated as an indicator of a normal biologic process, pathogenic process, or response to intervention. These are most useful when they are directly proportional to the change in status or amount of injury that has occurred. Multiple sensitive and specific cardiac biomarkers have been evaluated in a healthy patients and patients with various cardiac diseases in cats including N-terminal pro-Brain type natriuretic peptide (NT-proBNP), cardiac troponin I (cTnI), and recently, galectin-3 (Gal-3).[28–32]

The most widely used biomarker to aid in the diagnosis of HCM is NT-proBNP. B-type natriuretic peptide (BNP) is a hormone, released by cardiomyocytes, resulting in natriuresis, diuresis, and vasodilation.[33] The secretion of BNP is significantly upregulated in cardiac disease and heart failure in response to myocyte stress and stretch from increased volume and pressure.[34] The hormone BNP is secreted as a prohormone (proBNP) and cleaved by furin into the active BNP hormone and an inactive NT-proBNP.[33] The more stable analyte, NT-proBNP, has a significantly longer half-life than BNP or proBNP and thus is the more ideal diagnostic marker to assess the magnitude of myocardial wall stress or stretch.[35] In feline patients, quantitative NT-proBNP has been used in the clinical setting to differentiate between cardiac and pulmonary disease for patients presenting with respiratory signs and to increase the likelihood of identifying patients with moderate-to-severe preclinical or occult cardiac disease.[26,27,36,37] Several studies have investigated the ability of NT-proBNP to identify cats with subclinical disease and have determined that a cutoff of greater than 100 pmol/L yields the most clinically useful results.[37] Furthermore, an NT-proBNP concentration greater than 270 pmol/L can accurately distinguish between cardiogenic and noncardiogenic causes of respiratory clinical signs.[28] Although this biomarker can be an asset to any veterinarian, its sensitivity and specificity and ultimately negative and positive predictive values are substantially improved by patient selection (see "Physical examination" risk factors section). Importantly, indiscriminate testing of all apparently healthy cats, especially those without a risk factor, should be avoided because the rate of false-positive results, and thus normal echocardiograms, is increased due to the lower prevalence of HCM within the population. Rather, it is recommended to use targeted testing of cats with an increased likelihood of disease, based risk factors, to reduce the rate of false positives and improve the positive predict value of the test. **Table 1** summarizes the current use of NT-proBNP in the clinical setting. Although NT-proBNP is elevated in cats with occult or overt HCM, it is not specific to HCM and a confirmatory test, such as echocardiography or cardiac MRI (CMR), will be necessary to make the final determination as to the underlying cardiomyopathy.

Although NT-proBNP has become the most widely used and available biomarker for HCM screening, a significant amount of research has gone into the study of cTnI in the assessment of cardiac diseases in cats.[38–40] Cats with HCM have significantly higher serum cTnI concentrations than do healthy control cats, and a correlation exists between left ventricular free wall thickness and the serum concentration of cTnI.[39–42]

Table 1
Current use for the cardiac biomarker N-terminal pro-Brain type natriuretic peptide in the clinical setting for both quantitative and SNAP enzyme-linked immunosorbent assay (ELISA) assays

Clinical Indication	NT-proBNP Result	SNAP Result	Interpretation
Cat with respiratory signs possibly attributable to heart failure	<100	Normal	Heart failure *not* supported
	100–270	Abnormal	Heart failure possible and additional testing or therapeutic trial should be pursued
	>270		Heart failure highly likely
Asymptomatic cat with cardiac risk factors (eg, murmur, arrhythmia, gallop heart sound)	<100	Normal	Heart disease should not be considered
	>100	Abnormal	Heart disease highly likely, recommend confirmatory testing (eg, echocardiogram, MRI)

High sensitivity cTnI assays compare favorably with NT-proBNP as a screening test to differentiate healthy cats and cats with HCM. A proposed cutoff of greater than 0.06 ng/mL provides a high degree of sensitivity and specificity at differentiating healthy cats from cats with HCM.[42] As such, cTnI is useful in identifying patients who should undergo further cardiac evaluation and severely elevated cTnI is a predictor of adverse cardiac outcomes in cats with HCM.[43]

FUTURE DIRECTIONS
Cardiac Magnetic Resonance Imaging

Echocardiography is the noninvasive reference standard for the diagnosis of HCM in cats; however, it does have 2 major limitations. Due to the 2D nature of echocardiography, focal regions of hypertrophy or thinning can be missed during routine echocardiography. Moreover, echocardiography has little to no value in assessing myocardial fibrosis, an important prognostic indicator in people with HCM. The final common endpoint of irreversible fibrosis has been linked to an increased risk of cardiac complications.[44] This link has not been established in cats with HCM at this time. Cardiac magnetic resonance imaging (CMR) can be used to noninvasively assess myocardial fibrosis using late gadolinium enhancement (LGE); however, quantitative evaluation is limited.[45–48] Calculation of LGE and myocardial contrast enhancement has been performed in 26 Maine coon cats with mild-to-severe HCM without heart failure and 10 normal control cats. Only one cat with HCM had obvious evidence of delayed enhancement, and there was no difference in myocardial contrast enhancement between normal cats and cats with HCM.[49] This study supports the conclusion that contrast-enhanced sequences can detect myocardial fibrosis if there is a large focal area; however, identification and characterization of enhancement patterns is subjective and susceptible to interobserver and intraobserver variability in quantitative analysis.[50] Traditional LGE images are most useful for evaluation of focal diseases, where normal myocardium can be used as a standard of reference and a pattern of enhancement can be detected (**Fig. 4**). Diffuse fibrosis may go undetected on qualitative images if gadolinium uptake is uniform.[45]

One method to overcome the limitation of LGE to detect diffuse fibrosis is quantitative myocardial mapping. T1 mapping measures the longitudinal or spin-lattice relaxation time, which is determined by how rapidly protons reequilibrate their spins after an excitation radiofrequency pulse. All tissues have inherent T1 relaxation times that are based on a composite of their cellular and interstitial components (eg, water, protein, fat, and iron content).[45] At a fixed magnetic field strength, the native T1 values of normal tissues fall within a predictable range.[51] The 2 most important biological determinants of an increase in native T1 values are edema from increased tissue water and increased interstitial space from fibrosis.[52] Native T1 values are a composite signal of myocytes and extracellular volume (ECV), whereas contrast-enhanced T1 mapping can specifically calculate the ECV fraction (**Fig. 5**). Gadolinium-based contrast agents are distributed throughout the extracellular space and shorten T1 relaxation times of the myocardium proportional to the local concentration for gadolinium.[53] Areas of fibrosis and scar will therefore exhibit shorter T1 relaxation times, particularly after contrast administration.[54] Estimation of the ECV (interstitium and extracellular matrix) requires measurement of myocardial and blood T1 values before and after the administration of contrast agents, as well as the patient's hematocrit value according to the formula:

$$ECV = (1 - haematocrit) \frac{\frac{1}{post\ contrast\ T1\ myo} - \frac{1}{native\ T1\ myo}}{\frac{1}{post\ contrast\ T1\ blood} - \frac{1}{native\ T1\ blood}}$$

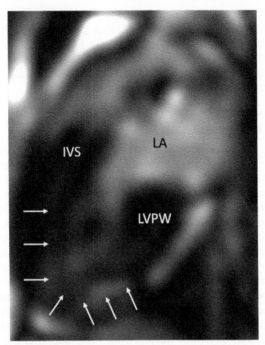

Fig. 4. LGE obtained via CMR in a 11-year-old Sphynx cat with preclinical HCM. The pattern demonstrates a discrete area of midwall enhancement (*arrows*) in the interventricular septum, left ventricular apex, and posterior free-wall at the midventricular 4-chamber view. IVS; interventricular septum, LA; left atrium, LVPW; left ventricular posterior wall.

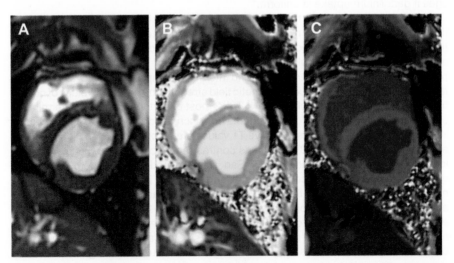

Fig. 5. CMR of the left ventricle, obtained in short-axis at the level of the papillary muscles at end-diastole. (*A*) Balanced steady-state precession, (*B*) T1 native map of the left ventricle, and (*C*) T1 postcontrast map of the left ventricle. These images can be used to noninvasively quantify ECV fraction (ie, interstitial fibrosis).

Normal ECV values have been reported in healthy individuals and in humans with a variety of myocardial diseases. Apart from amyloid, which has not been reported in cats, an increased ECV is most often due to excessive collagen deposition and is thus a more robust measure of diffuse or focal myocardial fibrosis than LGE.[52] Furthermore, ECV is highly correlated with histologic measures of collagen and fibrosis eliminating the need for invasive myocardial biopsy.[55]

The use of CMR to evaluate HCM in people has determined that native T1 values are prolonged in HCM and correlate with wall thickness, suggesting that it is a marker of disease severity.[56,57] Patients with HCM have reduced myocardial $T1_{post}$ values consistent with the presence of diffuse interstitial fibrosis outside areas of LGE. Interestingly, ECV can be used in the differential diagnosis of HCM versus athletic remodeling, particularly in those subjects in the gray zone of wall thickness.[58] Additionally, abnormal T1 values have been correlated with an increased ventricular filling pressure measured noninvasively with echocardiography in HCM, suggesting that diffuse fibrosis may play an important role in the pathophysiology of diastolic dysfunction.[59,60] Increased ECV has been shown to correlate with impaired diastolic function in patients with HCM but not systolic heart failure, suggesting a more predominant role of interstitial fibrosis in diastolic dysfunction.[61] T1 mapping and ECV assessment have the advantage of assessing fibrosis noninvasively and can detect diffuse fibrosis more accurately than LGE. One recent study demonstrated that CMR measures of the cardiac fibrosis (native T1 and ECV) are obtainable in cats, with acceptable repeatability, and are significantly different between healthy and HCM cats[22] (**Fig. 6**). In this study, cats with HCM had increased native T1 times and ECV compared with normal cats, and ECV was significantly correlated with diastolic function and left atrial size. Unlike in humans, markers of fibrosis derived from CMR were not correlated with wall thickness. In cats, fibrosis was independent of LV mass and echocardiographic derived wall thickness, illustrating the importance of fibrosis on diastolic function and the inability of linear wall thickness measurements from echocardiography to predict diffuse fibrosis. The relationship between ECV and diastolic dysfunction occurs in

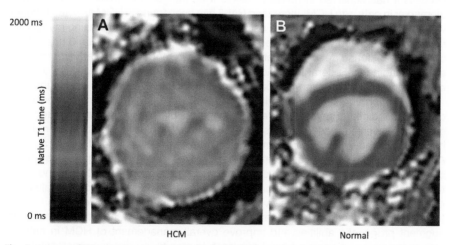

Fig. 6. Image of T1 mapping results in 2 cats with high-native versus low-native T1 values. (A) T1 map in a cat with hypertrophic cardiomyopathy, the T1 time is 1240 milliseconds, the ECV is 32.3%, and the left ventricular mass is 15.3 g. (B) T1 map in a healthy cat, the T1 time is 1132 milliseconds, the ECV is 23.4%, and left ventricular mass is 7.5 g.

people with clinical heart failure and asymptomatic HCM.[60,62,63] Additionally, in humans abnormal ECV values have been correlated with increased ventricular filling pressure measured noninvasively with echocardiography in HCM, suggesting that diffuse fibrosis plays an important role in the pathophysiology of diastolic dysfunction.[59,60] Although this study establishes CMR has a viable diagnostic modality for the evaluation of HCM in cats, larger prospective studies are necessary to validate the effect of ECV on prognosis and its ability to improve early screening for cats with HCM.

Galectin-3

Although CMR has promise as a diagnostic modality in the diagnosis and prognosis of HCM, its considerable technical expertise, cost, and availably will limit its widespread use. New biomarkers such as gelctin-3 (Gal-3) show promise in additional evaluation of cats with HCM. It remains to be seen what the role of Gal-3 in feline HCM will be. In humans with HCM, increasing myocardial fibrosis has been associated with worse outcomes in HCM, including increased risk of congestive heart failure, hospitalization events, and mortality.[64] Evaluation of myocardial fibrosis in humans is accomplished with both CMR and cardiac biomarkers. Gal-3 has been found to be correlated with myocardial fibrosis as determined by LGE and ECV using CMR, making it useful as a biomarker for risk-stratification of patients with known heart disease.[65–71] To date, no such biomarker exists in cats.

Gal-3 is a beta-galactoside binding lectin secreted by macrophages and is thought to play a role in the continued pathogenesis of HCM by promoting profibrotic pathways and stimulation of cardiac fibroblast proliferation and extracellular matrix deposition.[72,73] Gal-3 is thought to be a mediator of aldosterone-induced vascular and myocardial fibrosis and is upregulated in response to aldosterone secretion.[74,75] Maladaptive activation of the renin-angiotensin-aldosterone axis is a well-known component of the pathophysiology of heart failure and cardiac remodeling.[8] Blunting this response is an important part of the management of heart failure in both humans and veterinary species. Gal-3 has only recently been evaluated in cats, and the clinical success it has achieved in humans makes it an intriguing candidate as a potential biomarker in cats with HCM. Increased Gal-3 has been found in HCM affected humans with myocardial fibrosis confirmed using CMR.[65,66] In humans, increasing myocardial fibrosis is associated with worsened outcomes in heart failure, and Gal-3 has subsequently been found to be predictive of cardiac remodeling and adverse cardiac events, leading to Federal Drug Administration (FDA)-approval of Gal-3 as a useful biomarker in identifying high-risk patients as part of an initial cardiac evaluation.[64]

Current approaches to risk-stratifying cats with HCM largely depends on echocardiographic indices of myocardial remodeling, particularly ones that are already suggestive of severe disease, such as severe left atrial dilation, regional left ventricular hypokinesis, and evidence of thrombus formation within the auricle of the left atrium.[2] Although these findings are useful in late stages of disease, monitoring progression requires repeated echocardiographic studies, which is frequently a financial and practical obstacle for owners. Furthermore, even with echocardiographic evaluation, prognostication is still imprecise. A biomarker reflecting the progression of underlying fibrosis, which cannot be evaluated by echocardiography, has the potential to augment prognostic abilities and improve overall management of HCM in cats as well as permit a nonimaging-based approach to monitoring disease progression.

In a recent pilot study of 80 cats, Gal-3 was expressed in cats and could discriminate between cats with underlying HCM and cats with structurally normal hearts. There was a significant correlation between CMR-derived measurements of ECV and circulating Gal-3 levels mirroring earlier studies conducted in humans[32] (**Fig. 7**). Thus, Gal-3 seems to have potential value as a cardiac biomarker in patients with HCM and future studies evaluating the relationship between Gal-3 and myocardial fibrosis and most importantly patient outcomes are warranted.

Advanced Echocardiography

Echocardiographic diagnosis of HCM is straightforward when the disease is severe; however, even skilled operators may not agree on the diagnosis for patients who are mildly or moderately affected. This is because the diagnosis relies on measurements that require excellent repeatability and reliability. In awake cats, it has been established that both intraobserver and interobserver variation is common with echocardiography and can vary by up to 20% among colleagues.[76] Furthermore, the heterogeneity of the left ventricular wall thickness can make echocardiographic assessment challenging, possibly resulting in misdiagnoses and those with borderline left ventricular wall thicknesses labeled as equivocal. Upper limits for normal left ventricular diastolic wall thickness are commonly debated, and it is generally accepted that an average-sized adult cat should have a left ventricular free wall and interventricular septum of less than 5 mm, and any measurement of 6 mm or greater is considered affected.[9] Importantly, veterinary cardiology does not have an established echocardiography protocol for cats with known or suspected HCM, unlike in human cardiology, and diagnosis may be improved if such guidelines were followed.

Repeatable and reliable measurements of the left ventricular wall can be difficult to obtain due to irregularities of the endocardial wall, intracavitary structures, and prominent papillary muscles. Contrast-enhanced echocardiography has been used in human patients with HCM to optimize visualization of the left ventricular wall boundaries and has been shown to provide greater accuracy than standard echocardiography when compared with CMR for certain HCM phenotypes (**Fig. 8**). Additionally, contrast-enhanced echocardiography demonstrated superior intraobserver and interobserver variability compared with standard echocardiography.[77] Left ventricular contrast agents such as Lumason (sulfur hexafluoride lipid-type A microspheres) are readily available and have been safely used in healthy and HCM cats, including cats with congestive heart failure.[78–80] Studies are needed to determine if these contrast agents can increase the sensitivity of echocardiography while improving the repeatability and reproducibility of wall thickness measurements.

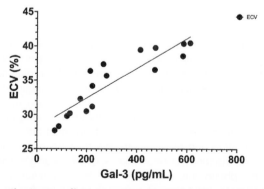

Fig. 7. Linear regression scatter diagram comparing ECV fraction with serum Gal-3 levels in cats with preclinical hypertrophic cardiomyopathy. There was a strong positive relationship ($r^2 = 0.81$, $P < .0001$). ECV; extracellular volume fraction, Gal-3; galectin-3.

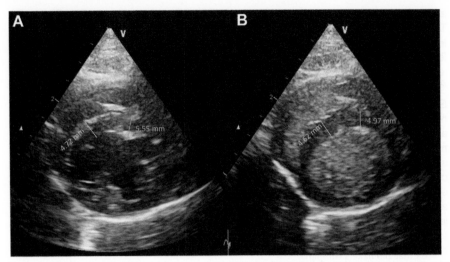

Fig. 8. Right parasternal, short-axis view of the left ventricle using 2D transthoracic (*A*) and contrast-enhanced (*B*) imaging at the level of the papillary muscles. The interventricular septum measured thicker, leading to a diagnosis of equivocal in the standard echocardiogram compared with contrast-enhanced measurements.

Strain imaging is used to determine the focal lengthening, shortening, or thickening of a myocardial segment at a specific time point during the cardiac cycle. Speckle-tracking echocardiography measures myocardial deformation using the natural acoustic markers in gray scale echocardiographic images, which form speckles in the myocardium. The displacement of these speckles can be measured frame by frame in an angle-independent manner, and as a result, a displacement curve can be produced for any specific myocardial segment during a complete cardiac cycle. Myocardial strain and strain rate can be quantified successfully in longitudinal, radial, and circumferential directions.[4] Although speckle-tracking strain has been implemented in cats with HCM, opportunities exist to explore the prognostic value of this imaging modality.[81] In humans, lower longitudinal strain is associated with an increased risk of sudden cardiac death, heart failure, ventricular dyssynchrony, and ventricular arrhythmias.

SUMMARY

Many cats with HCM are asymptomatic and identified incidentally or because of screening. Although many cats with HCM have a systolic murmur, physical examination findings are often not sufficient to rule in or out HCM. Cardiac biomarkers, most notably NT-proBNP, have significantly improved the nonimaging-based screening practices in primary care and referral veterinary centers. However, cardiac imaging plays an essential role in diagnosis and clinical decision-making for cats with HCM. Echocardiography is the primary imaging modality in most cats, with CMR offering complementary information and as an alternative to echocardiography for selected cats in whom the echocardiogram is inconclusive. CMR imaging is well suited for characterizing the diverse phenotypic expressions of HCM, providing diagnosis, tissue characterization, and potentially a novel approach to risk prediction. Important information to be gained from imaging includes establishing the diagnosis (or excluding alternative diagnoses), evaluating the severity of the phenotype, and evaluating for concomitant structural and functional cardiac abnormalities (eg, systolic, diastolic, valvular function). Documentation of the maximal wall thickness, cardiac chamber dimensions, systolic function, and the presence of left atrial thrombus or spontaneous echo-contrast all inform phenotype severity and risk stratification. Advances in echocardiography, such as tissue speckle-tracking and contrast-enhanced imaging, show promise in improving the diagnostic accuracy and potentially allowing for earlier diagnosis of HCM in cats. The hope is that with continued research and development of new modalities for evaluating HCM, our knowledge gap will reduce and allow for improvements in diagnosis, risk-stratification, clinical trial development, and therapeutics.

CLINICS CARE POINTS

- Echocardiography is required for the diagnosis of HCM.
- Mild subclinical disease is difficult to distinguish from normal in many cats.
- Cardiac biomakers compliment but cannot replace imaging for the diagnosis HCM.
- The phenotype of primary genetic HCM and secondary HCM is identical, therefore additional diagnostics such as blood pressure and thyroxine levels should be performed concurrently.

DISCLOSURE

I have no relevant disclosures.

FUNDING

Everycat Health Foundation, Wycoff NJ (Grant # MT21-006); Winn Feline Foundation, Wycoff NJ (Grant # MTW19-009, MTW17-009, W18-031); Doberman Pinscher Health Foundation, Vancouver, WA (Grant # DPHF 105340).

SUPPLEMENTARY DATA

Supplementary data related to this article can be found online at https://doi.org/10.1016/j.cvsm.2023.05.010.

REFERENCES

1. Paige CF, Abbott JA, Elvinger F, et al. Prevalence of cardiomyopathy in apparently healthy cats. J Am Vet Med Assoc 2009;234(11):1398–403.
2. Payne JR, Borgeat K, Connolly DJ, et al. Prognostic indicators in cats with hypertrophic cardiomyopathy. J Vet Intern Med 2013;27(6):1427–36.
3. Fox PR, Liu SK, Maron BJ. Echocardiographic assessment of spontaneously occurring feline hypertrophic cardiomyopathy. An animal model of human disease. Circulation 1995;92(9):2645–51.
4. Meurs KM, Sanchez X, David RM, et al. A cardiac myosin binding protein C mutation in the Maine Coon cat with familial hypertrophic cardiomyopathy. Hum Mol Genet 2005;14(23):3587–93.
5. Meurs KM, Norgard MM, Ederer MM, et al. A substitution mutation in the myosin binding protein C gene in ragdoll hypertrophic cardiomyopathy. Genomics 2007;90(2):261–4.

6. Liu SK, Roberts WC, Maron BJ. Comparison of morphologic findings in spontaneously occurring hypertrophic cardiomyopathy in humans, cats and dogs. Am J Cardiol 1993;72(12):944–51.

7. Martos R, Baugh J, Ledwidge M, et al. Diastolic heart failure: evidence of increased myocardial collagen turnover linked to diastolic dysfunction. Circulation 2007; 115(7):888–95.

8. Weber KT, Brilla CG. Pathological hypertrophy and cardiac interstitium. Fibrosis and renin-angiotensin-aldosterone system. Circulation 1991;83(6):1849–65.

9. Luis Fuentes V, Abbott J, Chetboul V, et al. ACVIM consensus statement guidelines for the classification, diagnosis, and management of cardiomyopathies in cats. J Vet Intern Med 2020;34(3):1062–77.

10. Fox PR, Keene BW, Lamb K, et al. International collaborative study to assess cardiovascular risk and evaluate long-term health in cats with preclinical hypertrophic cardiomyopathy and apparently healthy cats: The REVEAL Study. J Vet Intern Med 2018;32(3):930–43.

11. Fox PR, Keene BW, Lamb K, et al. Long-term incidence and risk of noncardiovascular and all-cause mortality in apparently healthy cats and cats with preclinical hypertrophic cardiomyopathy. J Vet Intern Med 2019;33(6):2572–86.

12. Longeri M, Ferrari P, Knafelz P, et al. Myosin-binding protein C DNA variants in domestic cats (A31P, A74T, R820W) and their association with hypertrophic cardiomyopathy. J Vet Intern Med 2013;27(2):275–85.

13. Granström S, Godiksen MTN, Christiansen M, et al. Genotype-phenotype correlation between the cardiac myosin binding protein C mutation A31P and hypertrophic cardiomyopathy in a cohort of Maine Coon cats: a longitudinal study. J Vet Cardiol 2015;17(Suppl 1):S268–81.

14. Payne JR, Brodbelt DC, Luis Fuentes V. Cardiomyopathy prevalence in 780 apparently healthy cats in rehoming centres (the CatScan study). J Vet Cardiol 2015;17(Suppl 1):S244–57.

15. Côté E, MacDonald KA, Meurs KM, et al. Hypertrophic cardiomyopathy. In: Feline cardiology. Ames, IA, USA: John Wiley & Sons, Ltd; 2011. p. 101–75.

16. Reference intervals and allometric scaling of echocardiographic measurements in Bengal cats - PubMed. https://pubmed.ncbi.nlm.nih.gov/26776586/. Accessed March 14, 2023.

17. Häggström J, Andersson ÅO, Falk T, et al. Effect of Body Weight on Echocardiographic Measurements in 19,866 Pure-Bred Cats with or without Heart Disease. J Vet Intern Med 2016;30(5):1601–11.

18. Karsten S, Stephanie S, Vedat Y. Reference intervals and allometric scaling of two-dimensional echocardiographic measurements in 150 healthy cats. J Vet Med Sci 2017;79(11):1764–71.

19. Parato VM, Antoncecchi V, Sozzi F, et al. Echocardiographic diagnosis of the different phenotypes of hypertrophic cardiomyopathy. Cardiovasc Ultrasound 2016;14:30.

20. Takano H, Isogai T, Aoki T, et al. Feasibility of radial and circumferential strain analysis using 2D speckle tracking echocardiography in cats. J Vet Med Sci 2015;77(2):193–201.

21. Wess G, Sarkar R, Hartmann K. Assessment of Left Ventricular Systolic Function by Strain Imaging Echocardiography in Various Stages of Feline Hypertrophic Cardiomyopathy. J Vet Intern Med 2010;24(6):1375–82.

22. Fries RC, Kadotani S, Keating SCJ, et al. Cardiac extracellular volume fraction in cats with preclinical hypertrophic cardiomyopathy. J Vet Intern Med 2021;35(2): 812–22.

23. Swoboda PP, McDiarmid AK, Erhayiem B, et al. Effect of cellular and extracellular pathology assessed by T1 mapping on regional contractile function in hypertrophic cardiomyopathy. J Cardiovasc Magn Reson 2017;19(1):16.

24. Rickers C, Wilke NM, Jerosch-Herold M, et al. Utility of Cardiac Magnetic Resonance Imaging in the Diagnosis of Hypertrophic Cardiomyopathy. Circulation 2005;112(6):855–61.

25. Massera D, McClelland RL, Ambale-Venkatesh B, et al. Prevalence of Unexplained Left Ventricular Hypertrophy by Cardiac Magnetic Resonance Imaging in MESA. J Am Heart Assoc 2019;8(8):e012250.

26. Hezzell MJ, Rush JE, Humm K, et al. Differentiation of Cardiac from Noncardiac Pleural Effusions in Cats using Second-Generation Quantitative and Point-of-Care NT-proBNP Measurements. J Vet Intern Med 2016;30(2):536–42.

27. Humm K, Hezzell M, Sargent J, et al. Differentiating between feline pleural effusions of cardiac and non-cardiac origin using pleural fluid NT-proBNP concentrations. J Small Anim Pract 2013;54(12):656–61.

28. Fox PR, Oyama MA, Reynolds C, et al. Utility of plasma N-terminal pro-brain natriuretic peptide (NT-proBNP) to distinguish between congestive heart failure and non-cardiac causes of acute dyspnea in cats. J Vet Cardiol 2009;11(Suppl 1): S51–61.

29. Machen MC, Oyama MA, Gordon SG, et al. Multi-centered investigation of a point-of-care NT-proBNP ELISA assay to detect moderate to severe occult (pre-clinical) feline heart disease in cats referred for cardiac evaluation. J Vet Cardiol 2014;16(4):245–55.

30. Mainville CA, Clark GH, Esty KJ, et al. Analytical validation of an immunoassay for the quantification of N-terminal pro–B-type natriuretic peptide in feline blood. J Vet Diagn Invest 2015;27(4):414–21.

31. Harris AN, Estrada AH, Gallagher AE, et al. Biologic variability of N-terminal pro-brain natriuretic peptide in adult healthy cats. J Feline Med Surg 2017;19(2): 216–23.

32. ACVIM Forum On Demand Research Abstract Program. J Vet Intern Med 2020; 34(6):2830–989.

33. Hall C. Essential biochemistry and physiology of (NT-pro)BNP. Eur J Heart Fail 2004;6(3):257–60.

34. Castiglione V, Aimo A, Vergaro G, et al. Biomarkers for the diagnosis and management of heart failure. Heart Fail Rev 2022;27(2):625–43.

35. Ala-Kopsala M, Magga J, Peuhkurinen K, et al. Molecular heterogeneity has a major impact on the measurement of circulating N-terminal fragments of A- and B-type natriuretic peptides. Clin Chem 2004;50(9):1576–88.

36. Connolly DJ, Soares Magalhaes RJ, Fuentes VL, et al. Assessment of the diagnostic accuracy of circulating natriuretic peptide concentrations to distinguish between cats with cardiac and non-cardiac causes of respiratory distress. J Vet Cardiol 2009;11(Suppl 1):S41–50.

37. Fox PR, Rush JE, Reynolds CA, et al. Multicenter evaluation of plasma N-terminal probrain natriuretic peptide (NT-pro BNP) as a biochemical screening test for asymptomatic (occult) cardiomyopathy in cats. J Vet Intern Med 2011;25(5): 1010–6.

38. Borgeat K, Connolly DJ, Luis Fuentes V. Cardiac biomarkers in cats. J Vet Cardiol 2015;17:S74–86.

39. Connolly DJ, Cannata J, Boswood A, et al. Cardiac troponin I in cats with hypertrophic cardiomyopathy. J Feline Med Surg 2003;5(4):209–16.

40. Herndon WE, Kittleson MD, Sanderson K, et al. Cardiac troponin I in feline hypertrophic cardiomyopathy. J Vet Intern Med 2002;16(5):558–64.

41. Hori Y, Iguchi M, Heishima Y, et al. Diagnostic utility of cardiac troponin I in cats with hypertrophic cardiomyopathy. J Vet Intern Med 2018;32(3):922–9.

42. Hertzsch S, Roos A, Wess G. Evaluation of a sensitive cardiac troponin I assay as a screening test for the diagnosis of hypertrophic cardiomyopathy in cats. J Vet Intern Med 2019;33(3):1242–50.

43. Borgeat K, Sherwood K, Payne JR, et al. Plasma cardiac troponin I concentration and cardiac death in cats with hypertrophic cardiomyopathy. J Vet Intern Med 2014;28(6):1731–7.

44. Adabag AS, Maron BJ, Appelbaum E, et al. Occurrence and frequency of arrhythmias in hypertrophic cardiomyopathy in relation to delayed enhancement on cardiovascular magnetic resonance. J Am Coll Cardiol 2008;51(14):1369–74.

45. Hamlin SA, Henry TS, Little BP, et al. Mapping the future of cardiac MR imaging: case-based review of T1 and T2 mapping techniques. Radiographics 2014;34(6):1594–611.

46. Choudhury L, Mahrholdt H, Wagner A, et al. Myocardial scarring in asymptomatic or mildly symptomatic patients with hypertrophic cardiomyopathy. J Am Coll Cardiol 2002;40(12):2156–64.

47. Moon JCC, Reed E, Sheppard MN, et al. The histologic basis of late gadolinium enhancement cardiovascular magnetic resonance in hypertrophic cardiomyopathy. J Am Coll Cardiol 2004;43(12):2260–4.

48. Wilson JM, Villareal RP, Hariharan R, et al. Magnetic resonance imaging of myocardial fibrosis in hypertrophic cardiomyopathy. Tex Heart Inst J 2002;29(3):176–80.

49. MacDonald KA, Wisner ER, Larson RF, et al. Comparison of myocardial contrast enhancement via cardiac magnetic resonance imaging in healthy cats and cats with hypertrophic cardiomyopathy. Am J Vet Res 2005;66(11):1891–4.

50. Cummings KW, Bhalla S, Javidan-Nejad C, et al. A pattern-based approach to assessment of delayed enhancement in nonischemic cardiomyopathy at MR imaging. Radiographics 2009;29(1):89–103.

51. Messroghli DR, Radjenovic A, Kozerke S, et al. Modified Look-Locker inversion recovery (MOLLI) for high-resolution T1 mapping of the heart. Magn Reson Med 2004;52(1):141–6.

52. Haaf P, Garg P, Messroghli DR, et al. Cardiac T1 Mapping and Extracellular Volume (ECV) in clinical practice: a comprehensive review. J Cardiovasc Magn Reson 2016;18(1):89.

53. Parsai C, O'Hanlon R, Prasad SK, et al. Diagnostic and prognostic value of cardiovascular magnetic resonance in non-ischaemic cardiomyopathies. J Cardiovasc Magn Reson 2012;14:54.

54. Taylor AJ, Salerno M, Dharmakumar R, et al. T1 Mapping: Basic Techniques and Clinical Applications. JACC Cardiovasc Imaging 2016;9(1):67–81.

55. Sibley CT, Noureldin RA, Gai N, et al. T1 Mapping in cardiomyopathy at cardiac MR: comparison with endomyocardial biopsy. Radiology 2012;265(3):724–32.

56. Dass S, Suttie JJ, Piechnik SK, et al. Myocardial tissue characterization using magnetic resonance noncontrast t1 mapping in hypertrophic and dilated cardiomyopathy. Circ Cardiovasc Imaging 2012;5(6):726–33.

57. Puntmann VO, Voigt T, Chen Z, et al. Native T1 mapping in differentiation of normal myocardium from diffuse disease in hypertrophic and dilated cardiomyopathy. JACC Cardiovasc Imaging 2013;6(4):475–84.

58. Swoboda PP, McDiarmid AK, Erhayiem B, et al. Assessing Myocardial Extracellular Volume by T1 Mapping to Distinguish Hypertrophic Cardiomyopathy From Athlete's Heart. J Am Coll Cardiol 2016;67(18):2189–90.

59. Ho CY, Abbasi SA, Neilan TG, et al. T1 Measurements Identify Extracellular Volume Expansion in Hypertrophic Cardiomyopathy Sarcomere Mutation Carriers With and Without Left Ventricular Hypertrophy. Circulation: Cardiovascular Imaging 2013;6(3):415–22.

60. Ellims AH, Iles LM, Ling LH, et al. Diffuse myocardial fibrosis in hypertrophic cardiomyopathy can be identified by cardiovascular magnetic resonance, and is associated with left ventricular diastolic dysfunction. J Cardiovasc Magn Reson 2012;14:76.

61. Su MYM, Lin LY, Tseng YHE, et al. CMR-Verified Diffuse Myocardial Fibrosis Is Associated With Diastolic Dysfunction in HFpEF. JACC (J Am Coll Cardiol): Cardiovascular Imaging 2014;7(10):991–7.

62. Iles L, Pfluger H, Phrommintikul A, et al. Evaluation of diffuse myocardial fibrosis in heart failure with cardiac magnetic resonance contrast-enhanced T1 mapping. J Am Coll Cardiol 2008;52(19):1574–80.

63. Nucifora G, Muser D, Gianfagna P, et al. Systolic and diastolic myocardial mechanics in hypertrophic cardiomyopathy and their link to the extent of hypertrophy, replacement fibrosis and interstitial fibrosis. Int J Cardiovasc Imaging 2015;31(8):1603–10.

64. O'Hanlon R, Grasso A, Roughton M, et al. Prognostic significance of myocardial fibrosis in hypertrophic cardiomyopathy. J Am Coll Cardiol 2010;56(11):867–74.

65. Hu DJ, Xu J, Du W, et al. Cardiac magnetic resonance and galectin-3 level as predictors of prognostic outcomes for non-ischemic cardiomyopathy patients. Int J Cardiovasc Imaging 2016;32(12):1725–33.

66. Yakar Tülüce S, Tülüce K, Çil Z, et al. Galectin-3 levels in patients with hypertrophic cardiomyopathy and its relationship with left ventricular mass index and function. Anatol J Cardiol 2016;16(5):344–8.

67. Lok DJ, Lok SI, Bruggink-André de la Porte PW, et al. Galectin-3 is an independent marker for ventricular remodeling and mortality in patients with chronic heart failure. Clin Res Cardiol 2013;102(2):103–10.

68. Lok DJA, Van Der Meer P, de la Porte PWBA, et al. Prognostic value of galectin-3, a novel marker of fibrosis, in patients with chronic heart failure: data from the DEAL-HF study. Clin Res Cardiol 2010;99(5):323–8.

69. Ho JE, Liu C, Lyass A, et al. Galectin-3, a marker of cardiac fibrosis, predicts incident heart failure in the community. J Am Coll Cardiol 2012;60(14):1249–56.

70. Chen H, Chen C, Fang J, et al. Circulating galectin-3 on admission and prognosis in acute heart failure patients: a meta-analysis. Heart Fail Rev 2020;25(2):331–41.

71. Kanukurti J, Mohammed N, Sreedevi NN, et al. Evaluation of Galectin-3 as a Novel Diagnostic Biomarker in Patients with Heart Failure with Preserved Ejection Fraction. J Lab Physicians 2020;12(2):126–32.

72. Sharma UC, Pokharel S, van Brakel TJ, et al. Galectin-3 marks activated macrophages in failure-prone hypertrophied hearts and contributes to cardiac dysfunction. Circulation 2004;110(19):3121–8.

73. Yu L, Ruifrok WPT, Meissner M, et al. Genetic and pharmacological inhibition of galectin-3 prevents cardiac remodeling by interfering with myocardial fibrogenesis. Circ Heart Fail 2013;6(1):107–17.

74. Martínez-Martínez E, Calvier L, Fernández-Celis A, et al. Galectin-3 blockade inhibits cardiac inflammation and fibrosis in experimental hyperaldosteronism and hypertension. Hypertension 2015;66(4):767–75.

75. Calvier L, Miana M, Reboul P, et al. Galectin-3 mediates aldosterone-induced vascular fibrosis. Arterioscler Thromb Vasc Biol 2013;33(1):67–75.

76. Chetboul V, Concordet D, Pouchelon JL, et al. Effects of inter- and intra-observer variability on echocardiographic measurements in awake cats. J Vet Med A Physiol Pathol Clin Med 2003;50(6):326–31.

77. Urbano-Moral JA, Gonzalez-Gonzalez AM, Maldonado G, et al. Contrast-Enhanced Echocardiographic Measurement of Left Ventricular Wall Thickness in Hypertrophic Cardiomyopathy: Comparison with Standard Echocardiography and Cardiac Magnetic Resonance. J Am Soc Echocardiogr 2020;33(9):1106–15.

78. Streitberger A, Hocke V, Modler P. Measurement of pulmonary transit time in healthy cats by use of ultrasound contrast media "Sonovue®": feasibility, reproducibility, and values in 42 cats. J Vet Cardiol 2013;15(3):181–7.

79. Streitberger A, Modler P, Häggström J. Increased normalized pulmonary transit times and pulmonary blood volumes in cardiomyopathic cats with or without congestive heart failure. J Vet Cardiol 2015;17(1):25–33.

80. Gleason HE, Phillips H, Fries R, et al. Ala vestibuloplasty improves cardiopulmonary and activity-related parameters in brachycephalic cats. Vet Surg. Published online March 2023;7.

81. Spalla I, Boswood A, Connolly DJ, et al. Speckle tracking echocardiography in cats with preclinical hypertrophic cardiomyopathy. J Vet Intern Med 2019;33(3):1232–41.

Mitral Valve Repair–The Development and Rise of Options in the Veterinary World

Poppy Bristow, MVetMed, PGCertVetEd, FHEA, MRCVS, DipECVS[a],*,
Lauren E. Markovic, DVM, DACVIM (Cardiology)[b]

KEYWORDS

- Edge-to-edge • Degenerative • Canine • Transcatheter • Surgery
- Minimally invasive

KEY POINTS

- Surgical correction of canine degenerative mitral valve disease is performed under cardio-pulmonary bypass whereas transcatheter edge-to-edge MVR is performed with a beating-heart hybrid intervention.
- Advanced imaging techniques are vital to patient selection, pre-procedural planning, and for intra-operative steps.
- Further MVR training and expertise across the world is necessary to help the millions of dogs with degenerative mitral valve disease.

 Video content accompanies this article at http://www.vetsmall.theclinics.com.

INTRODUCTION

In 1923, Dr. Elliot Cutler and team performed the first successful mitral valve repair (MVR), in a child with mitral stenosis.[1] This was a closed technique and used for only a short period of time, but is hailed as a milestone in human cardiac surgery. The evolution and practice of MVR continued, albeit slowly, with the next major surgical breakthrough not until 1957, when Dr Walton Lillehei and team performed the first MVR for mitral insufficiency in 1957. Further progress to MVR came in the 1980s following publication by Dr. Alain Carpentier of an article classifying lesions of the mitral valve and sharing methods on achieving successful outcome with MVR due to degenerative mitral valve disease (DMVD).[1]

[a] Dick White Referrals, Linnaeus and Mars Veterinary Health, Station Farm, London Road, Cambridgeshire CB8 0UH, UK; [b] Department of Small Animal Medicine and Surgery, University of Georgia, College of Veterinary Medicine, 2200 College Station Road, Athens, GA 30602, USA
* Corresponding author.
E-mail address: poppy.bristow@dwr.co.uk

Vet Clin Small Anim 53 (2023) 1343–1352
https://doi.org/10.1016/j.cvsm.2023.07.001
0195-5616/23/© 2023 Elsevier Inc. All rights reserved.

The successful use and then refinement of cardiopulmonary bypass (CPB) in humans from 1953 onwards however, truly enabled the field of open heart surgery to progress in leaps and bounds in the latter half of the 20th century, resulting in today's success rates of almost 100% for open MVR in human medicine.[2]

The field has further progressed to percutaneous MVR now being approved in the 21st century as an alternative to open MVR.[3] To date there is growing experience of successful use of transcatheter therapies for mitral regurgitation (MR) in humans, with edge-to-edge repair the current treatment of choice for transcatheter intervention,[4] improving mitral valve leaflet coaptation as the mechanism of reducing MR.[5] Although open MVR remains the current gold standard technique for MVR in human patients,[6–9] percutaneous techniques are being progressed and refined, and are becoming more commonplace. Interventional edge-to-edge mitral valve techniques have now started to be performed in dogs in a small number of centers worldwide.[10] Recent literature has shown that alongside the advancements in technology and techniques, the success of modern MVR is also dependent upon a collaborative network of cardiologists, cardiac surgeons, anesthesiologists, and critical care specialists working together to achieve a common goal.[1,11]

Etiology of Mitral Regurgitation

Mitral regurgitation (MR) is classified into two broad categories: primary (organic or degenerative) or secondary (ischemic or functional), which are important to differentiate in order to guide appropriate clinical decision making. In primary (degenerative/myxomatous) MR, there is a primary abnormality of one or more components of the mitral valve apparatus, for example, the mitral valve leaflets or chordae tendineae.[12] Secondary (functional) MR occurs due to a disease affecting the left ventricle and includes pathology such as dilated cardiomyopathy and myocardial infarction.[13] With secondary MR, there is an imbalance between the closing of the valve itself and tethering forces on the valve due to alterations in the geometry of the left ventricle, rather than a primary problem with the valve apparatus.[14] The focus of this article will be on primary regurgitation secondary to degenerative mitral valve disease (DMVD), which is the most common cardiac disease in dogs, affecting millions worldwide.[15]

Surgical Therapy

Surgical therapy for DMVD is becoming increasingly popular in the veterinary field, though is still rarely used when the population of potential surgical candidates is considered, mainly due to the current lack of availability worldwide. The field of open heart surgery in veterinary medicine has very much lagged behind its human counterpart for many reasons, including the cost of equipment, the requirement for expertise in multiple disciplines, as well as the differences between dogs and humans, resulting in a direct translation across these two species not being possible. Additionally, there was historical opinion in the veterinary world by some that small dogs (those under 20 lbs.), would not be able to tolerate CPB, a necessity for open MVR. Consequently, for many years, the only open heart surgeries performed in dogs were congenital repairs such as for tricuspid valve dysplasia and pulmonary valve stenosis, due to their propensity for some of the larger canine breeds.[16] However, as some of these conditions are rare, the number of heart surgeries performed by those few centers was very low, resulting in an inhibition of progress.

A major turning point in veterinary open heart surgery was with the publications by Professor Uechi and team in 2012.[17,18] They showed for the first time in veterinary medicine, in a large population, that use of CPB in small dogs can be successful; simultaneously showing that open MVR in dogs also resulted in sustained excellent long-term results. As DMVD is the most common acquired heart condition in dogs,[15] this has opened up huge possibilities for the advancement of this field in veterinary medicine. As with all interventions and techniques, a learning curve exists, and it is imperative that procedures are performed on a regular basis for sustained success and progress.

Surgical Technique

The technique for MVR for DMVD in dogs is based on described human techniques, consisting of placement of artificial chordae tendineae and an annuloplasty[12,13,19]; these two steps enable a significant reduction in MR. Expanded polytetrafluorethylene (GoreTex) suture material is used for artificial chords, as well as for the annuloplasty, due to its low thrombogenicity and pliability.[20] Artificial chords are anchored in the tips of the papillary muscles, at the closest point to the native chords, and then anchored in the edge of the valve segments (**Figs. 1** and **2**). The annuloplasty used by most centers is termed as a partial annuloplasty, and is an older human technique, using two rows of a continuous suture pattern from one trigone round to the other.[19] (**Fig. 3**) In human MVR, annuloplasty techniques have advanced substantially in the last few decades, in part helped by the advancement of imaging techniques which have enabled 4D geometric mapping of the mitral valve annuloplasty. On the shelf annuloplasty rings are available in humans which saves time and restores annular anatomy to a much higher level than a sutured annuloplasty, thereby reducing MR as much as is possible. Due to the average dog size undergoing MVR, human annuloplasty rings cannot be used, and would be cost-prohibitive even in the minority of patients where a good fit might be possible. Furthermore, this would add further foreign material which could result in a higher degree of thromboembolic complications post-operatively and would

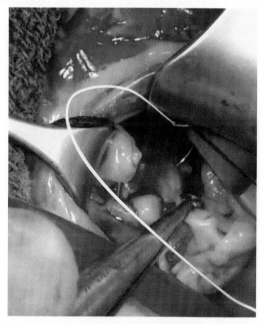

Fig. 1. Intra-operative view looking past the mitral valve into the left ventricle. The ringed forceps are gently grasping native chords and the needle is about to be passed into the tip of the papillary muscle to secure an artificial chord. (Courtesy of Dr. Anne Kurosawa.).

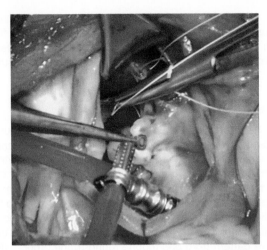

Fig. 2. Intra-operative view of the mitral valve. The ringed forceps are gently grasping the edge of the thickened mitral valve, with the needle about to be passed 2 mm from its edge. Note the presence of two suction tips to enable a clear field and to recirculate blood back into the cardiopulmonary bypass machine.

therefore need to be trialed cautiously before widespread use, even if specific designs for canine patients became available in the future.

A common misnomer is that only those chords that are stretched or ruptured are replaced however as this is a degenerative condition, it is important that all main valve segments are supported with the placement of artificial chords, these chords are evenly distributed throughout all main valve segments as depicted in **Fig. 4**.[17,18,21] The use of an annuloplasty is essential as by the time surgery is performed typically in ACVIM stage C of disease, annular dilation is a major contributor to the degree of MR seen.[21] Therefore, only placing artificial chords would very unlikely result in enough reduction in MR to enable a good long-, or even short-term outcome. This is an important differentiation when considering the use of interventional human

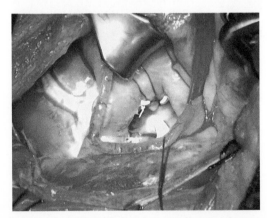

Fig. 3. Intra-operative view through the left atriotomy, showing the annuloplasty which has now been tied. The two pledgets, also made from expanded tetrafluoroethylene, at the start and end of the annuloplasty can be seen in close approximation to each other.

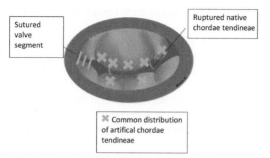

Fig. 4. Schematic of birds eye view of the mitral valve from the atrial surface depicting placement of artificial chordae tendineae in an average case. (Image courtesy of Dr Anne Kurosawa.)

techniques in dogs, as due to the extremely high success rates in human heart surgery, it is common to intervene very early in the disease process.

Therefore, with human candidates for surgical repair of primary mitral valve disease, secondary annular dilation is typically not a major contributor to the degree of MR, resulting in good outcomes with minimally invasive techniques that do not address this component of MR; only the prolapse of valve segments.

Intra-operatively, four-dimensional TEE is used to further quantify the primary abnormalities causing the degree of MR in each individual patient in order to guide the surgery team, as well as to assess the repair whilst the patient is on CPB.[21] (Videos 1–3). Just as cardiac remodeling can be seen with the administration of pimobendan in ACVIM stage B2, remodeling also occurs following successful MVR, even if a trivial or mild amount of MR remains (Video 4), enabling pimobendan to be discontinued in almost all patients within 3 months post-operatively. Diuretic medications are discontinued immediately following MVR in almost all patients, with a significant reduction in cardiac medications seen even by 1 month post-operatively.[22] As well as good short- and long-term survival rates seen in established veterinary centers, health-related quality of life has also been shown to significantly improve by 1 month post-operatively, and is sustained in the long term.[17,18,21,22]

Advancements in Mitral Valve Repair

Advancement in MVR in dogs since 2012,[12,18] is mainly as a result of refinements in the use of CPB in dogs and post-operative care, and in a smaller part due to subtle refinements of surgical techniques. The use of CPB in dogs is an area where direct translation from the human field is not possible. Although of course we are leaps and bounds ahead of where our human colleagues had to start, with the invention and then refinement of the equipment alone, major differences in canine tolerances and drug interactions are important to be aware of and familiar with before embarking on the use of this technique, even when an experienced human perfusionist is used. Fortunately, as opposed to certain aspects of surgery, there are some aspects of CPB that dogs do tolerate better than humans, for example, the ability to perfuse adequately at much lower mean pressures. This is an important contributor to being able to use CPB in small dogs, as due to smaller vessel diameters, venous return is typically proportionally poorer. Unfortunately, on the other hand, the use of protamine, a necessary drug to reverse the effects of heparin, has a much poorer tolerance canine patients, resulting in higher levels of mortality and morbidity both intra-operatively, and if not able to be used to its full dose, in the short term post-operative period as well.[21]

Other than small body size, a key difference in surgical technique between dogs and humans is the fragility of the vascular tissues, namely the canine aorta, compared to the human aorta, another important factor to consider when transferring human techniques.

Despite the refinements seen to date with CPB in dogs, it remains one of the major contributors to morbidity in both humans and dogs, and alongside its high initial cost and need for expertise, it is one of the main drivers behind the desire for less invasive techniques to be further developed.

To date, the surgical technique advancements in canine MVR have been due to increasing individual and collaborative experience, enabling refinement of certain aspects of the repair. As well as appropriate handling of cardiovascular structures, an aspect that comes primarily with increasing experience is the correct length of artificial chordae tendineae. Our smaller patient size makes use of human measuring devices difficult to use, thereby tying them to an appropriate length is more subjective. A further balance comes from weighing up the time taken to perfect the MVR versus the disadvantage of increasing cross-clamp times. In human medicine, there is an increase in a mortality rate of 2% per every 1 minute of cross-clamp time.[23] Although this has not been interrogated yet in canine patients, it is unlikely to be dissimilar. An advantage we do have, though not one to be overused, is that as canine life expectancy is so much shorter than in humans, and due to patients undergoing MVR for DMVD being middle-age to older, a degree of mild residual MR post-repair has not been seen to progress to a future clinical problem in dogs.[12,13] Therefore, balancing the need for a perfect repair with use of additional minor cleft suture techniques or additional chords for example, needs to be carefully weighed up with the inevitable prolongation of cross-clamp time.

Currently, there is a lack of veterinary publications and textbooks available in the field of open heart surgery, which in addition to the scarcity of training programs, are major reasons for the lack of progress in terms of more centers being able to offer this technique. It is a tricky field to navigate as with the existence of a handful of successful centers, to open new centers from scratch, without prior training is somewhat controversial due to the inevitable learning curve that will occur at a slower rate when prior experience is not in existence. Fortunately, with the presence of now at least some established centers, it should not be necessary to start a new center from the very beginnings with no prior training, though the availability of this training does of course still make this extremely challenging.

Despite it being over 10 years since the publication of a large cohort of dogs undergoing MVR under CPB with high success rates, the option of this treatment strategy remains to this day largely unknown in the veterinary field, and as a result, largely unoffered to many owners of dogs who would otherwise be surgical candidates, inhibiting them from making an informed decision. Of course, this is not helped by the lack of publications in recent years on center success rates, something which will inevitably change in the coming years. With the use of CPB, high equipment costs and the need for a high level of expertise, costs will of course remain prohibtive to many; however this cost is typically lower than preconceptions, as an in conference survey recently found.

MVR is inevitably many years behind human medicine, and we are lacking a large amount of veterinary data as a result which leads to a degree of a vicious cycle in terms of enabling refinement and meaningful improvements. The last 10 years have enabled a small handful of centers to develop, refine their techniques, and become established. Now that this is the case, publications and further interrogation of data will be possible within the next few years, furthering center success rates and hopefully thereby helping other centers to establish, without the need for as long a learning curve. Surgical success rates, though high,[17,18,21] are unlikely to ever be equivalent to human medicine due in part to the difference in clinical severity between dogs and humans when undergoing MVR, something which ethically, is unlikely to ever match in veterinary medicine.

Rise of Interventional Therapy

Minimally invasive MVR has become a routine treatment for MR in humans, and is a developing method in veterinary medicine. Novel interventional therapy for mitral valve disease has been on the horizon more recently, and is currently being performed in dogs with MR secondary to DMVD in a small handful of centers. One percutaneous MVR technique, MitraClip, mimics the surgical edge-to-edge Alfieri technique through the mechanical coaptation of the mitral leaflets.[5] In humans the MitraClip system is commonly used technology and currently recommended for transcatheter mitral valve edge-to-edge repair for symptomatic, grade 3+ mitral regurgitation.[24] Another edge-to-edge device, known as the ValveClamp, was first reported in a porcine model in 2018.[25] Two years later, the ValveClamp was reported effective at reducing the severity of MR in eight dogs with naturally occurring DMVD.[26] The most recent version of the device for edge-to-edge transcatheter repair in the dog is currently known as the V-Clamp, and the device is currently being used at select centers worldwide.

The V-Clamp is a newer device that is placed transapically via a beating-heart hybrid intervention, with teams that typically include one or more cardiologists, surgeons, and anesthesiologists. Large scale clinical research in veterinary medicine investigating the effectiveness and safety of transcatheter MVR devices, including the V-clamp, are lacking, making the knowledge of optimal candidates for these interventions currently unknown.

The technological advancements in imaging techniques have additionally helped revolutionize interventional therapies for MVR. Advanced imaging techniques, including 3- and 4-dimensional transthoracic and transesophageal echocardiography, have proved to be essential to not only pre-procedural planning but also to optimizing intra-procedural techniques including device deployment. Cardiac Computed Tomography (CT) is considered vital to pre-procedural planning for transcatheter MVR in humans,[4] and a CT scanner with enhanced resolution and appropriate cardiac packages should be considered when starting an interventional MVR program in dogs. Fluoroscopy and transesophageal echocardiography are used in combination for the deployment of the V-clamp (edge-to-edge) technique in dogs. Transesophageal echocardiography of the mitral annulus and left heart should additionally be optimized to help guide the surgeon during transapical access into the left ventricle. Communication among all of the hybrid team members, particularly the interventionalist and echocardiographer, is essential during transcatheter MVR, especially given the need for the use of multiple imaging techniques simultaneously, in order to guide these procedures. As with many new interventions, there is a learning curve to transcatheter MVR and operators with the most experience as well as medical device vendors should be contacted for questions and ideally visited, when embarking on the learning deployment technique.[10]

Multidisciplinary Heart Team

Successful surgical and interventional therapy for MVR requires a multidisciplinary heart team approach as the patient journey involves many disciplines from cardiac assessment, through to post-operative care.[11,27] Success of MVR is dependent in a large part upon the ability to use a team approach to assessment and care. The heart team consists of cardiologists, surgeons, anesthesiologists, critical care specialists, technicians, and client care specialists. Multidisciplinary meetings should be held to assist in organized preparation and planning, with the goal of improving the quality of care of each animal undergoing MVR. The authors recommend pre-procedural planning meetings as well as debriefing after each procedure to enable continued progress, refinement and to give all team members a space to voice any concerns or suggestions.

Suitability for Mitral Valve Repair and Patient Selection

Currently, candidates are considered suitable for open MVR in an established center when in ACVIM stage C or D. Mitral valve repair is also being performed in ACVIM stage B2, though as dogs can have a good quality of life in stage B2 for a prolonged period time, and/or may never enter stage C, these candidates need to be very carefully considered and MVR in this stage should only be performed by an experienced team in the authors' opinion. Other factors than simply stage of disease that need to be considered include co-morbidities, age, and degree of pulmonary hypertension. For both open MVR and the current hybrid transcatheter edge-to-edge technique, published comprehensive veterinary guidelines will likely be available in the coming years. Criteria is being developed for use of transcatheter edge-to-edge MVR in dogs, with the most recent talks citing the following guidelines for selection: ACVIM Stage B2 or Stage C,[10] meeting current guidelines from ACC/AHA and ASE for mitral valve interventions in humans,[28,29] and supportive criteria for severe mitral regurgitation as well as anatomy suitable for edge-to-edge MVR as previously described.[10] One of the difficulties as mentioned above, is that TEER does not address the annular dilation directly. In addition, selective patient criteria are needed due to the device deployment, with some dogs in ACVIM stage C or D having mitral valve anatomy that might not be favorable for success, for example, flail leaflet, multiple segments of prolapse or multiple regurgitant jets.[10] However, there are still many dogs that would fit current selection criteria, especially given how many dogs have DMVD. At some centers, the cost of TEER is relatively equivocal to open MVR, therefore further adding to the complexity when weighing the two options. When considering either option, it is important to consider the stage of disease with ACVIM stage B2 (unless advanced), difficult for most centers to justify currently without randomized clinical trials. Hopefully with increasing experience resulting in further refinements, this will change over time. Additionally, the long-term success of interventional procedures that do not directly address the annular dilation which is a contributor to MR in advanced patients with DMVD, is currently unknown.

SUMMARY

Surgical and interventional therapies for MVR due to DMVD are on the rise in veterinary medicine. Given the numbers of dogs with DMVD across the world, ongoing development of surgical, transcatheter, and hybrid techniques are inevitable with undoubtedly future improvements to outcomes in all management options.

CLINICS CARE POINTS

- Dogs are considered candidates for MVR in ACVIM C, D or advanced B2 disease.

- Anticoagulants (typically aspirin, clopidogrel or rivaroxaban or a combination), are continued for three months after open MVR.
- Pimobendan is continued postoperatively until the cardiac dimensions have normalised following open MVR in the authours centre.

DISCLOSURE

Dr Bristow is an employee of Linnaeus and Mars Veterinary Health. No funding was obtained for either author for the purposes of this article.

SUPPLEMENTARY DATA

Supplementary data to this article can be found online at https://doi.org/10.1016/j.cvsm.2023.07.001.

REFERENCES

1. Cohn LH, Tchantchaleishvili V, Rajab TK. Evolution of the concept and practice of mitral valve repair. Ann Cardiothorac Surg 2015;4:315–21.
2. Gillinov AM, Cosgrove DM, Blackstone EH, et al. Durability of mitral valve repair for degenerative disease. J Thorac Cardiovasc Surg 1998;116:734–43.
3. Stewart MH, Jenkins JS. The Evolving Role of Percutaneous Mitral Valve Repair. Ochsner J 2016;16:270–6.
4. Hensey M, Brown RA, Lal S, et al. Transcatheter Mitral Valve Replacement: An Update on Current Techniques, Technologies, and Future Directions. JACC Cardiovasc Interv 2021;14:489–500.
5. Wan B, Rahnavardi M, Tian DH, et al. A meta-analysis of MitraClip system versus surgery for treatment of severe mitral regurgitation. Ann Cardiothorac Surg 2013; 2:683–92.
6. Meyer MA, von Segesser LK, Hurni M, et al. Long-term outcome after mitral valve repair: a risk factor analysis. Eur J Cardio Thorac Surg 2007;32:301–7.
7. Zhou YX, Leobon B, Berthoumieu P, et al. Long-term outcomes following repair or replacement in degenerative mitral valve disease. Thorac Cardiovasc Surg 2010; 58:415–21.
8. Chikwe J, Goldstone AB, Passage J, et al. A propensity score-adjusted retrospective comparison of early and mid-term results of mitral valve repair versus replacement in octogenarians. Eur Heart J 2011;32:618–26.
9. Mick SL, Keshavamurthy S, Gillinov AM. Mitral valve repair versus replacement. Ann Cardiothorac Surg 2015;4:230–7.
10. Orton EC, Potter B. Transcatheter edge-to-edge mitral valve repair. 2022 ACVIM forum proceedings. USA. Greenwood Village, Colorado: ACVIM; 2022.
11. Jonik S, Marchel M, Huczek Z, et al. An Individualized Approach of Multidisciplinary Heart Team for Myocardial Revascularization and Valvular Heart Disease-State of Art. J Pers Med 2022;12. https://doi.org/10.3390/jpm12050705.
12. Van Praet KM, Stamm C, Sundermann SH, et al. Minimally Invasive Surgical Mitral Valve Repair: State of the Art Review. Interv Cardiol 2018;13:14–9.
13. Ciarka A, Van de Veire N. Secondary mitral regurgitation: pathophysiology, diagnosis, and treatment. Heart 2011;97:1012–23.
14. Baumgartner H, Falk V, Bax JJ, et al. 2017 ESC/EACTS Guidelines for the management of valvular heart disease. Eur Heart J 2017;38:2739–91.

15. Markby G, Summers KM, MacRae VE, et al. Myxomatous Degeneration of the Canine Mitral Valve: From Gross Changes to Molecular Events. J Comp Pathol 2017;156:371–83.
16. Oliveira P, Domenech O, Silva J, et al. Retrospective review of congenital heart disease in 976 dogs. J Vet Intern Med 2011;25:477–83.
17. Uechi M. Mitral valve repair in dogs. J Vet Cardiol 2012;14:185–92.
18. Uechi M, Mizukoshi T, Mizuno T, et al. Mitral valve repair under cardiopulmonary bypass in small-breed dogs: 48 cases (2006-2009). J Am Vet Med Assoc 2012; 240:1194–201.
19. Carpentier AAD, Filsoufi F. In: carpentier's reconstructive valve surgery. 1st Edition. Philadelphia: WB Saunders; 2010.
20. Di Mauro M, Bonalumi G, Giambuzzi I, et al. Mitral valve repair with artificial chords: Tips and tricks. J Card Surg 2022;37:4081–7.
21. Bristow P, Kurosawa A. Mitral valve repair: Experience to date. 2021 ACVIM Forum Proceedings; 2021 June 9 - 12; Available at: acvim.org.
22. Pennington C, Kurosawa TA, Navarro-Cubas X, et al. Use of the Functional Evaluation of Cardiac Health questionnaire to assess health-related quality of life before and after mitral valve repair in dogs with myxomatous mitral valve disease. J Am Vet Med Assoc 2022;260:1806–12.
23. Al-Sarraf NTL, Hughes A, Houlihan M, et al. Cross-clamp time is an independent predictor of mortality and morbidity in low- and high-risk cardiac patients. Int J Surg 2011;9:104–9.
24. Feldman T, Foster E, Glower DD, et al. Percutaneous repair or surgery for mitral regurgitation. N Engl J Med 2011;364:1395–406.
25. Pan W, Pan C, Jilaihawi H, et al. A novel user-friendly transcatheter edge-to-edge mitral valve repair device in a porcine model. Catheter Cardiovasc Interv 2019; 93:1354–60.
26. Liu B, Leach SB, Pan W, et al. Preliminary Outcome of a Novel Edge-to-Edge Closure Device to Manage Mitral Regurgitation in Dogs. Front Vet Sci 2020;7: 597879.
27. Archbold A, Akowuah E, Banning AP, et al. Getting the best from the Heart Team: guidance for cardiac multidisciplinary meetings. Heart 2022;108:e2.
28. Otto CM, Nishimura RA, Bonow RO, et al. 2020 ACC/AHA Guideline for the Management of Patients With Valvular Heart Disease: A Report of the American College of Cardiology/American Heart Association Joint Committee on Clinical Practice Guidelines. Circulation 2021;143:e72–227.
29. Zoghbi WA, Adams D, Bonow RO, et al. Recommendations for Noninvasive Evaluation of Native Valvular Regurgitation: A Report from the American Society of Echocardiography Developed in Collaboration with the Society for Cardiovascular Magnetic Resonance. J Am Soc Echocardiogr 2017;30:303–71.

Beyond Angiotensin-Converting Enzyme Inhibitors

Modulation of the Renin–Angiotensin–Aldosterone System to Delay or Manage Congestive Heart Failure

Marisa K. Ames, DVM, DACVIM (Cardiology)[a],*,
Darcy B. Adin, DVM, DACVIM (Cardiology)[b], James Wood, DVM[a]

KEYWORDS

- Diuretics • Angiotensin 1,7 • Angiotensin-converting enzyme 2
- Angiotensin converting enzyme inhibitor • Angiotensin receptor blocker
- Mineralocorticoid receptor antagonist

KEY POINTS

- The renin–angiotensin–aldosterone system (RAAS) consists of a classical arm (angiotensin-converting enzyme, angiotensin II, and its type I receptor and aldosterone) which promotes vasoconstriction, sodium retention, increased thirst and is pro-fibrotic and inflammatory) and an alternative arm (angiotensin-converting enzyme 2, angiotensin 1,7, and its Mas receptor) which tends to oppose these effects. Newer technologies are allowing for high-throughput assays that comprehensively evaluate circulating and tissue RAAS activity.
- Most evaluation of the comprehensive circulating RAAS has been performed in dogs with myxomatous mitral valve disease (MMVD). Estimated angiotensin-converting enzyme (ACE2) activity is higher in dogs with more advanced MMVD (American College of Veterinary Internal Medicine [ACVIM] Stage B2) as compared with normal dogs. Dogs with heart failure have significant RAAS activation (likely due in part to diuretic administration) as compared with normal dogs and dogs with preclinical MMVD.

Continued

---

[a] Department of Medicine and Epidemiology, School of Veterinary Medicine, University of California - Davis, 1 Shields Avenue, Davis, CA 95616, USA; [b] University of Florida, College of Veterinary Medicine, 2015 Southwest 16th Avenue, Gainesville, FL 32608, USA
* Corresponding author.
E-mail address: mkames@ucdavis.edu

Vet Clin Small Anim 53 (2023) 1353–1366
https://doi.org/10.1016/j.cvsm.2023.05.015
0195-5616/23/© 2023 Elsevier Inc. All rights reserved.

Continued

- Clinical studies have not been able to show conclusive benefit of RAAS suppression before the onset of congestive heart failure, but both advanced disease and diuretic medications administered to dogs with congestive heart failure induce RAAS activation. Suppression of the RAAS should be comprehensive (mineralocorticoid receptor antagonist paired with a medication that blocks the action of or reduces the formation of angiotensin II) to prevent aldosterone breakthrough.
- Genetic polymorphisms in the RAAS have been documented, including a functional polymorphism in the ACE gene. The pharmacogenomics of the RAAS is an ongoing area of research.
- Future pharmacotherapy of cardiovascular and kidney disease will likely include a multimodal modulation of the RAAS that aims to enhance its alternative arm and blunt its classical arm.

INTRODUCTION

The renin–angiotensin–aldosterone system (RAAS) plays a key role during development and in the day-to-day maintenance of blood pressure, sodium, and electrolyte homeostasis. The RAAS is constitutively active with capacity to upregulate in response to stressors such as hypovolemia, hypotension, inadequate sodium intake, and sustained sympathetic nervous system activation. Cardiovascular disease leads to activation of this system,[1–8] which is associated with physiologic (sodium retention, water intake, and vasoconstriction) and pathophysiologic (hypertrophy, fibrosis, and oxidative stress) responses.[9–12] The suppression of RAAS therefore remains a key treatment strategy for chronic cardiovascular diseases. However, current therapies do not always prolong survival or reduce morbidity.[13–15] Redundancy in this system and inadvertent suppression of beneficial components may reduce the benefits of our medical therapy. The development of future medical therapies for cardiovascular diseases will require a better understanding of how this entire system changes with disease and during therapy.

DISCUSSION
The Classical and Alternative Renin–Angiotensin System and Aldosterone

The renin–angiotensin system (RAS) is made up of angiotensin peptides (APs), enzymes, and receptors (**Fig. 1**). Angiotensin II (AngII) is the major effector molecule of this system and is produced from the degradation of angiotensinogen (AGT) to angiotensin I (AngI) by renin and degradation of AngI to AngII by the angiotensin-converting enzyme (ACE). The fluid and sodium retentive, vasoconstrictive, pro-inflammatory, and pro-fibrotic effects of RAS are primarily mediated by AngII acting at the angiotensin type 1 receptor (AT_1R). AngII also stimulates aldosterone secretion from the zona glomerulosa of the adrenal gland, which potentiates the physiologic and pathophysiologic effects of AngII.

AP and receptor combinations that lead to vasodilation and counteract or inhibit inflammation, fibrosis, and apoptosis include angiotensin 1,7 (Ang1,7) binding its Mas receptor and AngII binding its type 2 receptor (AT_2R).[16] The ACE2, ACE, and neprilysin (NEP) are responsible for the formation of Ang1,7 from AngI (via angiotensin 1,9) and AngII. Because of the counter regulatory actions of these AP receptors, and enzymes, the ACE2, Ang1,7, Mas pathway, and the AT_2R have been classified as an alternative pathway, differentiating them from the classical pathway of the core RAS (AngI, ACE, AngII, and AT_1R). Newly described alamandine, a metabolite of Ang1,7 or angiotensin

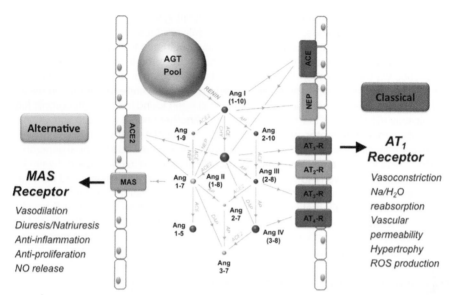

Fig. 1. The peptides, enzymes, and receptors of the renin–angiotensin system. The sphere sizes are quantitative and represent the amount of peptide determined by high-performance liquid chromatography tandem mass spectrometry. Red indicates that the peptide or receptor leads to vasoconstriction and can cause pathologic remodeling. Green indicates that the peptide or receptor has vasodilatory and/or anti-pathologic remodeling effects. Blue represents intermediate or metabolite peptides that do not, themselves, exert actions. Orange represents peptides whose effects are currently under investigation. Enzymes that metabolize or interact with angiotensin peptides are shown in blue connectors. ACE, angiotensin-converting enzyme; ACE2, angiotensin-converting enzyme 2; AGT, angiotensinogen; Ang, angiotensin peptide; AP, aminopeptidase; AT_1R, AT_2R, angiotensin II type 1 and 2 receptors; AT_3R, angiotensin III receptor; AT_4R, angiotensin IV receptor; CHY, chymase; DAP, dipeptidyl aminopeptidase IV; NO, nitric oxide; ROS, reactive oxygen species. (Figure reproduced with permission from Attoquant Diagnostics, GmbH.)

A (which is another metabolite of AngII) seems to confer counterregulatory (primarily vasodilatory) effects when binding to the G-protein coupled receptor member D.[17]

Circulating and Tissue Renin–Angiotensin Systems

The RAS was historically viewed as primarily an endocrine system where renin, released into the blood in a highly controlled manner from the juxtaglomerular apparatus of the kidney, encounters constitutively produced hepatic AGT and forms AngI. AngI contacts ACE on the surface of vascular endothelial cells and is converted to AngII, which acts at the AT_1R and AT_2R. The AT_1R is the predominant AngII receptor type in adult organisms and is widely distributed, occurring in the vasculature, kidney, adrenal gland, brain, and elsewhere.[18] Enzymes such as ACE, chymase, ACE2, prolyl-carboxy-peptidase (PCP), prolyl-endo-peptidase (PEP), and NEP then degrade AngII into its various metabolites including angiotensin A, 1,9; 1,7; 1,5; III, and IV with most of these metabolites having activity. In this endocrine model, APs reach the tissues via the circulation. However, local (tissue) formation of AngI and AngII occurs in the heart, kidneys, brain, and vascular tissue, which amplifies the effects of this system. The enzymes of the RAS (ACE, chymase, ACE2, PCP, PEP, NEP, and others) are also present, and all AP metabolites of the RAS are also formed locally in the tissues. Whether the generation of renin (the rate limiting step within RAS) and AGT occurs de novo in the tissues, or the circulation delivers these to the tissues remains controversial. It is likely that in health, most renin originates from the juxtaglomerular apparatus of the kidney and most AGT originates from the liver and is delivered to the tissues via the circulation.[19,20] However, tissue production of renin and AGT may mediate some disease processes (eg, hypertension) independently of the circulating RAS.[21] Higher AGT transcription levels have also been found in cats with chronic kidney disease (CKD) as compared with controls.[22] Another source of tissue activation of RAS is the prorenin receptor, which binds the precursor of renin (prorenin) and renders it active, bypassing the rate limiting step and initiating the cascade for local generation of APs.[23] The local enzyme environment also affects the overall balance between the classical and alternative RAS (see **Fig. 1**).[24] The balance of the classical and the alternative arms is a therapeutic target, and the ideal RAS modulating drug/drug combination will increase the alternative RAS activity and decrease the classical RAS activity. The serine protease chymase is also capable of catalyzing AngII production from AngI in the tissues independently of ACE. If chymase is confirmed as a potent mechanism for AngII formation in tissues, it would be a promising therapeutic target.

Quantification of the Renin–Angiotensin–Aldosterone System

Circulating angiotensin peptide quantification

Components of the RAS can be measured separately via a variety of assay types (radioimmunoassay [RIA], enzyme-linked immunosorbent assay, fluorescent assays, and liquid chromatography tandem mass spectrometry [LC-MS/MS]). The simultaneous measurement of multiple APs and aldosterone via LC-MS/MS (eg, the RAS Fingerprint [Attoquant Diagnostics GmbH, Vienna, Austria]) is a sensitive, specific, and efficient way to comprehensively profile this system in both the blood and tissues. Quantification of AP concentrations via LC-MS/MS is performed using two approaches: (1) immediate protease inhibition of a whole blood sample and subsequent analysis of plasma or (2) analysis of untreated serum or plasma. Protease inhibition provides an instantaneous quantification of AP concentrations that the moment the sample was taken. Equilibrium dialysis incubates the serum or plasma at body temperature for 1 hour and applies the concept that AGT concentrations greatly exceed that of "down-stream" metabolites, leading to a constant formation of AngI. As angiotensin metabolizing enzymes are still active in the sample and exceed the concentrations of metabolites, there is an establishment of stable equilibrium levels of downstream APs, where formation and degradation rates become equal. Serum aldosterone and AGT quantification complete the comprehensive assessment of the RAAS. Aldosterone does not require protease inhibition and is measured in routinely handled serum or plasma. AngI and II concentrations quantified via the equilibrium dialysis method are highly correlated to directly measure (using protease inhibition) concentrations in the dog.[8]

Enzymes and ratios

Comprehensive quantification of the RAS has expanded our understanding of the relationships between RAS metabolites and the balance between classical and alternative pathways, which is largely controlled by enzyme availability. Surrogates of enzyme activities show good correlation with direct enzyme measurements.[25,26] For example, the sum of Ang I and II correlates well with direct renin activity and is considered a surrogate of plasma renin activity (PRA_{surr}).[26] The ratio of angiotensin 1,5 (Ang1,5) to AngII is a surrogate of ACE2 activity ($ACE2_{surr}$) because it accounts for both the substrate (AngII) and degradation product (Ang1,5) of the formation product of ACE2 (Ang1,7).[8] Using the formation and degradation of metabolites to estimate enzyme activities is not as accurate as direct enzyme quantification when multiple enzyme pathways exist. For example, the ratio of AngII to AngI is considered a surrogate of ACE activity (ACE_{surr}) except when chymases are also contributors to AngII formation.[1] In this situation, ACE activity is more accurately estimated by the formation rate of AngII in the presence and absence of both ACE and chymase inhibitors.

Metabolite ratios provide insight into the overall balance of RAS activity (**Table 1**). For example, the ratio of the alternative RAS pathway metabolites (Ang1,7 and 1,5) indexed to the sum of these alternative metabolites and classical metabolites (AngI and II) allows interpretation of the alternative metabolites relative to overall RAS activation (ALT_{surr}).[27] The ratio of Ang1,7 to AngI has also been proposed as a reflection of alternative RAS balance.[28] In this situation, indexing the major alternative metabolite (Ang1,7) to the most proximal metabolite (AngI) accounts for the possibility of different pathways for Ang1,7 production which might be altered in some patients with genetic variants. The ratio of aldosterone to AngII provides an estimate of adrenal responsiveness to AngII, which can help our understanding of aldosterone production in the setting of RAAS stimulation.[1] These ratios require more study to understand their precision and predictive value. Some of these enzyme surrogates and metabolite ratios have potential as biomarkers of disease (eg, ACE2, ALT_{surr}, Ang1,7/AngII) and are active areas of investigation.[25,29,30]

Quantification of the tissue renin–angiotensin system

Methods for localizing and quantifying RAS activity in the tissues include immunohistochemistry, LC-MS/MS, and reverse transcription and quantitative polymerase chain reaction. APs are rapidly cleaved by tissue enzymes postmortem, and AP quantification must be performed on tissues that are harvested and frozen antemortem or immediately after death. Because this is difficult in clinical patients, an alternative approach is to measure the tissue synthesis rates of AngII and Ang1,7 in the presence and absence of specific inhibitors.[24] The relative contributions of enzymes such as ACE2, NEP, PEP, and PCP to Ang1,7 formation and the relative contributions of ACE and chymase to AngII formation are then determined.[31] Greater AngII synthesis as compared with Ang1,7 synthesis provides evidence for RAS dysregulation. Immunohistochemistry allows for visualization of enzyme expression patterns. The presence of ACE2 within canine kidney and myocardial tissues has been proven via this method.[2] The intrarenal RAS has been evaluated in cats with CKD using reverse transcriptase and quantitative polymerase chain reaction and LC-MS/MS.[22]

Urine aldosterone-to-creatinine ratio

The urine aldosterone-to-creatinine ratio (UAldo:C) is used as an indicator of RAAS activation. One study showed that the UAldo:C from a single sample was correlated

Table 1
Renin–angiotensin–aldosterone system ratios and enzyme surrogates

Abbreviation	Formula
PRA_{surr}	AngI + AngII[26]
ACE_{surr}	AngII/AngI[1]
$ACE2_{surr}$	Ang1,5/AngII[8]
ALT_{surr}	(Ang1,5 + Ang1,7)/(Ang1,5 + Ang1,7 + AngI + AngII)[27]
Ang1,7/AngI	Ang1,7/AngI[28]
Ang1,7/AngII	Ang1,7/AngII[25]
$AA2_{surr}$	Aldosterone/AngII[26,52]

to the 24-hour UAldo:C in normal dogs and the UAldo:C values mirrored circulating APs and aldosterone concentrations during diuretic administration.[32] A limitation of the UAldo:C is that drugs such as RAAS suppressants and diuretics may affect the clearance of aldosterone from the kidney and it is not known if this needs to be considered when interpreting the UAldo:C. Also, the detection of urinary aldosterone metabolites is difficult in cats.[33]

Week-to-week variation

The RAS Fingerprint assay coefficient of variation is less than 10% within reference intervals and less than 15% when close to the lower limit of quantification for all covered analytes. The coefficients of variation in normal dogs for the week-to-week variation of AngI, AngII, and Ang1,7 in one study were 29%, 38%, and 29%, respectively.[8] In this same study, the coefficient of variation for the ALT_{surr}, which represents the overall balance of the classical and alternative arms, was 10%. The higher week-to-week variation in AP concentrations may reflect stress level, timing of the sample, and the most recent meal, hydration, and dietary sodium intake. The lower variation of the ALT surrogate suggests that the balance of alternative versus classical (ie, ACE2 vs ACE) enzyme activity remains more stable as compared with the individual AP concentrations. The ALT surrogate may serve as a more reliable indicator of a patient's RAS "balance" and may have prognostic value. With current RIAs, the UAldo:C has moderate day-to-day variation which limits the use of this test as a point of care biomarker. Serial UAldo:C or a UAldo:C determined from pooled urine samples may make this test more useful.

The Renin–Angiotensin–Aldosterone System in Cardiovascular Disease

Several studies have quantified the comprehensive RAS in dogs and cats with naturally occurring cardiovascular and kidney disease using the RAS Fingerprint. In a recent study, no differences were found in circulating AP concentrations when dogs with American College of Veterinary Internal Medicine (ACVIM) stage B1 and B2 myxomatous mitral valve disease (MMVD) (naïve to cardiac medications) were compared with normal dogs.[8] However, the balance of the alternative to classical RAS changed with MMVD progression, as evidenced by a significantly greater $ACE2_{surr}$ in B2 as compared with normal dogs. This may result from increased activity of other alternative enzymes (NEP) or increased cleavage of ACE2 from the tissues, which enhances its presence in the circulation. The latter phenomenon is hypothesized to be a pathologic displacement of the protective ACE2 enzyme from tissues mediated by the protease ADAM17 (also called tumor necrosis factor-alpha-converting enzyme).[34] Once heart failure due to MMVD develops and furosemide therapy is initiated, circulating RAAS activation increases significantly.[1,2]

The comprehensive RAAS has been compared between cats with systemic hypertension, cats with cardiomyopathy (including preclinical disease and cats with acute and chronic heart failure), and age- and sex-matched controls.[7] In this study, the incidence of CKD in control cats, hypertensive cats, and cats with cardiomyopathy was 43%, 57%, and 60%, respectively. In the subset of cats with cardiomyopathy not yet receiving furosemide, circulating RAAS activity was higher when compared with controls, whereas RAAS activity in cats with systemic hypertension not yet receiving amlodipine did not differ significantly from controls. Treatment with the diuretic furosemide or amlodipine was associated with RAAS activation. In another study, circulating AP concentrations did not differ between healthy controls and cats with cardiomyopathy (two of which were receiving furosemide).[27]

The intrarenal RAS may be upregulated in cats with CKD.[22] When compared with healthy controls, cats with CKD had increased AGT and decreased ACE transcript levels. Concentrations of AngII from kidney tissue homogenates were higher in the CKD group as compared with controls, yet this did not reach significance.

Clinical Trials Investigating Renin–Angiotensin–Aldosterone System Suppression in Dogs with Mitral Valve Disease

Preclinical disease

The usefulness of ACEi to delay disease progression in MMVD before the onset of congestive heart faliure (CHF) has been called into question by the results of several large clinical trials that were unable to show conclusive benefit. Although one study showed promising results, the difference in time to onset of CHF was not statistically significantly different between dogs receiving enalapril and dogs not receiving enalapril.[15] Other studies clearly failed to demonstrate benefit to ACEi use in preclinical disease in cats[35] and dogs.[14]

Congestive heart failure

Clinical studies evaluating ACEi in dogs with CHF demonstrated morbidity and mortality reductions over background therapy of furosemide.[36–38] These studies support the benefit of RAAS suppression in the setting of CHF treated solely with diuretics. Subsequent studies demonstrated superiority of pimobendan over ACEi for the treatment of CHF, but the trial design does not reflect clinical practice where both medications are typically administered together without a need to make a choice between them.[39,40] The BESST study demonstrated end point benefit for CHF dogs given comprehensive RAAS suppression (benazepril and spironolactone) compared with benazepril alone,[41] which supports the concept that aldosterone breakthrough (ABT) is important to outcomes; however, pimobendan was not part of the study design which limits its applicability to practical clinical approaches. Finally, a recent study concluded that there was no additive benefit of ramipril in dogs with CHF treated with pimobendan and furosemide.[42] Unlike earlier studies,[36–38] this study included pimobendan[42] which is now standard of care for dogs with CHF. However, the study design did not evaluate comprehensive RAAS suppression with an aldosterone antagonist (eg, spironolactone) in addition to ACEi, and the impact of ABT is unknown.[42]

Explanations for neutral study results in preclinical disease

One explanation for negative or neutral study results of ACEi in dogs is the phenomenon of ABT, which is defined by high blood aldosterone or AngII concentrations after appropriate ACEi use.[43] General causes of ABT include, persistent AngII production (AngII breakthrough), upregulation of other aldosterone secretagogues, and decreased aldosterone metabolism and clearance.[43,44] To address ABT, the DELAY study evaluated comprehensive RAAS suppression using benazepril and spironolactone together in dogs with preclinical MMVD; however, this study also failed to find a benefit regarding time to onset of CHF when compared with benazepril treatment alone.[13] Despite the lack of primary end point benefit, the DELAY study found reductions in cardiac size and biomarkers in the benazepril and spironolactone group compared with the benazepril only group.[13] Another explanation for neutral study results may be that the RAAS is not activated or dysregulated "enough" in the preclinical stage of disease. Finally, multiple modifiers of the RAAS likely contribute to individual heterogeneity in regard to basal RAAS activity and response to pharmacotherapy (**Box 1**).

Knowledge gaps

Despite the standard use of, and recommendation for multimodal therapy involving pimobendan, ACEi, spironolactone, and loop diuretics in dogs with CHF,[45] there are

---

Box 1
Potential modifiers of the renin–angiotensin–aldosterone system

Medications (eg, diuretics, vasodilators, ACEi, angiotensin receptor blockers, spironolactone, beta blockers)[32,50,52–55]

Cardiac disease[1,13,54,56]

Renal disease[57]

Inflammation[58]

Sex[28,59,60]

Breed[49,50,59]

Genetic variants[48,50,61]

Diet[62,63]

Age[59]

Exercise[64]

Biologic and temporal variability[8,65]

Supplements[66]

---

no clinical trials evaluating the efficacy of these medications used together in dogs with CHF. Additional clinical trials will be needed to better define the appropriate use and timing of RAAS inhibitors in dogs with heart disease. The effect of current RAS inhibitors on the tissue RAS is also not well understood and the mechanisms by which the tissue RAS can break through suppression warrant further investigation.

The Genetics of the Renin–Angiotensin–Aldosterone System

Meurs and colleagues showed that polymorphisms in the RAAS occur in dogs and cats and are similar to those described in people.[46] These included polymorphisms in ACE, AGT, and the AT_2R. A polymorphism in the canine ACE gene is the best studied to date. Certain breeds have a high prevalence of this variant (Cavalier King Charles Spaniels, Dachshunds, Irish Wolfhounds, and Doberman Pinschers).[28,47–49]

Although dogs with the ACE polymorphism were shown to have a lower baseline ACE activity when compared with wild type dogs, there was no difference between these groups in regard to suppression of ACE activity with ACEi therapy.[47,50] A more recent study using RAS Fingerprint analysis showed no difference in RAAS profiles and the ACE_{surr} with respect to this polymorphism.[48] This discordant finding may have been due to the different methodologies of determining ACE activity. In one study, ABT was more common in dogs with the ACE polymorphism, likely occurring via mechanisms other than altered ACE activity or AngII levels.[48] The effect of RAAS polymorphisms on long-term cardiovascular outcomes and further evaluation of functionality of the ACE and other polymorphisms warrants further study. It is likely that genetic variation influences baseline RAAS activity and response of this system to disease progression and pharmacotherapy.

FUTURE APPROACHES TO RENIN–ANGIOTENSIN–ALDOSTERONE SYSTEM MODULATION

With a more complete understanding of the RAAS and more comprehensive quantification methods, various strategies of modulating the system seem beneficial (**Fig. 2**).

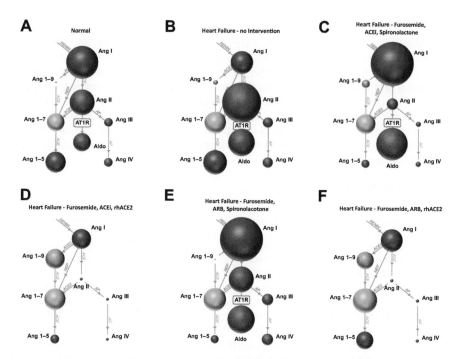

Fig. 2. Hypothetical circulating renin–angiotensin–aldosterone system (RAAS) profiles. See **Fig. 1** for explanation of sphere size and color. (*A*) The relative balance of angiotensin peptides in normal dogs. (*B*) RAAS is activated in the untreated heart failure patient, leading to increased angiotensin peptide concentrations. Angiotensin II is a secretagogue of aldosterone, which is also increased. (*C*) Although diuretics further stimulate the release of renin, and cause an increase in angiotensin I concentrations, concurrent angiotensin-converting enzyme inhibitor (ACEi) therapy leads to an overall reduction angiotensin II concentrations, whereas spironolactone (a mineralocorticoid receptor antagonist) leads to an increase in aldosterone. The blockade of ACE leads to accumulation of angiotensin I, which is metabolized to angiotensin I,7. The ACEi prevents further degradation of angiotensin 1,7 to 1,5. (*D*) The addition of human recombinant ACE2 should increase the degradation of angiotensin I and II (reducing concentrations of these peptides) to angiotensin 1,9, and 1,7 (increasing concentrations of these peptides). These changes are supported by one study that added human recombinant ACE2 to the plasma of dogs with advanced myxomatous mitral valve disease who were receiving an ACEi.[51] Aldosterone is removed from this diagram for simplicity. (*E*) Diuretic and vasodilator (angiotensin receptor blocker [ARB]) therapy likely contributes to RAAS activation and increased production of angiotensin I. Treatment with an ARB also leads to accumulation of angiotensin II due to blockade of its angiotensin type 1 receptor.[51] (*F*) The addition of human recombinant ACE2 should increase the metabolism of angiotensin I and II (reducing concentrations of these peptides) to angiotensin 1,9, and 1,7 (increasing concentrations of these peptides). In the absence of ACEi, angiotensin 1,7 is further degraded to angiotensin 1,5. These changes are supported by one study that added human recombinant ACE2 to the plasma of dogs with advanced myxomatous mitral valve disease who were receiving an ARB.[51] Aldosterone is removed from this diagram for simplicity. (Figure reproduced with permission from Attoquant Diagnostics, GmbH.)

SUMMARY

The RAAS consists of bioactive APs, enzymatic pathways, receptors, and the steroid hormone aldosterone. The RAAS regulates blood pressure, sodium, and electrolyte homeostasis and mediates pathologic disease processes. Within this system is an alternative arm that counterbalances the vasoconstrictive, sodium and water retentive, and pro-fibrotic and inflammatory effects of the classical arm. Improved biochemical methodologies in RAAS quantification are elucidating how this complex system changes in health and disease. Future treatments for cardiovascular and kidney disease will likely involve a more nuanced manipulation of this system rather than simple blockade.

CLINICS CARE POINTS

- When added to furosemide therapy, the combination of spironolactone and benazepril is superior to benazepril alone in the management of congestive heart failure due to myxomatous mitral valve disease in dogs. Whether or not this benefit remains when pimobendan is added to the backgroud therapy remains unknown.

- On balance, studies to date evaluating renin-angiotensin-aldosterone system (RAAS) blockade in pre-clinical myxomatous mitral valve disease have yielded neutral results. Future studies will likely involve a more strategic modulation of the RAAS using inhibitors while supplementing beneficial alternative angiotensin peptides and enzymes.

- Quantification of renin-angiotensin system (RAS) peptides and enzyme activities are not yet used in daily clinical decision making. Ratios such as the 'alternative surrogate' (ALT$_{surr}$) that reflect the balance between the alternative and classical RAS have potential as future biomarkers.

DISCLOSURE

Dr M.K. Ames is a consultant for Ceva Animal Health. She has also received research support, travel reimbursement, gifts, and honoraria fromCeva Animal Health (directly and in support of the Translational RAAS Interest Group) and Boehringer Ingelheim. Dr D. Adin is a consultant for Ceva and Boehringer Ingelheim. She has also received research support, travel reimbursement, gifts, and honoraria from Ceva Animal Health (directly and in support of the Translational RAAS Interest Group) and Boehringer Ingelheim. Dr J. Wood has received travel reimbursement and research support from Ceva Animal Health through the Translational RAAS Interest Group.

REFERENCES

1. Adin D, Kurtz K, Atkins C, et al. Role of electrolyte concentrations and renin-angiotensin-aldosterone activation in the staging of canine heart disease. J Vet Intern Med 2020;34(1):53–64.
2. Larouche-Lebel É, Loughran KA, Oyama MA, et al. Plasma and tissue angiotensin-converting enzyme 2 activity and plasma equilibrium concentrations of angiotensin peptides in dogs with heart disease. J Vet Intern Med 2019;33(4):1571–84.
3. Tidholm A, Häggström J, Hansson K. Effects of dilated cardiomyopathy on the renin-angiotensin-aldosterone system, atrial natriuretic peptide activity, and thyroid hormone concentrations in dogs. Am J Vet Res 2001;62(6):961–7.
4. O'Sullivan ML, O'Grady MR, Minors SL. Plasma big endothelin-1, atrial natriuretic peptide, aldosterone, and norepinephrine concentrations in normal Doberman

Pinschers and Doberman Pinschers with dilated cardiomyopathy. J Vet Intern Med 2007;21(1):92–9.

5. MacDonald KA, Kittleson MD, Larson RF, et al. The effect of ramipril on left ventricular mass, myocardial fibrosis, diastolic function, and plasma neurohormones in Maine Coon cats with familial hypertrophic cardiomyopathy without heart failure. J Vet Intern Med 2006;20(5):1093–105.

6. Jensen J, Henik RA, Brownfield M, et al. Plasma renin activity and angiotensin I and aldosterone concentrations in cats with hypertension associated with chronic renal disease. Am J Vet Res 1997;58(5):535–40.

7. Ward JL, Guillot E, Domenig O, et al. Circulating renin-angiotensin-aldosterone system activity in cats with systemic hypertension or cardiomyopathy. J Vet Intern Med 2022;36(3):897–909.

8. Hammond H, Ames M, Domenig O, et al. The classical and alternative circulating renin-angiotensin system in normal dogs and dogs with stage B1 and B2 myxomatous mitral valve disease. J Vet Intern Med 2023;37(3):875–86.

9. Weber KT, Brilla CG. Pathological hypertrophy and cardiac interstitium. Fibrosis and renin-angiotensin-aldosterone system. Circulation 1991;83(6):1849–65.

10. Waanders F, de Vries LV, van Goor H, et al. Aldosterone, from (patho)physiology to treatment in cardiovascular and renal damage. Curr Vasc Pharmacol 2011; 9(5):594–605.

11. Schiffrin EL. Effects of aldosterone on the vasculature. Hypertension 2006;47(3): 312–8.

12. Chappell MC. Biochemical evaluation of the renin-angiotensin system: the good, bad, and absolute? Am J Physiol Heart Circ Physiol 2016;310(2):H137–52.

13. Borgarelli M, Ferasin L, Lamb K, et al. DELay of Appearance of sYmptoms of Canine Degenerative Mitral Valve Disease Treated with Spironolactone and Benazepril: the DELAY Study. J Vet Cardiol 2020;27:34–53.

14. Kvart C, Häggström J, Pedersen HD, et al. Efficacy of enalapril for prevention of congestive heart failure in dogs with myxomatous valve disease and asymptomatic mitral regurgitation. J Vet Intern Med 2002;16(1):80–8.

15. Atkins CE, Keene BW, Brown WA, et al. Results of the veterinary enalapril trial to prove reduction in onset of heart failure in dogs chronically treated with enalapril alone for compensated, naturally occurring mitral valve insufficiency. J Am Vet Med Assoc 2007;231(7):1061–9.

16. Santos RAS, Sampaio WO, Alzamora AC, et al. The ACE2/Angiotensin-(1-7)/MAS Axis of the Renin-Angiotensin System: Focus on Angiotensin-(1-7). Physiol Rev 2018;98(1):505–53.

17. Lautner RQ, Villela DC, Fraga-Silva RA, et al. Discovery and characterization of alamandine: a novel component of the renin-angiotensin system. Circ Res 2013;112(8):1104–11.

18. Carey RM, Padia SH. Chapter 1: Physiology and Regulation of the Renin-Angiotensin-Aldsoterone System. In: Singh A, Williams GH, editors. Textbook of nephroendocrinology. 2nd edition. London: Elsevier/Academic Press; 2009. p. 1–25. https://doi.org/10.1016/B978-0-12-803247-3.12001-X.

19. Matsusaka T, Niimura F, Shimizu A, et al. Liver angiotensinogen is the primary source of renal angiotensin II. J Am Soc Nephrol 2012;23(7):1181–9.

20. de Lannoy LM, Danser AH, van Kats JP, et al. Renin-angiotensin system components in the interstitial fluid of the isolated perfused rat heart. Local production of angiotensin I. Hypertension 1997;29(6):1240–51.

21. Davisson RL, Ding Y, Stec DE, et al. Novel mechanism of hypertension revealed by cell-specific targeting of human angiotensinogen in transgenic mice. Physiol Genomics 1999;1(1):3–9.
22. Lourenço BN, Coleman AE, Berghaus RD, et al. Characterization of the intrarenal renin-angiotensin system in cats with naturally occurring chronic kidney disease. J Vet Intern Med 2022;36(2):647–55.
23. Hennrikus M, Gonzalez AA, Prieto MC. The prorenin receptor in the cardiovascular system and beyond. Am J Physiol Heart Circ Physiol 2018;314(2):H139–45.
24. Kovarik JJ, Kaltenecker CC, Kopecky C, et al. Intrarenal Renin-Angiotensin-System Dysregulation after Kidney Transplantation. Sci Rep 2019;9(1):9762.
25. Basu R, Poglitsch M, Yogasundaram H, et al. Roles of Angiotensin Peptides and Recombinant Human ACE2 in Heart Failure. J Am Coll Cardiol 2017;69(7):805–19.
26. Pavo N, Goliasch G, Wurm R, et al. Low- and High-renin Heart Failure Phenotypes with Clinical Implications. Clin Chem 2018;64(3):597–608.
27. Huh T, Larouche-Lebel É, Loughran KA, et al. Effect of angiotensin receptor blockers and angiotensin-converting enzyme 2 on plasma equilibrium angiotensin peptide concentrations in cats with heart disease. J Vet Intern Med 2021;35(1):33–42.
28. Adin DB, Hernandez JA. Influence of sex on renin-angiotensin-aldosterone system metabolites and enzymes in Doberman Pinschers. J Vet Intern Med 2023;37(1):22–7.
29. Kintscher U, Slagman A, Domenig O, et al. Plasma Angiotensin Peptide Profiling and ACE (Angiotensin-Converting Enzyme)-2 Activity in COVID-19 Patients Treated With Pharmacological Blockers of the Renin-Angiotensin System. Hypertension 2020;76(5):e34–6.
30. Resende MM, Mill JG. Alternate angiotensin II-forming pathways and their importance in physiological or physiopathological conditions. Arq Bras Cardiol 2002;78(4):425–38.
31. Weitzhandler E, Ames M, Domenig O. Tissue renin-angiotensin system enzyme activity in canine post-mortem myocardial and kidney samples. J Vet Intern Med 2022;36(6):2414–5 (abstract).
32. Potter BM, Ames MK, Hess A, et al. Comparison between the effects of torsemide and furosemide on the renin-angiotensin-aldosterone system of normal dogs. J Vet Cardiol 2019;26:51–62.
33. Syme HM, Fletcher MG, Bailey SR, et al. Measurement of aldosterone in feline, canine and human urine. J Small Anim Pract 2007;48(4):202–8.
34. Patel VB, Clarke N, Wang Z, et al. Angiotensin II induced proteolytic cleavage of myocardial ACE2 is mediated by TACE/ADAM-17: a positive feedback mechanism in the RAS. J Mol Cell Cardiol 2014;66:167–76.
35. King JN, Martin M, Chetboul V, et al. Evaluation of benazepril in cats with heart disease in a prospective, randomized, blinded, placebo-controlled clinical trial. J Vet Intern Med 2019;33(6):2559–71.
36. Controlled clinical evaluation of enalapril in dogs with heart failure: results of the Cooperative Veterinary Enalapril Study Group. The COVE Study Group. J Vet Intern Med 1995;9(4):243–52.
37. Acute and short-term hemodynamic, echocardiographic, and clinical effects of enalapril maleate in dogs with naturally acquired heart failure: results of the Invasive Multicenter PROspective Veterinary Evaluation of Enalapril study. The IMPROVE Study Group. J Vet Intern Med 1995;9(4):234–42.

38. Ettinger SJ, Benitz AM, Ericsson GF, et al. Effects of enalapril maleate on survival of dogs with naturally acquired heart failure. The Long-Term Investigation of Veterinary Enalapril (LIVE) Study Group. J Am Vet Med Assoc 1998;213(11):1573–7.
39. Häggström J, Boswood A, O'Grady M, et al. Effect of pimobendan or benazepril hydrochloride on survival times in dogs with congestive heart failure caused by naturally occurring myxomatous mitral valve disease: the QUEST study. J Vet Intern Med 2008;22(5):1124–35.
40. Lombard CW, Jöns O, Bussadori CM. Clinical efficacy of pimobendan versus benazepril for the treatment of acquired atrioventricular valvular disease in dogs. J Am Anim Hosp Assoc 2006;42(4):249–61.
41. Coffman M, Guillot E, Blondel T, et al. Clinical efficacy of a benazepril and spironolactone combination in dogs with congestive heart failure due to myxomatous mitral valve disease: The BEnazepril Spironolactone STudy (BESST). J Vet Intern Med 2021;35(4):1673–87.
42. Wess G, Kresken JG, Wendt R, et al. Efficacy of adding ramipril (VAsotop) to the combination of furosemide (Lasix) and pimobendan (VEtmedin) in dogs with mitral valve degeneration: The VALVE trial. J Vet Intern Med 2020;34(6):2232–41.
43. Ames MK, Atkins CE, Eriksson A, et al. Aldosterone breakthrough in dogs with naturally occurring myxomatous mitral valve disease. J Vet Cardiol 2017;19(3):218–27.
44. Lefebvre H, Duparc C, Naccache A, et al. Paracrine Regulation of Aldosterone Secretion in Physiological and Pathophysiological Conditions. Vitam Horm 2019;109:303–39.
45. Keene BW, Atkins CE, Bonagura JD, et al. ACVIM consensus guidelines for the diagnosis and treatment of myxomatous mitral valve disease in dogs. J Vet Intern Med 2019;33(3):1127–40.
46. Meurs KM, Chdid L, Reina-Doreste Y, et al. Polymorphisms in the canine and feline renin-angiotensin-aldosterone system genes. Anim Genet 2015;46(2):226.
47. Meurs KM, Stern JA, Atkins CE, et al. Angiotensin-converting enzyme activity and inhibition in dogs with cardiac disease and an angiotensin-converting enzyme polymorphism. J Renin Angiotensin Aldosterone Syst 2017;18(4). 1470320317737184.
48. Adin D, Atkins C, Domenig O, et al. Renin-angiotensin aldosterone profile before and after angiotensin-converting enzyme-inhibitor administration in dogs with angiotensin-converting enzyme gene polymorphism. J Vet Intern Med 2020;34(2):600–6.
49. Adin DB, Atkins CE, Friedenberg SG, et al. Prevalence of an angiotensin-converting enzyme gene variant in dogs. Canine Med Genet 2021;8(1):6.
50. Meurs KM, Olsen LH, Reimann MJ, et al. Angiotensin-converting enzyme activity in Cavalier King Charles Spaniels with an ACE gene polymorphism and myxomatous mitral valve disease. Pharmacogenet Genomics 2018;28(2):37–40.
51. Larouche-Lebel É, Loughran KA, Huh T, et al. Effect of angiotensin receptor blockers and angiotensin converting enzyme 2 on plasma equilibrium angiotensin peptide concentrations in dogs with heart disease. J Vet Intern Med 2021;35(1):22–32.
52. Adin D, Atkins C, Wallace G, et al. Effect of spironolactone and benazepril on furosemide-induced diuresis and renin-angiotensin-aldosterone system activation in normal dogs. J Vet Intern Med 2021;35(3):1245–54.
53. Ames MK, Atkins CE, Lantis AC, et al. Evaluation of subacute change in RAAS activity (as indicated by urinary aldosterone:creatinine, after pharmacologic provocation) and the response to ACE inhibition. J Renin Angiotensin Aldosterone Syst 2016;17(1). 1470320316633897.

54. Ames MK, Atkins CE, Pitt B. The renin-angiotensin-aldosterone system and its suppression. J Vet Intern Med 2019;33(2):363–82.

55. Olson RD, Nies AS, Gerber JG. Beta adrenergically mediated release of renin in the dog is not confined to either beta-1 or beta-2 adrenoceptors. J Pharmacol Exp Ther 1982;222(3):606–11.

56. Pedersen HD, Koch J, Poulsen K, et al. Activation of the renin-angiotensin system in dogs with asymptomatic and mildly symptomatic mitral valvular insufficiency. J Vet Intern Med 1995;9(5):328–31.

57. Pouchelon JL, Atkins CE, Bussadori C, et al. Cardiovascular-renal axis disorders in the domestic dog and cat: a veterinary consensus statement. J Small Anim Pract 2015;56(9):537–52.

58. Junho CVC, Trentin-Sonoda M, Panico K, et al. Cardiorenal syndrome: long road between kidney and heart. Heart Fail Rev 2022;27(6):2137–53.

59. Galizzi A, Bagardi M, Stranieri A, et al. Factors affecting the urinary aldosterone-to-creatinine ratio in healthy dogs and dogs with naturally occurring myxomatous mitral valve disease. BMC Vet Res 2021;17(1):15.

60. O'Donnell E, Floras JS, Harvey PJ. Estrogen status and the renin angiotensin aldosterone system. Am J Physiol Regul Integr Comp Physiol 2014;307(5): R498–500.

61. Zakrzewski-Jakubiak M, de Denus S, Dubé MP, et al. Ten renin-angiotensin system-related gene polymorphisms in maximally treated Canadian Caucasian patients with heart failure. Br J Clin Pharmacol 2008;65(5):742–51.

62. Mochel JP, Fink M, Bon C, et al. Influence of feeding schedules on the chronobiology of renin activity, urinary electrolytes and blood pressure in dogs. Chronobiol Int 2014;31(5):715–30.

63. Freeman LM, Rush JE, Markwell PJ. Effects of dietary modification in dogs with early chronic valvular disease. J Vet Intern Med 2006;20(5):1116–26.

64. Holbrook T, Lester G, Sleeper M, et al. Renin-angiotensin-aldosterone system profilling in horses before and after exercise. 2021;35(6):2975-2976 (abstract).

65. Mochel JP, Fink M, Peyrou M, et al. Chronobiology of the renin-angiotensin-aldosterone system in dogs: relation to blood pressure and renal physiology. Chronobiol Int 2013;30(9):1144–59.

66. Ito T, Schaffer S, Azuma J. The effect of taurine on chronic heart failure: actions of taurine against catecholamine and angiotensin II. Amino Acids 2014;46(1):111–9.

The Role of Autoantibodies in Companion Animal Cardiac Disease

Luís Dos Santos, DVM, PhD[a],*, Ashley L. Walker, DVM[b]

KEYWORDS

- Inflammation • Autoimmunity • Functional antibodies • Dilated cardiomyopathy
- Arrhythmogenic right ventricular cardiomyopathy • Canine

KEY POINTS

- Familial cardiomyopathies in dogs may be linked to inflammation and immune responses.
- Functional autoantibodies (AABs) are a newer class of AABs that act as agonists to G-protein coupled receptors and induce pathologic intracellular signaling and conditions.
- Functional AABs are increasingly accepted as playing a role in the pathogenesis of several cardiomyopathies including dilated cardiomyopathy and Chagas cardiomyopathy.

INTRODUCTION/BACKGROUND

Inflammation has historically been linked to cardiac diseases, especially in advanced cardiac stages or in patients with congestive heart failure.[1–3] Because of this, clinical studies of the roles that autoimmune diseases (ADs) play in cardiac dysfunction have become increasingly common in both human and veterinary literature.[1,4] ADs are characterized by aberrant immune responses to healthy cells of a specific organ; this can occur because of genetic predisposition, environmental influences, or both.[5] Because increasing evidence have described the aberrant activation and trafficking of immune cells into the heart, new discoveries have revealed that affected cardiomyocytes can have intrinsic inflammatory signaling pathways activated, which results in tissue pathology and remodeling.[6] In addition, specific circulating autoantibodies (AABs) and inflammatory cytokines have been linked to the development and/or deterioration of specific cardiomyopathies, including dilated cardiomyopathy (DCM), arrhythmogenic right ventricular cardiomyopathy (ARVC), Chagas cardiomyopathy, and feline hypertrophic cardiomyopathy (HCM).[7,8] In this article, we will

[a] Department of Veterinary Clinical Sciences, Purdue University, College of Veterinary Medicine, 625 Harrison Street, West Lafayette, IN 47907, USA; [b] William R. Pritchard Veterinary Medical Teaching Hospital, University of California, Davis, 1 Garrod Drive, Davis, CA 9561, USA
* Corresponding author.
E-mail address: dossantos@purdue.edu

Vet Clin Small Anim 53 (2023) 1367–1377
https://doi.org/10.1016/j.cvsm.2023.05.018
vetsmall.theclinics.com

summarize the recent literature about AABs and their role in cardiac diseases of small animals.

CURRENT EVIDENCE IN VETERINARY CARDIOLOGY
Dilated Cardiomyopathy

DCM is the second most common cardiac disease in dogs and the most common in large breed dogs.[9,10] Clinically, DCM is characterized by left ventricular dilatation, systolic dysfunction, and arrhythmias.[10,11] The pathologic phenotype, disease progression, and histologic findings are similar in the canine and human form of DCM.[12] A genetic basis for the development of DCM is known or suspected in several canine breeds and in approximately 20% to 35% of human patients with DCM; however, in many cases the cause is unclear.[11,12] Other proposed causes include nutritional deficiencies and nontraditional diets infectious agents, drugs and toxins, and inflammatory and metabolic disorders.[10] Yet another cause, autoimmunity, is increasingly accepted as playing a role in the pathogenesis of human DCM and as a possible avenue for targeted patient therapy.[13,14] Given these new insights and the similarities in disease across species, this has sparked more recent research into the role of AABs in canine DCM.

AABs to the adrenergic, beta-1 receptor (β1-AABs) and the muscarinic receptor 2 (M2-AABs) have been documented in both human and canine DCM.[4,15–17] Unlike classic AABs that induce inflammation and cellular or tissue damage, these AABs are considered "functional autoantibodies" that bind to G-protein coupled receptors (GPCR-AABs) on cell surfaces and have been implicated as playing an important role in DCM.[18,19] GPCRs are integral cell membrane receptors that work in cooperation with intracellular G-proteins (guanine nucleotide binding proteins)—ligand binding of a GPCR results in a conformational change that induces activation or inactivation of the G-protein and downstream pathways. They comprise the largest family of proteins in biology and are the most important regulators of cardiac function, acting as a switch for intracellular signaling cascades.[20] This newer class of AABs was first discovered in the 1970s when studying Chagas cardiomyopathy in people.[21] Acting as a ligand on the cell surface and binding to GPCRs, these AABs are thought to induce disturbed metabolic balance and pathologic conditions intracellularly.[19] Unlike physiologic and pharmacologic ligands, these GPCR-AABs are not subject to receptor downregulation and desensitization, removing the checks and balances of normal physiology that prevent such pathologic conditions. Interestingly, there is some evidence that a diseased state such as hypoxia, ischemia, or inflammation may be needed to activate these GPCR-AABs but this requires further elucidation.[18]

Fig. 1 illustrates the downstream effects of β1-AAB and M2-AAB binding to GPCRs. Specifically, for β1-AABs, binding results in excessive G-protein activation and subsequent activation of adenylate cyclase. Adenylate cyclase works to increase cyclic AMP production, which in turn activates protein kinase A and results in phosphorylation of plasma membrane L-type calcium channels. The apparent result is increased calcium influx and prolongation of the action potential duration; however, stimulation of beta-adrenergic GPCRs plays a varied and important role in cell proliferative signaling, and this pathologic activation by β1-AABs has also been shown to result in mitochondrial and membrane potential changes, cell death and apoptosis, degranulation of cardiac mast cells, and myocardial hypertrophy.[18,22–25] Alternatively, binding of M2-AABs results in deactivation of the same G-protein cascade, resulting in decreased calcium influx and reduced inotropy and chronotropy. Additionally, this results in increased

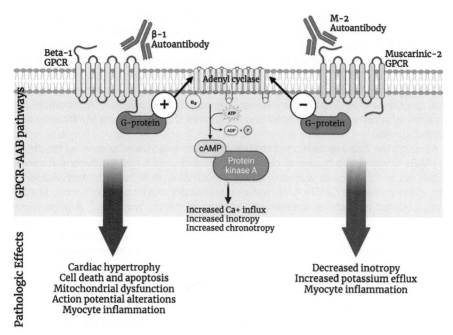

Fig. 1. GPCR-AAB pathways and pathologic effects. The top panel shows how beta-1 and muscarinic-2 receptor AABs work on their respective GPCRs and the downstream intracellular effects. The bottom panel lists the main pathologic effects that these AABs have been shown to cause.

potassium efflux out of the cells and may induce a proarrhythmic state. Finally, M2-AABs have also been shown to interfere with the cycloogenase-2 enzyme (COX-2) and induce proinflammatory conditions. Experimentally, laboratory animals immunized against the 2 receptors or given IgG preparations of β1-AABs and M2-AABs developed a cardiomyopathy phenotype with left ventricular hypertrophy and systolic dysfunction.[26,27]

Studies in human DCM have shown that 26% to 95% and 15% to 50% of the studied patients possessed β1-AABs and M2-AABs, respectively.[18,28] The presence of β1-AABs has been shown to be predictive of disease development in healthy relatives of DCM patients and treatment with immunoadsorption therapy has resulted in an improved left ventricular ejection fraction and New York Heart Association functional classification.[29,30] These developments have sparked recent research into the role of GPCR-AABs in Doberman Pinschers with DCM and the possibility for them to serve as a target for therapy. The first of these studies demonstrated the presence of β1-AABs in almost 70% of the studied Dobermans with DCM but also in a similar proportion of their control cohort.[4] However, 9 of the 19 dogs initially in the control cohort developed DCM in the study period and 8 out of 9 were β1-AABs positive. Reassigning these dogs to the DCM group revealed a more pronounced difference between the groups. M2-AABs were found at a much lower prevalence in both the DCM and control groups.

As mentioned, people with DCM that are GPCR-AAB positive have improved outcomes when treated with therapeutic plasma exchange or immunoadsorption to remove these AABs. Due to the expensive and logistic burden of such therapies, recent focus has been on the development of in vivo methods to bind and neutralize these AABs. A newly favored strategy is the use of aptamers, a single-strand DNA or RNA oligonucleotide that is developed to bind and neutralize GPCR-ABBs by mimicking the extracellular domain of GPCRs that the AABs would otherwise bind to.[18,31] One aptamer, named BC 007, was developed to bind and neutralize β1-AABs and M2-AABs.[26] A follow-up clinical trial in DCM-afflicted Dobermans tested BC 007 showing its ability to neutralize β1-AABs in vivo and subsequent improved cardiac function and left ventricular volumes compared with controls.[32] Additionally, the aptamer infusion was well tolerated and the treated Dobermans had significantly prolonged survival.

Although the 2 abovementioned studies in Dobermans yielded promising results for β1-AABs to serve as a marker of disease progression and target for therapy in canine DCM, further longitudinal studies in other breeds have yet to be performed. Additionally, measurement of GPCR-AABs remains logistically challenging with many studies using cultured neonatal spontaneously beating rat cardiomyocytes.[18] A large multicenter trial in people treated with BC 007 is currently underway and more research in canine DCM is expected.[33] For now, however, the measurement and treatment of AABs in canine DCM remains within the realm of research with no widespread clinical applications to date.

Arrhythmogenic Right Ventricular Cardiomyopathy

ARVC is an inherited myocardial disease reported in dogs, cats, and humans.[34,35] It is particularly common and well known in the Boxer breed, where it manifests as malignant ventricular arrhythmias, cardiac dilation, systolic dysfunction, and sudden death. Accordingly, the Boxer breed is considered an important, spontaneous model of ARVC in humans.[36–38] Although multiple mechanisms have been implicated in the pathogenesis of the disease, ARVC can be a complex diagnosis because there is no reference standard antemortem diagnostic test in dogs or people.[37,39–42]

A common feature identified in ARVC is that it seems to be a "disease of the desmosome," because, in humans, it is predominantly associated with mutations in genes encoding or related to desmosomal proteins (component of intercellular junctions/intercalated disc between cardiomyocytes).[39,43,44] In the veterinary literature, a mutation of the striatin gene (which produces a protein that colocalizes with 3 desmosomal proteins) in Boxers is the only genetic mutation currently known to be associated with ARVC.[39] Notably, however, this mutation is inconsistently associated with disease phenotype in Boxers—not all individuals with the mutation will show signs and others without the mutation commonly show signs—weakening diagnostic value of genetic screening and suggesting nongenetic factors in shaping the ARVC phenotype.[45,46]

Although the specifics of the early pathophysiology of ARVC remain unknown, immune cells have been consistently detected in the myocardium of people, dogs, and cats with varying stages of ARVC severity.[35,47,48] Inflammatory infiltrates consisting of T-lymphocytes were reported in cats with advanced ARVC, reinforcing that the immune microenvironment exists even in the late course of disease.[35] Similarly, in murine experimental models, inflammatory cells and cytokine production seem to persist in chronic disease phases.[49] However, it is unknown the extent to which inflammation and immune activation causes pathology at the disease onset and in different stages of the disease.[40,50–52] Given this context, investigation of immune modulation as a potential therapeutic for ARVC could potentially be a fruitful area of future research.

Investigations in human subjects have shown increased serum levels of antiheart and antidesmosomal (anti-desmoglein-2 [anti-DSG-2]) antibodies in clinically affected patients with ARVC, reinforcing the theory that autoimmune response against intercalated disk components is involved in ARVC pathogenesis.[8,28] Documenting these circulating antiheart AABs has been considered as a promising avenue to evaluate cardiac inflammatory component frequently identified in ARVC. Anti-DSG-2 antibodies were present in ARVC-afflicted human subjects regardless of the underlying genetic variant, suggesting that a final common pathway can underlie gene-elusive ARVC cases.[53] The same study also demonstrated that AABs can be detected in nonhuman mammalian species with good correlation to disease phenotype, as serum anti-DSG-2 were present in 10 out of 10 Boxer dogs with ARVC and absent in 18 out of 18 Boxer dogs without the disease, implicating anti-DSG-2 as a potentially sensitive and specific biomarker for ARVC in Boxers. It should be noted, however, that this finding was not replicated in 2 recent prospective cohort studies undertaken by the authors of this article, both of which assessed Boxers with ARVC and healthy control Boxers for the presence of circulating anti-DSG-2 antibodies.[54,55] Data from both studies showed that circulating anti-DSG-2 antibodies did not discriminate between normal and affected Boxer dogs but a positive correlation between the quantity and complexity of ventricular arrhythmias and anti-DSG2 was observed within the afflicted groups.[54,55] Additionally, one of these studies also evaluated non-Boxer dogs, including Doberman Pinschers with DCM, dogs with myxomatous mitral valve disease and healthy dogs, and found anti-DSG-2 antibodies to be present in all the dogs studied, calling into question the specificity of such antibodies to ARVC.[55] Interestingly, in addition to the complexity of ventricular arrhythmias, a positive correlation between the degree of left ventricular remodeling and anti-DSG-2 antibody expression was also found when assessing all dogs with cardiac disease (ARVC, DCM, and myxomatous mitral valve disease).[55] Therefore, whether anti-DSG-2 antibodies play a role in the pathogenesis of Boxer ARVC or are rather a sequelae of cardiomyocyte death and damage from any cardiac disease remains unclear. Although circulating antiDSG-2 antibodies may not consistently be correlated with ARVC-status, it is unknown whether tissue-bound cardiac AABs in the myocardium can be indicative of disease status. Further studies are needed to assess the functional activity and clinical utility of AABs as potential biomarkers for ARVC in dogs.

Chagas Cardiomyopathy

Chagas disease or American trypanosomiasis, caused by the zoonotic protozoan parasite *Trypanosoma cruzi*, is an important cause of morbidity and mortality in both dogs and people.[56] In dogs, clinical manifestations often include a similar cardiomyopathy to that seen in humans, characterized by an acute or chronic myocarditis with or without arrhythmias and a DCM phenotype chronically.[56] In both species, histopathology of the myocardium from affected patients reveals mononuclear cell infiltration, perivasculitis, and significant fibrosis but rarely the presence of the parasite itself.[56,57] This lack of parasitic infiltration into the myocardium have led to a suggestion that autoimmunity is playing a role in the pathogenesis of Chagas cardiomyopathy.[57]

Studies in people with Chagas disease have demonstrated the presence of anticardiac myosin, anticardiac troponin T, and GPCR AABs.[18] One study showed that there was a correlation between anticardiac myosin and anticardiac troponin T AAB titers and left ventricular ejection fraction in patients with chronic Chagas cardiomyopathy, with ejection fractions being reduced in those patients with increased AAB titers.[58] Studies have also shown a very-high frequency of GPCR-AABs in patients with Chagas cardiomyopathy, including β1-AAB and M2-AAB, as well as AABs to the beta-2 receptor (β2-AAB).[59,60] The degree of positivity of these AABs were significantly elevated in patients with Chagas cardiomyopathy compared with healthy controls or asymptomatic AAB-positive patients but no study has found a correlation between GPCR-AAB levels and clinical parameters of cardiac disease or disease outcome.[19,59,60]

A recent study evaluated Beagle dogs experimentally infected with 2 strains of *T cruzi* and subsequently assayed them for the presence of β1-AABs, β2-AABs, and M2-AABs.[57] All of the dogs infected with *T cruzi* developed AABs to all 3 receptors. Furthermore, none of the healthy age-matched control dogs was found to have any of these 3 GPCR-AABs. Although interesting, further research is required to investigate the role of GPCR-AABs in dogs with naturally occurring Chagas cardiomyopathy. In particular, the relationship between circulating GPCR-AABs titers, severity of disease, and outcome should be assessed before any clinical applications can be investigated.

Feline Hypertrophic Cardiomyopathy

HCM is the most common cardiomyopathy in cats and may affect up to approximately 15% of the domestic feline population.[61] Although the pathologic manifestation of feline HCM has traditionally been focused on cardiac hypertrophy, fibrosis, and myocyte disarray, the role of inflammatory and vascular components has not been historically addressed as part of pathophysiology of the disease. Similarly, the contribution of early inflammation to human HCM has not been elucidated either. In contrast to DCM, where serum concentrations of β1-AAb and M2-AAb have been closely associated to DCM in humans and dogs, AABs relating to HCM have only rarely been reported in people and, to the authors' knowledge, not studied in cats yet.[4,14] The first study performed in people evaluated the occurrence of circulating GCPR-AABs and their relation to the clinical manifestation of HCM.[62] Those results suggested that the existence of circulating AABs could be associated with an advanced stage or a severe manifestation of the disease. More recently, another study measured serum concentrations of β1-AAb and M2-AAb in human subjects with different stages of HCM, and their results revealed that concentration of AABs reflected diastolic dysfunction to some extent and might be involved in arrhythmogenesis.[63]

Inflammatory changes and remodeling processes have been investigated in cats with HCM. Recently, data assessing the transcription pattern of a broad range of inflammatory and remodeling markers have provided further information on the pathogenesis of HCM in cats. One study evaluated transcription of extracellular remodeling enzymes in the myocardium of 26 cats aged between 2 and 19 years that had died with noncardiac diseases.[64] Interestingly, the myocardium of young and male cats seemed to be in a proinflammatory state, whereas in older and female cats, the myocardium exhibits a reduced inflammatory reaction to systemic disease.

As HCM is more predominant in older cats, it is unclear if the inflammatory state seen in younger cats in this study may have led to HCM had they lived longer. When assessing HCM hearts, the same research group documented increased macrophage population and several inflammatory and profibrotic mediators, suggesting that HCM is a progressive process of diffuse expansion of the interstitium by macrophages, collagen, and repair processes triggered by a still-unknown cause.[64] In an attempt to elucidate the connection between inflammatory markers and HCM, cytokines both inflammatory—interleukin (IL)-1, IL-2, IL-4, IL-6, IL-8, IL-10, IL-12, IL-18, TNF-α, and interferon-γ—and profibrotic—transforming growth factor ß; matrix metalloproteinase (MMP)-2, MMP-3, MMP-9, MMP-13; and tissue inhibitor of matrix metalloproteinase (TIMP)-1, TIMP-2, and TIMP-3—were assayed in different populations of cats.[65] Interestingly, the results showed that active inflammation was not present in structural cardiac remodeling during the advanced stage of HCM in cats, which is the opposite of what is seen in other advanced cardiomyopathies in humans and dogs. Although some cats were reported to have more myocardial inflammatory activity at younger age, it is possible that this inflammation, while not present in late disease, could set HCM into motion.[66] In cats defined as "preclinical HCM" stage, histology of the left ventricular myocardium revealed multifocal regions containing neutrophils, dense populations of lymphocytes, plasma cells, and macrophages in 4 out of 6 animals.[67] Although inflammatory infiltrates may be present, it is unclear if this ultimately causes myocyte injury and death. Further analysis using transcriptomics to better characterize the role of inflammation in the pathogenesis of HCM at preclinical stage is lacking, probably at least partially due to the difficulty in identifying preclinical HCM. Even though several studies support a proinflammatory environment in the pathogenesis of feline HCM, results show predominance of extracellular matrix remodeling affecting structural and functional myocardial changes instead of cell death pathways in the myocardium.

DISCUSSION

Increasing attention is being given to the role of immunologic mechanisms in the development of cardiomyopathies. Unfortunately, despite the emerging evidence that AABs and cell signaling between immune cells and cardiomyocytes can play a role in different cardiac diseases, we are far from understanding how to translate this knowledge of autoimmunity to successful immunomodulation and improvement of cardiac health. Prospective, longitudinal studies correlating autoantibody presence and levels to disease progression are required to further elucidate their role in the pathogenesis of cardiac diseases. Additionally, recent novel promising therapeutics from DCM dogs have yet to be evaluated in ARVC or Chagas disease. Further research is needed on both the potential use of AABs and inflammatory cytokine assays in the diagnosis of small animal cardiomyopathies as well as on immunomodulatory therapy in treatment. Posttranslational molecular mechanisms and complex genomic analysis from spontaneous animal models of human diseases might provide better understanding of autoimmune components of cardiac disease. If the negative influence of AABs in companion animal cardiac disease is consistently confirmed, a new class of drugs and therapy with plasma might serve as potential future therapeutic options.

CLINICS CARE POINTS

- AABs may represent future targets for diagnosis, monitoring, and novel therapeutics for patients.
- AABs likely play a role in the pathogenesis of some companion animal cardiac diseases; however, current understanding is incomplete and requires further study.
- The current lack of commercially available assays to measure AABs limits their use clinically.

DISCLOSURE

The authors have nothing to disclose.

REFERENCES

1. Carrillo-Salinas FJ, Ngwenyama N, Anastasiou M, et al. Heart Inflammation. Am J Pathol 2019;189(8):1482–94.

2. Fiordelisi A, Iaccarino G, Morisco C, et al. NFkappaB is a Key Player in the Cross-talk between Inflammation and Cardiovascular Diseases. Int J Mol Sci 2019; 20(7):1599.
3. Moskalik A, Niderla-Bielińska J, Ratajska A. Multiple roles of cardiac macrophages in heart homeostasis and failure. Heart Fail Rev 2022;27(4):1413–30.
4. Wess G, Wallukat G, Fritscher A, et al. Doberman pinschers present autoimmunity associated with functional autoantibodies: A model to study the autoimmune background of human dilated cardiomyopathy. PLoS One 2019;14(7). https://doi. org/10.1371/journal.pone.0214263.
5. Mazzone R, Zwergel C, Artico M, et al. The emerging role of epigenetics in human autoimmune disorders. Clin Epigenet 2019;11(1):34.
6. Dobrev D, Heijman J, Hiram R, et al. Inflammatory signalling in atrial cardiomyocytes: a novel unifying principle in atrial fibrillation pathophysiology. Nat Rev Cardiol 2022. https://doi.org/10.1038/s41569-022-00759-w.
7. Satta N, Vuilleumier N. Auto-Antibodies As Possible Markers and Mediators of Ischemic, Dilated, and Rhythmic Cardiopathies. Curr Drug Targets 2014;16(4): 342–60.
8. Reichart D, Lindberg EL, Maatz H, et al. Pathogenic variants damage cell composition and single cell transcription in cardiomyopathies. Science 2022;377(6606): eabo1984.
9. O'Grady MR, O'Sullivan ML. Dilated cardiomyopathy: An update. Vet Clin N Am Small Anim Pract 2004;34(5):1187–207.
10. Tidholm A, Häggström J, Borgarelli M, et al. Canine Idiopathic Dilated Cardiomyopathy. Part I: Aetiology, Clinical Characteristics, Epidemiology and Pathology. Vet J 2001;162(2):92–107.
11. Stern JA, Ueda Y. Inherited cardiomyopathies in veterinary medicine. Pflügers Archiv 2019;471(5):745–53.
12. Simpson S, Edwards J, Ferguson-Mignan TFN, et al. Genetics of human and canine dilated cardiomyopathy. Int J Genomics 2015;2015. https://doi.org/10. 1155/2015/204823.
13. Dandel M, Wallukat G, Potapov E, et al. Role of β 1-adrenoceptor autoantibodies in the pathogenesis of dilated cardiomyopathy. Immunobiology 2012;217(5): 511–20.
14. Hong W, Tang W, Naga Prasad SV. Autoantibodies and cardiomyopathy: focus on beta-1 adrenergic receptor autoantibodies. J Cardiovasc Pharmacol 2022; 80(3):354–63.
15. Nikolaev VO, Boivin V, Störk S, et al. A novel fluorescence method for the rapid detection of functional beta1-adrenergic receptor autoantibodies in heart failure. J Am Coll Cardiol 2007;50(5):423–31.
16. Wallukat G, Nissen E, Morwinski R, et al. Autoantibodies against the beta- and muscarinic receptors in cardiomyopathy. Herz 2000;25(3):261–6.
17. Jahns R, Boivin V, Siegmund C, et al. Autoantibodies activating human 1-adrenergic receptors are associated with reduced cardiac function in chronic heart failure. Circulation 1999;. http://www.circulationaha.org.
18. Becker NP, Müller J, Göttel P, et al. Cardiomyopathy — An approach to the autoimmune background. Autoimmun Rev 2017;16(3):269–86.
19. Becker NP, Goettel P, Mueller J, et al. Functional autoantibody diseases: Basics and treatment related to cardiomyopathies. Front Biosci Landmark Ed 2019;24: 48–95.
20. Katz AM. Physiology of the heart. 5th edition. Philadelphia PA: Wolters Kluwer Health/Lippincott Williams & Wilkins Health; 2011.

21. Cossio PM, Diez C, Szarfman A, et al. Chagasic cardiopathy demonstration of a serum gamma globulin factor which reacts with endocardium and vascular structures. Circulation 1974;49(1). 13-21.
22. Christ T, Wettwer E, Dobrev D, et al. Autoantibodies against the β1-adrenoceptor from patients with dilated cardiomyopathy prolong action potential duration and enhance contractility in isolated cardiomyocytes. J Mol Cell Cardiol 2001;33(8): 1515–25.
23. Wang L, Lu K, Hao H, et al. Decreased autophagy in rat heart induced by anti-β1-adrenergic receptor autoantibodies contributes to the decline in mitochondrial membrane potential. PLoS One 2013;8(11).
24. Staudt Y, Mobini R, Fu M, et al. β1-adrenoceptor antibodies induce apoptosis in adult isolated cardiomyocytes. Eur J Pharmacol 2003;466(1–2):1–6.
25. Okruhlicova L, Morwinski R, Schulze W, et al. Autoantibodies against G-protein-coupled receptors modulate heart mast cells. Cell Mol Immunol 2007;127–33.
26. Matsui S, Fu M, Hayase M, et al. Transfer of immune components from rabbit autoimmune cardiomyopathy into severe combined immunodeficiency (SCID) mice induces cardiomyopathic changes. Autoimmunity 2006;39(2):121–8.
27. Jahns R, Boivin V, Hein L, et al. Direct evidence for a β1-adrenergic receptor–directed autoimmune attack as a cause of idiopathic dilated cardiomyopathy. J Clin Invest 2004;113(10):1419–29.
28. Caforio ALP, Re F, Avella A, et al. Evidence From Family Studies for Autoimmunity in Arrhythmogenic Right Ventricular Cardiomyopathy: Associations of Circulating Anti-Heart and Anti-Intercalated Disk Autoantibodies With Disease Severity and Family History. Circulation 2020;141(15):1238–48.
29. Caforio ALP, Mahon NG, Baig MK, et al. Prospective familial assessment in dilated cardiomyopathy: Cardiac autoantibodies predict disease development in asymptomatic relatives. Circulation 2007;115(1):76–83.
30. Reinthaler M, Empen K, Herda LR, et al. The effect of a repeated immunoadsorption in patients with dilated cardiomyopathy after recurrence of severe heart failure symptoms. J Clin Apher 2015;30(4):217–23.
31. Haberland A, Wallukat G, Dahmen C, et al. Aptamer neutralization of beta1-adrenoceptor autoantibodies isolated from patients with cardiomyopathies. Circ Res 2011;109(9):986–92.
32. Werner S, Wallukat G, Becker NP, et al. The aptamer BC 007 for treatment of dilated cardiomyopathy: evaluation in Doberman Pinschers of efficacy and outcomes. ESC Heart Fail 2020;7(3):844–55.
33. Becker NP, Haberland A, Wenzel K, et al. A Three-Part, Randomised Study to Investigate the Safety, Tolerability, Pharmacokinetics and Mode of Action of BC 007, Neutraliser of Pathogenic Autoantibodies Against G-Protein Coupled Receptors in Healthy, Young and Elderly Subjects. Clin Drug Investig 2020;40(5): 433–47.
34. Basso C, Fox PR, Meurs KM, et al. Arrhythmogenic Right Ventricular Cardiomyopathy Causing Sudden Cardiac Death in Boxer Dogs: A New Animal Model of Human Disease. Circulation 2004;109(9):1180–5. https://doi.org/10.1161/01. CIR.0000118494.07530.65.
35. Fox PR, Maron BJ, Basso C, et al. Spontaneously Occurring Arrhythmogenic Right Ventricular Cardiomyopathy in the Domestic Cat: A New Animal Model Similar to the Human Disease. Circulation 2000;102(15):1863–70. https://doi. org/10.1161/01.CIR.102.15.1863.
36. Meurs KM, Spier AW, Miller MW, et al. Familial ventricular arrhythmias in Boxers pedigree evaluation. J Vet Intern Med 1999;13:437–9.

37. Cunningham SM, Rush JE, Freeman LM, et al. Echocardiographic ratio indices in overtly healthy boxer dogs screened for heart disease. J Vet Intern Med 2008; 22(4):924–30.

38. Cunningham SM, Dos Santos L. Arrhythmogenic right ventricular cardiomyopathy in dogs. J Vet Cardiol 2022;40:156–69.

39. Meurs KM, Mauceli E, Lahmers S, et al. Genome-wide association identifies a deletion in the 3 untranslated region of Striatin in a canine model of arrhythmogenic right ventricular cardiomyopathy. Hum Genet 2010;128(3):315–24.

40. Basso C, Thiene G. Adipositas cordis, fatty infiltration of the right ventricle, and arrhythmogenic right ventricular cardiomyopathy. Just a matter of fat? Cardiovasc Pathol 2005;14(1):37–41.

41. Cunningham SM, Aona BD, Antoon K, et al. Echocardiographic assessment of right ventricular systolic function in Boxers with arrhythmogenic right ventricular cardiomyopathy. J Vet Cardiol 2018;20(5):343–53.

42. Corrado D, Zorzi A, Cipriani A, et al. Evolving Diagnostic Criteria for Arrhythmogenic Cardiomyopathy. J Am Heart Assoc 2021;10(18):e021987.

43. Te Riele ASJM, James CA, Philips B, et al. Mutation-positive arrhythmogenic right ventricular dysplasia/cardiomyopathy: The triangle of dysplasia displaced. J Cardiovasc Electrophysiol 2013;24(12):1311–20.

44. Delmar M, Alvarado FJ, Valdivia HH. Desmosome-Dyad Crosstalk: An Arrhythmogenic Axis in Arrhythmogenic Right Ventricular Cardiomyopathy. Circulation 2020;141(18):1494–7.

45. Meurs KM, Stern JA, Reina-Doreste Y, et al. Natural History of Arrhythmogenic Right Ventricular Cardiomyopathy in the Boxer Dog: A Prospective Study. J Vet Intern Med 2014;28(4):1214–20.

46. Cattanach BM, Dukes-McEwan J, Wotton PR, et al. Paper: A pedigree-based genetic appraisal of Boxer ARVC and the role of the Striatin mutation. Vet Rec 2015; 176(19):492.

47. Basso C, Corrado D, Valente M, et al. Arrhythmogenic right ventricular cardiomyopathy: Dysplasia, dystrophy or myocarditis? J Am Coll Cardiol 1996;27(2):394.

48. Asimaki A, Tandri H, Duffy ER, et al. Altered Desmosomal Proteins in Granulomatous Myocarditis and Potential Pathogenic Links to Arrhythmogenic Right Ventricular Cardiomyopathy. Circ Arrhythm Electrophysiol 2011;4(5):743–52.

49. Lubos N, van der Gaag S, Gerçek M, et al. Inflammation shapes pathogenesis of murine arrhythmogenic cardiomyopathy. Basic Res Cardiol 2020;115(4):42.

50. Chimenti C, Pieroni M, Maseri A, et al. Histologic findings in patients with clinical and instrumental diagnosis of sporadic arrhythmogenic right ventricular dysplasia. J Am Coll Cardiol 2004;43(12):2305–13.

51. Asimaki A, Tandri H, Huang H, et al. A New Diagnostic Test for Arrhythmogenic Right Ventricular Cardiomyopathy. N Engl J Med 2009;360(11):1075–84.

52. Ollitrault P, Al Khoury M, Troadec Y, et al. Recurrent acute myocarditis: An under-recognized clinical entity associated with the later diagnosis of a genetic arrhythmogenic cardiomyopathy. Front Cardiovasc Med 2022;9:998883.

53. Chatterjee D, Fatah M, Akdis D, et al. An autoantibody identifies arrhythmogenic right ventricular cardiomyopathy and participates in its pathogenesis. Eur Heart J 2018;39(44):3932–44.

54. Dos Santos L, Cunningham S, Hamilton R, et al. Anti-desmosomal antibody as a potential biomarker of arrhythmia burden in Boxers with arrhythmogenic ventricular cardiomyopathy. ACVIM Forum Res Abstr Program; 2022.

55. Walker AL, Li RHL, Nguyen N, et al. Evaluation of autoantibodies to desmoglein-2 in dogs with and without cardiac disease. Sci Rep 2023;13(1):5044.

56. Barr SC. Canine Chagas' Disease (American Trypanosomiasis) in North America. Vet Clin N Am Small Anim Pract 2009;39(6):1055–64.
57. Wallukat G, Botoni FA, Rocha MO da C, et al. Functional antibodies against G-protein coupled receptors in Beagle dogs infected with two different strains of Trypanosoma cruzi. Front Immunol 2022;13:926682.
58. Nunes DF, Guedes PM da M, de Mesquita Andrade C, et al. Troponin T autoantibodies correlate with chronic cardiomyopathy in human Chagas disease. Trop Med Int Health 2013;18(10):1180–92.
59. Talvani A, Rocha MOC, Ribeiro AL, et al. Levels of anti-M2 and anti-β1 autoantibodies do not correlate with the degree of heart dysfunction in Chagas' heart disease. Microbes Infect 2006;8(9–10):2459–64.
60. Wallukat G, Muñoz Saravia SG, Haberland A, et al. Distinct Patterns of Autoantibodies Against G-Protein-Coupled Receptors in Chagas' Cardiomyopathy and Megacolon. Their Potential Impact for Early Risk Assessment in Asymptomatic Chagas' Patients. J Am Coll Cardiol 2010;55(5):463–8.
61. Kittleson MD, Côté E. The Feline Cardiomyopathies: 2. Hypertrophic cardiomyopathy. J Feline Med Surg 2021;23(11):1028–51.
62. Peukert S, Fu MLX, Eftekhari P, et al. The Frequency of Occurrence of Anticardiac Receptor Autoantibodies and their Correlation with Clinical Manifestation in Patients with Hypertrophic Cardiomyopathy. Autoimmunity 1999;29(4):291–7.
63. Duan X, Liu R, Luo X, et al. The relationship between β_1-adrenergic and M_2-muscarinic receptor autoantibodies and hypertrophic cardiomyopathy. Exp Physiol 2020;105(3):522–30.
64. Kitz S, Fonfara S, Hahn S, et al. Feline Hypertrophic Cardiomyopathy: The Consequence of Cardiomyocyte-Initiated and Macrophage-Driven Remodeling Processes? Vet Pathol 2019;56(4):565–75.
65. Fonfara S, Kitz S, Monteith G, et al. Myocardial transcription of inflammatory and remodeling markers in cats with hypertrophic cardiomyopathy and systemic diseases associated with an inflammatory phenotype. Res Vet Sci 2021;136:484–94.
66. Fonfara S, Hetzel U, Hahn S, et al. Age- and gender-dependent myocardial transcription patterns of cytokines and extracellular matrix remodelling enzymes in cats with non-cardiac diseases. Exp Gerontol 2015;72:117–23.
67. Khor KH, Campbell FE, Owen H, et al. Myocardial collagen deposition and inflammatory cell infiltration in cats with pre-clinical hypertrophic cardiomyopathy. Vet J 2015;203(2):161–8.

The Genetics of Canine Pulmonary Valve Stenosis

Samantha Kovacs, DVM, PhD[a],*, Brian A. Scansen, DVM, MS[b],
Joshua A. Stern, DVM, PhD[c]

KEYWORDS

- Congenital heart disease • Pulmonic stenosis • Bulldog • French Bulldog • Gene
- RAS/MAPK pathway • Transcription factor

KEY POINTS

- Pulmonary valve stenosis (PS) is one of the most common congenital heart diseases (CHDs) in dogs making up 20% to 32% of all CHDs and brachycephalic breeds are commonly affected.
- Canine pedigree studies support a recessive mode of inheritance although it is likely more complicated and influenced by genetic modifiers and environment. Within the same litter, the morphology and severity of PS may vary.
- In humans, many mutations in PS involve transcription factors related to heart development or cell signaling pathways such as the ras protein/mitogen-activated protein kinase (Ras/MAPK) pathway.
- In Bulldogs, a genome-wide association study followed by whole genome sequencing and multiplex genotyping identified a 22,270-bp deletion that truncated the transcription factor *ZNF446*.
- In French Bulldogs, a genome-wide association study identified a peak on Chromosome 34 that included the transcription factor *IRX4*.

INTRODUCTION

In dogs, pulmonary valve stenosis (PS) is one of the most common congenital heart diseases (CHDs), with a prevalence of 20% to 32% of all CHDs identified.[1–3] Importantly, certain breeds have a higher incidence, such as Bulldogs, which have 4% of their population affected by naturally occurring PS.[4] PS is caused by a narrowing of the right ventricular outflow tract due to thickened/fused/dysplastic valve leaflets and/or a narrowed

[a] Anatomic Pathology Service, School of Veterinary Medicine, University of California Davis, UC Davis VMTH, 1 Garrod Drive, Davis, CA 95616, USA; [b] College of Veterinary Medicine & Biomedical Sciences, Colorado State University, Veterinary Teaching Hospital, 300 West Drake Road, 1678 Campus Delivery, Fort Collins, CO 80523-1678, USA; [c] Department of Medicine and Epidemiology, School of Veterinary Medicine, University of California Davis, UC Davis VMTH, 1 Garrod Drive, Davis, CA 95616, USA
* Corresponding author.
E-mail address: skovacs@ucdavis.edu

Vet Clin Small Anim 53 (2023) 1379–1391
https://doi.org/10.1016/j.cvsm.2023.05.014

annulus, that may ultimately lead to complications such as right-sided congestive heart failure or sudden death (**Fig. 1**).[5] Although percutaneous balloon valvuloplasty is currently the standard of care, it does not return the valve to normal function, stenosis can reoccur, and this procedure may be contraindicated in some forms of the disease,[6–9] which is why an understanding of the genetics and pathogenesis is important.

Cardiovascular diseases have similar pathophysiology, lesions, and clinical findings between dogs and humans.[10] Many human CHDs have a genetic component, and the genetic evidence for CHDs in dogs is increasing.[11–14] In humans, most mutations in PS involve transcription factors related to heart development or cell signaling pathways such as the RAS/MAPK pathway.[15,16] To date in dogs, no genetic mutation has been definitively identified; if a genetic cause could be identified, it would increase our understanding of the molecular pathogenesis, which may lead to novel prevention and therapeutic strategies. The goal of this article is to present what is currently known about the genetics associated with PS in both species with the hopes of fostering further research in the field.

CANINE BREED PREDISPOSITIONS

PS is suspected to have a genetic predisposition in dogs because certain breeds have a higher incidence of this abnormality compared with others and purebreds are more susceptible than mixed-breeds.[1,17–22] Although any dog may develop PS, brachycephalic breeds are overrepresented.[4] In an Italian population of Boxers, the prevalence of PS increased from 2001 to 2009 indicating a need to identify the genetic basis of the disease to efficiently eliminate it from the breeding program.[23] Interestingly, breed screenings resulted in an increased prevalence of PS, whereas the frequency of severe cases went down suggesting genetic modifiers are involved. Further support of a genetic cause is the recognition that PS can develop in dog families where consanguineous mating is present despite the breed having a low incidence overall.[24]

MODE OF INHERITANCE

The most complete inheritance study of PS in dogs occurred in Beagles, although today Beagles are less commonly affected in clinical practice.[25] In Beagles, recessive

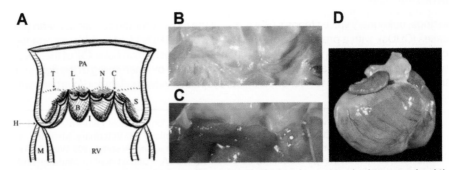

Fig. 1. Gross anatomy of pulmonary valve and secondary right ventricular hypertrophy. (*A*) The right ventricular outflow tract opened longitudinally with 1 of the 3 pulmonary valve leaflets cut in half to illustrate internal anatomy. (*B*) Normal pulmonary valve with thin, semitransparent leaflets. (*C*) Thickened pulmonary valve leaflets in a dog diagnosed with PS. (*D*) Severe right ventricular hypertrophy secondary to pulmonary valve stenosis. B, belly; C, commissure; H, hinge; I, interleaflet triangle; L, Lunula; M, myocardium; N, nodule of Arantius; PA, pulmonary artery; RV, right ventricle; S, sinus; T, sinotubular junction.

inheritance was suspected because *affected X normal crosses* failed to produce affected offspring and litters with the highest percentage of affected puppies had affected and related parents. A recessive form of inheritance has been described in other breeds.[4,21,26,27] Other informative pedigrees include Keeshonds, Boxers and Bulldogs, where clinically normal dogs produced PS affected offspring.[4,20,23] Although a recessive mode of inheritance is most likely, incomplete penetrance or very mild forms of the disease going undetected in the parents remain a possibility until a definitive mutation is identified.

X-linked inheritance is unlikely because in several canine studies, no male or female predisposition was found for PS.[3,25,28,29] Some studies have reported a male predisposition in certain breeds such as Bulldogs,[30,31] Boxers,[1,23] and Bullmastiffs[17] and in the canine species overall.[1,2,29,32,33] However, it is unclear whether the variability in sex predisposition is a function of differences in the mutations contained within the population studied or an artifact of sample size. The mode of inheritance of PS in humans is variable depending on the gene involved but autosomal dominant, autosomal recessive, and haploinsufficiency are common.

There is clinical variability among human patients with the same mutation suggesting environmental, epigenetic, and genetic modifiers influence disease presentation.[34,35] This is likely to be the same in dogs. Human patients with pulmonary valve dysplasia have been reported to have parents and/or siblings with a different phenotype of PS.[36] Similarly, in canines, full siblings can have variable severity and morphology (typical dome-shaped abnormality vs dysplastic thickened valve abnormality).[4,25,26] Future investigations into the possibility of a major effect gene with associated modifier genes, dosage alterations, or environmental influences is warranted.

HUMAN GENETICS

A database that curates literature on CHDs known as CHDBase lists numerous genetic associations with PS; with the exponential advancement of genetic techniques in recent years, more genetic associations are being identified.[37] There are currently 137 publications encompassing 57 syndromic-PS genes, 90 nonsyndromic-PS genes, and 40 genes associated with both syndromic and nonsyndromic cases summarized in **Table 1**.[37] In dogs, there are 2 publications describing a gene associated with PS: a dissertation[38] and an abstract[27] (see **Table 1**). Some of the genes are well studied, whereas others may represent the first case report of a novel player. Many of these mutations do not cause PS in isolation and instead cause it as part of a complex heart malformation such as Tetralogy of Fallot, double outlet right ventricle, or transposition of great arteries.[39] One of the challenges of identifying PS genes is the spectrum of phenotypes with which a single mutation can present.

The most referenced genes associated with PS according to CHDBase as of 2022 are as follows: *PTPN11*, *GATA4*, and *NKX2-5*. Most genes are part of the RAS/MAPK pathway such as *PTPN11*. This is a critical pathway to heart development that controls cell proliferation, differentiation, and survival.[40] Another large category of genes are cardiac transcription factors such as *GATA4* and *NKX2.5*, which are critical for regulating the precise orchestration of timing and dosages of proteins during development.[41] Additional mutations are associated with syndromes due to genes that have widespread effects on embryologic development.

RASopathies

RASopathies are caused by mutations in the RAS-MAPK pathway that lead to a disease syndrome, which may or may not include PS.[42,43] The RASopathy best associated with

Table 1
Genes, syndromes, and regions associated with pulmonary valve stenosis

RASopathies[15,40]	Transcription Factors	Syndromes

• *BRAF*
  ○ Cardiofaciocutaneous (CFC) syndrome[75]
  ○ Noonan syndrome
  ○ Leopard syndrome
• *HRAS*
  ○ Costello syndrome
• *KRAS*
  ○ Noonan syndrome
  ○ CFC syndrome
• *MAP2K1/MAP2K2*
  ○ CFC syndrome
• *NF1*[42]
  ○ Neurofibromatosis syndrome
• *NRAS*[76]
  ○ Noonan syndrome
• *PTPN11*[40,43,45,77,78]
  ○ Noonan syndrome
  ○ Leopard syndrome
  ○ Noonan-like multiple giant cell lesion syndrome
• *RAF1*[79,80]
  ○ Leopard syndrome
  ○ Noonan syndrome
• *RIT1*[81]
  ○ Noonan syndrome
	• *GATA4*[16,53,84-86]
	  ○ Deletion of 8p23.1
	• *HAND2/dHAND*[57,58,87]
	  ○ 4q deletion syndrome
	  ○ Nonsyndrome
	• *HEY2*[54]
	• *LZTR1*[40,43,66]
	  ○ 22q11 deletion syndrome; DiGeorge syndrome
	• *NKX2.5*[56,88]
	• *PITX*[89]
	• *TBX5*[55]
	  ○ Holt-Oram syndrome
	  ○ Non-Holt-Oram syndrome
	• *ZIC3*[90]
	Regions Associated in Dogs
	• Bulldogs[38]
	  ○ GWAS, WGS, MassArray
	  ○ Chr1: 100,196,786–100,219,056
	  ○ 22,270 bp deletion
	  ○ Possible gene *ZNF446*
	• French Bulldogs[27]
	  ○ GWAS
	  ○ Chr 34, 10–10.5Mbp
	  ○ Possible gene *IRX4*
		• Alagille syndrome[35,49]
		  ○ *JAG1*
		  ○ *NOTCH2*
		  ○ *NOTCH1*
		• Andersen syndrome[91]
		  ○ *KCNJ2*
		• CHIME syndrome[92]
		  ○ *PIGL*
		• Ellis-Van Creveld syndrome[93]
		  ○ *EVC*
		• Nephrotic syndrome[71,72]
		  ○ *NPHS2*
		  ○ *NPHS1*
		• Robinow syndrome[47]
		  ○ *DVL3*
		  ○ *WNT5A*
		  ○ *DVL1*
		• Simpson-Golabi-Behmel syndrome[94]
		  ○ *GPC3*
		• Williams-Beuren[67-70]
		  ○ 7q11.23-q21.11; *ELN*
		• Weill-Marchesani syndrome[52]
		  ○ *ADAMTS10*
		• Kleefstra/9qSTD syndrome[95,96]
		  ○ *EHMT1*

Potential Genes

- *ADAMST9*[97]
  - ○ Chr 3p14 deletion
- *CNOT1*[73]
- *GATA6*[98]
- *PBX1*[62,73]
- *SALL4*[63]
- *SMARCA4*[61]
- *TMED8*[73]
- *USP34*[73]
- *ZFPM2*[64]

- *RASA2*[81]
  - ○ Noonan syndrome
- *SHOC2*
  - ○ Noonan syndrome—like disorder
    with loose anagen hair
- *SOS1*[82]
  - ○ Noonan syndrome
- *SPRED1*[83]
  - ○ NF1-like syndrome
  - ○ Legius syndrome

Potential Regions

- Chr 1q21 deletion/duplication[34]
- Chr 6pter-p24deletion[89]
  - ○ CHARGE syndrome
- Trisomy9p[89]
- Chr 10q26.3 deletion[89]
- Terminal 18q deletion[89]
- Chr 14q23.3 deletion[99]
  - ○ Heart hand Syndrome
- Chr 17p deletion[100]
  - ○ Smith Magenis syndrome
- Chr 19p13.3-pter deletion[101–103]
  - ○ Mosaicism for ring 19

The list of genes in blue are those described in human literature to be associated with PS. Many cause RASopathies, various syndromes, and/or are transcription factors. The ones in red are genes/regions described in dogs to be associated with PS; both are transcription factors. Included are lists of genes and regions that should be investigated further.

PS is Noonan syndrome in humans.[44,45] Genes involved with Noonan syndrome and PS include *PTPN11*, *SHOC2*, *RIT1*, *RAF1*, *BRAF*, *KRAS*, and *SOS1*.[40,42,43] The *PTPN11* gene tends to cause severe PS, whereas *SOS1* mutations typically cause milder forms of PS.[43] Additional RASopathies include the following: Costello syndrome, cardiofaciocutaneous syndrome, neurofibromatosis type 1 syndrome, LEOPARD syndrome, and several "Noonan-like" syndromes.[11,15,40,42] Abnormalities that occur with these syndromes include but are not limited to short stature, abnormal facies, cardiovascular abnormalities, cryptorchidism, and pectus abnormalities.[40,42] It has been previously hypothesized that brachycephalic breeds such as the Bulldog may have a Noonan-like syndrome.[46]

ADDITIONAL SYNDROMES ASSOCIATED WITH PULMONARY VALVE STENOSIS

Although PS in dogs is not associated with a defined syndrome, it is possible that the phenotype selected for in certain breeds can be interpreted as a syndrome. For example, Robinow syndrome is caused by mutations in the WNT developmental pathway.[47,48] It is characterized by slow body growth, hypertelorism, low set ears, and ptosis of the eyelids.[47,48] Bulldogs are fixed for a mutation in a gene associated with Robinow syndrome, although its connection to PS in the breed has not been investigated.[48] Alagille syndrome, characterized by chronic cholestasis, butterfly vertebra, ocular changes, and specific facial features including broad forehead, pointed chin, bulbous nose, deep-set eyes, and hypertelorism, is caused by mutations in either the ligand (*JAG1*) or the receptor (*NOTCH2*) associated with the NOTCH pathway.[15,49–51] Weill-Marchesani syndrome characterized by short stature, short fingers and toes, and eye abnormalities is caused by several mutations in *ADAMTS10*.[52] Additional human syndromes where PS may be present are summarized in **Table 1**.

TRANSCRIPTION FACTORS

Transcription factors play a critical role in pathogenesis of PS as well as other complex CHDs.[41] This is to be expected because transcription factors help facilitate the precise timing and coordination of developmental events. The transcription factors that have been identified in humans with PS are as follows: *GATA4*,[16,53] *HEY2*,[54] *TBX5*,[55] *NKX2.5*,[56] *HAND2*,[57,58] and *LZTR1*.[40,43] Both *GATA4* and *NKX2.5* have been isolated and characterized in dogs, although screening in a limited number of canine families with various congenital heart defects did not identify a significant mutation.[59,60] A fascinating article that investigated the protein-transcription factor interactomes of *GATA4* and *TBX5* identified many genes (*SMARCA4*,[61] *PBX1*,[62] *SALL4*,[63] and *ZFPM2*[64]) that have been associated PS in individual cases reports.[41] This suggests that additional research is necessary in these genes.

There is evidence that transcription factors are associated with PS in Bulldogs and French Bulldogs.[27,38] A genome-wide association study of French Bulldogs with and without PS identified a region on canine chromosome 34 that contains the *IRX4* transcription factor.[27] *IRX4* is related to cardiomyocyte differentiation.[11] A genetic analysis of Bulldogs with and without PS that included genome-wide association study, whole genome sequencing, and multiplex genotyping identified a 22-kbp deletion that truncated the transcription factor *ZNF446*.[38] *ZNF446* is cloned from a human embryonic heart cDNA library and is associated with the MAPK pathway.[65] Although exciting, both these genes associated with PS need further validation and functional studies before their utilization as genetic screens.

MICRODELETIONS AND MICRODUPLICATIONS

Microdeletions and microduplications are commonly associated with PS (see **Table 1**) with several eventually having a causative gene identified. For example, *GATA4* was identified due to its localization in a Chr8p23.1 deletion syndrome.[53] However, not all larger structural variants associated with PS have a gene identified. The DiGeorge or 22q11 deletion syndrome is commonly associated with complex heart defects although *LZTR1* mentioned previously is contained in this deletion.[66] The *ELN* gene whose loci was associated with the William-Beuren syndrome's microdeletion at 7q11.23 has mounting case reports.[67–70] These regions serve as avenues for future research to identify the gene(s) responsible. These microdeletions and duplications are not limited to humans. In Bulldogs, a large 22-kbp deletion has been found associated with PS.[38]

FUTURE GENETIC WORK

There are additional genes that hold promise but need to be more intensely studied to understand their contribution to PS especially when there are limited case reports. Several articles have identified an association with *NPHS2* and *NPHS1*.[71,72] Whole exome sequencing identified mutations in *CNOT1*, *PBX1*, *TMED8*, and *USP34* in patients with PS.[73] As always, investigating genes contained in the same genetic family as previously associated genes may be important such as *GATA6*, *TBX*, and *ADAMTS19* genes.[74] If any mutations in these genes are identified in dogs with PS, it could provide stronger evidence of a causative effect because it crosses species.

SUMMARY

The genetics of PS is expanding rapidly with genes in the RAS/MAPK pathway and transcription factors most associated with PS in humans. Brachycephalic breeds have a predisposition to PS and preliminary genetic studies have similarly identified transcription factors associated with heart development. Future validation and functional studies are necessary to confirm these genetic associations.

CLINICS CARE POINTS

- Pulmonary valve stenosis (PS) is one of the most common congenital heart diseases in dogs and brachycephalic breeds are commonly affected. This stresses the importance of careful cardiac ausculation/evaluation of puppies and dogs used for breeding purposes.
- If a dog has pulmonic stenosis, the dog should not be used for breeding.
- If a dam and sire produced an offspring with pulmonic stenosis, the dam and sire should not be bred together in the future.

DISCLOSURE

The authors have no commercial or financial conflicts of interest.

REFERENCES

1. Oliveira P, Domenech O, Silva J, et al. Retrospective review of congenital heart disease in 976 dogs. J Vet Intern Med 2011;25(3):477–83.
2. Tidholm A. Retrospective study of congenital heart defects in 151 dogs. J Small Anim Pract 1997;38(3):94–8.

3. Schrope DP. Prevalence of congenital heart disease in 76,301 mixed-breed dogs and 57,025 mixed-breed cats. J Vet Cardiol 2015;17(3):192–202.

4. Ontiveros ES, Fousse SL, Crofton AE, et al. Congenital Cardiac Outflow Tract Abnormalities in Dogs: Prevalence and Pattern of Inheritance From 2008 to 2017. Front Vet Sci 2019;6:1–10.

5. MacDonald KA. Congenital Heart Diseases of Puppies and Kittens. Vet Clin Small Anim 2006;36:503–31.

6. Buchanan James W, Anderson James H, RIW. The 1st Balloon Valvuloplasty: An Historical Note. J Vet Intern Med 2002;16:116–7.

7. Kan JS, White RI Jr, Mitchell SEGT. Percutaneous Balloon Valvuloplasty: A new method for treating congenital pulmonary valve stenosis. N Engl J Med 1982; 307(9):540–2.

8. Scansen BA. Pulmonary Valve Stenosis. In: Weisse C, Berent A, editors. *Veterinary Image-Guided Interventions*. First. John Wiley and Sons Inc; 2015. p. 575–87.

9. Syamasundar Rao P. Percutaneous balloon pulmonary valvuloplasty: State of the art. Catheter Cardiovasc Interv 2007;69(5):747–63.

10. Loen V, Vos MA, van der Heyden MAG. The canine chronic atrioventricular block model in cardiovascular preclinical drug research. Br J Pharmacol 2022;179(5): 859–81.

11. Morton SU, Quiat D, Seidman JG, et al. Genomic frontiers in congenital heart disease. Nat Rev Cardiol 2022;19(1):26–42.

12. Pierpont ME, Basson CT, Benson DW, et al. Genetic Basis for Congenital Heart Defects: Current Knowledge. Circulation 2007;115(23):3015–38.

13. Parker HG, Meurs KM, Ostrander EA. Finding cardiovascular disease genes in the dog. J Vet Cardiol 2006;8(2):115–27.

14. Meurs KM. Genetics of cardiac disease in the small animal patient. Vet Clin North Am Small Anim Pract 2010;40:701–15.

15. Richards AA, Garge V. Genetics of congenital heart disease. Curr Cardiol Rev 2010;6:91–7.

16. Lahaye S. Genetics of Valvular Heart Disease. Curr Cardiol Rep 2014;16(6):487.

17. Malik R, Church DB, Hunt GB. Valvular pulmonic stenosis in bullmastiffs. J Small Anim Pract 1993;34(6):288–92.

18. Patterson DF. Epidemiologic and genetic studies of congenital heart disease in the dog. Circ Res 1968;23(2):171–202.

19. Mulvihill JJ, Priester WA. Congenital Heart Disease in Dogs : Epidemiologic Similarities to Man. Teratology 1973;7(1):73–7.

20. Detweiler DK, Patterson DF. The Prevalence and Types of Cardiovascular Disease in Dogs. Ann N Y Acad Sci 1965;127(1):481–516.

21. Patterson DF. Congenital heart disease in the dog. Ann N Y Acad Sci 1965;127: 541–69.

22. Buchanan JW. In: Philip R, Fox D, Sisson NSM David, editors. Prevalence of cardiovascular Disorders. W.B. Saunders; 1999.

23. Bussadori C, Pradelli D, Borgarelli M, et al. Congenital heart disease in boxer dogs: Results of 6years of breed screening. Vet J 2009;181(2):187–92.

24. Jacobs G, Mahaffey M, Rawlings CA. Valvular pulmonic stenosis in four Boykin spaniels. J Am Anim Hosp Assoc 1990;26(3):247–52.

25. Patterson DF, Haskins ME, Schnarr WR. Hereditary dysplasia of the pulmonary valve in beagle dogs. Pathologic and genetic studies. Am J Cardiol 1981;47(3): 631–41.

26. Patterson DF. Two hereditary forms of ventricular outflow obstruction in the dog: Pulmonary Valve dyspasia and discrete subaortic stenosis. In: Nora J, Takao A,

editors. Congenital heart disease: Causes and Processes. Mt. Kisco (NY): Future Publishing Co.; 1984. p. 43–63.

27. Toom ML, Szatmári V, Borgeat K, et al. ESV-O-6 Genome wide association study of congenital pulmonic stenosis in French Bulldogs. Research Communications of the 32 nd ECVIM-CA Online Congress. J Vet Intern Med 2022;36(6):2455–551.

28. Johnson MS, Martin M. Results of balloon valvuloplasty in 40 dogs with pulmonic stenosis. J Small Anim Pract 2004;45(3):148–53.

29. Fingland RB, Bonagura JD, Myer CW. Pulmonic stenosis in the dog: 29 cases (1975-1984). J Am Vet Med Assoc 1986;189(2):218–26. http://www.ncbi.nlm. nih.gov/pubmed/3744983.

30. Fox PR, Sisson D, Moise NS. Textbook of canine and Feline Cardiology: Principles and clinical practice. Second edition. Philadelphia: Saunders; 1998.

31. Buchanan JW. Causes and Prevalence of cardiovascular disease. In: Keene BW, editor. Kirks current Veterinary Therapy XI, Small Animal practice. Philedelphia, PA: Saunsers/Philadephia, PA; 1992. p. 647–55.

32. Ristic JME, Marin CJ, Baines EA, et al. Congenital Pulmonic Stenosis a Retrospective study of 24 cases seen between 1990-1999. J Vet Cardiol 2001;3(2):13–9.

33. Bussadori C, DeMadron E, Santilli RA, et al. Balloon Valvuloplasty in 30 Dogs with Pulmonic Stenosis: Effect of Valve Morphology and Annular Size on Initial and 1-Year Outcome. J Vet Intern Med 2001;15(6):553.

34. Digilio MC, Bernardini L, Consoli F, et al. Congenital heart defects in recurrent reciprocal 1q21.1 deletion and duplication syndromes: Rare association with pulmonary valve stenosis. Eur J Med Genet 2013;56(3):144–9.

35. Eldadah ZA, Hamosh A, Biery NJ, et al. Familial Tetralogy of Fallot caused by mutation in the jagged1 gene. Hum Mol Genet 2001;10(2):163–9.

36. Koretzky ED, Moller JH, Korns ME, et al. Congenital pulmonary stenosis resulting from dysplasia of valve. Circulation 1969;40(1):43–53.

37. Zhou W-Z, Li W, Shen H, et al. CHDbase: A Comprehensive Knowledgebase for Congenital Heart Disease-related Genes and Clinical Manifestations. bioRxiv 2022. https://doi.org/10.1101/2022.01.06.475217.

38. Kovacs SL. Genetics of Pulmonary Valve Stenosis in Bulldogs (Doctoral dissertation, UC Davis). 2022.

39. Saef JM, Ghobrial J. Valvular heart disease in congenital heart disease: A narrative review. Cardiovasc Diagn Ther 2021;11(3):818–39.

40. Aoki Y, Niihori T, Inoue S-I, et al. Recent advances in RASopathies. J Hum Genet 2016;61(1):33–9.

41. Gonzalez-Teran B, Pittman M, Felix F, et al. Transcription factor protein interactomes reveal genetic determinants in heart disease. Cell 2022;185(5):794–814.e30.

42. Bell JM, Considine EM, McCallen LM, et al. The Prevalence of Noonan Spectrum Disorders in Pediatric Patients with Pulmonary Valve Stenosis. J Pediatr 2021; 234:134–41.e5.

43. Leoni C, Blandino R, Delogu AB, et al. Genotype-cardiac phenotype correlations in a large single-center cohort of patients affected by RASopathies: Clinical implications and literature review. Am J Med Genet Part A 2022;188(2): 431–45.

44. Colquitt JL, Noonan JA. Cardiac Findings in Noonan Syndrome on Long-term Follow-up. Congenit Heart Dis 2014;9(2):144–50.

45. Roberts AE, Allanson JE, Tartaglia M, et al. Noonan syndrome. Lancet 2013; 381(9863):333–42.

46. Locatelli C, Spalla I, Domenech O, et al. Pulmonic stenosis in dogs: Survival and risk factors in a retrospective cohort of patients. J Small Anim Pract 2013;54(9): 445–52.

47. Soman C, Lingappa A. Robinow Syndrome: A Rare Case Report and Review of Literature. Int J Clin Pediatr Dent 2015;8(2):149–52.

48. Mansour TA, Lucot K, Konopelski SE, et al. Whole genome variant association across 100 dogs identifies a frame shift mutation in DISHEVELLED 2 which contributes to Robinow-like syndrome in Bulldogs and related screw tail dog breeds. PLoS Genet 2018;14(12):1–23.

49. Bauer RC, Laney AO, Smith R, et al. Jagged1 (JAG1) mutations in patients with tetralogy of fallot or pulmonic stenosis. Hum Mutat 2010;31(5):594–601.

50. McDaniell R, Warthen DM, Sanchez-Lara PA, et al. NOTCH2 mutations cause Alagille syndrome, a heterogeneous disorder of the notch signaling pathway. Am J Hum Genet 2006;79(1):169–73.

51. Turnpenny PD, Ellard S. Alagille syndrome: Pathogenesis, diagnosis and management. Eur J Hum Genet 2012;20(3):251–7.

52. Dagoneau N, Benoist-Lasselin C, Huber C, et al. ADAMTS10 mutations in autosomal recessive weill-marchesani syndrome. Am J Hum Genet 2004;75(5):801–6.

53. Pehlivan T, Pober BR, Brueckner M, et al. GATA4 haploinsufficiency in patients with interstitial deletion of chromosome region 8p23.1 and congenital heart disease. Am J Med Genet 1999;83(3):201–6.

54. Jordan VK, Rosenfeld JA, Lalani SR, et al. Duplication of HEY2 in Cardiac and Neurologic Development. Am J Med Genet 2015;167A:2145–9.

55. Marie Reamon-Buettner S, Borlak J. TBX5 Mutations in Non-Holt-Oram Syndrome (HOS) Malformed Hearts. Mutat Br Hum Mutat Mutat Br 2004;726. https://doi.org/10.1002/humu.9255.

56. Goldmuntz E, Geiger E, Benson DW. NKX2.5 mutations in patients with tetralogy of fallot. Circulation 2001;104(21):2565–8.

57. Sun YM, Wang J, Qiu XB, et al. A HAND2 loss-of-function mutation causes familial ventricular septal defect and pulmonary stenosis. G3 Genes, Genomes, Genet 2016;6(4):987–92.

58. Huang T, Lin AE, Cox GF, et al. Cardiac phenotypes in chromosome 4q- syndrome with and without a deletion of the dHAND gene. Genet Med 2002;4(6): 464–7.

59. Hyun C, Lavulo L, O'Leary C, et al. Isolation and characterization of the canine NKX2-5 gene. J Anim Breed Genet 2006;123(3):213–6.

60. Lee S, Lee S, Moon H, et al. Isolation , characterization and genetic analysis of canine GATA4 gene in a family of Doberman Pinschers with an atrial septal defect. J Genet 2007;86(3):241–7.

61. Tan RNGB, Witlox RSGM, Hilhorst-Hofstee Y, et al. Clinical and molecular characterization of an infant with a tandem duplication and deletion of 19p13. Am J Med Genet Part A 2015;167(8):1884–9.

62. Alankarage D, JO Szot, Pachter N, et al. Functional characterization of a novel PBX1 de novo missense variant identified in a patient with syndromic congenital heart disease. Hum Mol Genet 2020;29(7):1068–82.

63. Li B, Chen S, Sun K, et al. Genetic Analyses Identified a SALL4 Gene Mutation Associated with Holt–Oram Syndrome. DNA Cell Biol 2018;37(4):398–404.

64. Pulignani S, Vecoli C, Borghini A, et al. Targeted Next-Generation Sequencing in Patients with Non-syndromic Congenital Heart Disease. Pediatr Cardiol 2018; 39(4):682–9.

65. Liu F, Zhu C, Xiao J, et al. A novel human KRAB-containing zinc-finger gene ZNF446 inhibits transcriptional activities of SRE and AP-1. Biochem Biophys Res Commun 2005;333(1):5–13.

66. Momma K. Cardiovascular Anomalies Associated With Chromosome 22q11.2 Deletion Syndrome. Am J Cardiol 2010;105(11):1617–24.

67. Mizugishi K, Yamanaka K, Kuwajima K, et al. Interstitial deletion of chromosome 7q in a patient with Williams syndrome and infantile spasms. J Hum Genet 1998; 43(3):178–81.

68. Von Dadelszen P, Chitayat D, Winsor EJT, et al. De novo 46,XX,t(6;7)(q27;q11;23) associated with severe cardiovascular manifestations characteristic of supravalvular aortic stenosis and Williams syndrome. Am J Med Genet 2000;90(4):270–5.

69. Miura M, Sugayama S, Lúcia Moisés R, Wagënfur J, et al. Williams-Beuren Syndrome. Cardiovascular Abnormalities in 20 Patients Diagnosed with Fluorescence in Situ Hybridization. Arq Bras Cardiol 2003;81(5):468–73.

70. Jakob A, Unger S, Arnold R, et al. A family with a new elastin gene mutation: broad clinical spectrum, including sudden cardiac death. Cardiol Young 2011;21(1):62–5.

71. Frishberg Y, Feinstein S, Rinat C, et al. The Heart of Children with Steroid-Resistant Nephrotic Syndrome: Is It All Podocin? J Am Soc Nephrol 2006; 17(1):227–31.

72. Uysal B, Dönmez O, Uysal F, et al. Congenital nephrotic syndrome of NPHS1 associated with cardiac malformation. Pediatr Int 2015;57(1):177–9.

73. JO Szot, Cuny H, Blue GM, et al. A Screening Approach to Identify Clinically Actionable Variants Causing Congenital Heart Disease in Exome Data. Circ Genomic Precis Med 2018;11(3):1–11.

74. Wünnemann F, Ta-Shma A, Preuss C, et al. Loss of ADAMTS19 causes progressive non-syndromic heart valve disease. Nat Genet 2020;52(1):40–7.

75. Roberts A, Allanson J, Jadico SK, et al. The cardiofaciocutaneous syndrome. J Med Genet 2006;43(11):833–42.

76. You X, Ryu MJ, Cho E, et al. Embryonic Expression of NrasG 12 D Leads to Embryonic Lethality and Cardiac Defects. Front Cell Dev Biol 2021;9(February;0–2.

77. Bertola DR, Pereira AC, Oliveira PSL de, et al. Clinical variability in a Noonan syndrome family with a newPTPN11 gene mutation. Am J Med Genet 2004; 130A(4):378–83.

78. Sarkozy A, Obregon MG, Conti E, et al. A novel PTPN11 gene mutation bridges Noonan syndrome, multiple lentigines/LEOPARD syndrome and Noonan-like/multiple giant cell lesion syndrome. Eur J Hum Genet 2004;12(12):1069–72.

79. Fathallah M, Krasuski RA. Pulmonic Valve Disease: Review of Pathology and Current Treatment Options. Curr Cardiol Rep 2017;19(11).

80. Stout KK, Daniels CJ, Aboulhosn JA, et al. 2018 AHA/ACC Guideline for the Management of Adults With Congenital Heart Disease: A Report of the American College of Cardiology/American Heart Association Task Force on Clinical Practice Guidelines. J Am Coll Cardiol 2019;73(12):e81–192.

81. Chen P, Yin J, Yu H, et al. Next-generation sequencing identifies rare variants associated with Noonan syndrome. Proc Natl Acad Sci U S A 2014;111(31): 11473–8.

82. Roberts AE, Araki T, Swanson KD, et al. Germline gain-of-function mutations in SOS1 cause Noonan syndrome. Nat Genet 2007;39(1):70–4.

83. Brems H, Pasmant E, Van Minkelen R, et al. Review and update of SPRED1 mutations causing legius syndrome. Hum Mutat 2012;33(11):1538–46.

84. Garg V, Kathiriya IS, Barnes R, et al. GATA4 mutations cause human congenital heart defects and reveal an interaction with TBX5. Nature 2003;424:443–7.

85. Barber JCK, Maloney V, Hollox EJ, et al. Duplications and copy number variants of 8p23.1 are cytogenetically indistinguishable but distinct at the molecular level. Eur J Hum Genet 2005;13(10):1131–6.

86. Ang YS, Rivas RN, Ribeiro AJS, et al. Disease Model of GATA4 Mutation Reveals Transcription Factor Cooperativity in Human Cardiogenesis. Cell 2016;167(7): 1734–49.e22.

87. de Soysa TY, Ranade SS, Okawa S, et al. Single-cell analysis of cardiogenesis reveals basis for organ-level developmental defects. Nature 2019;572(7767): 120–4.

88. Chung IM, Rajakumar G. Genetics of congenital heart defects: The NKX2-5 gene, a key player. Genes 2016;7(2). https://doi.org/10.3390/genes7020006.

89. Hussein IR, Bader RS, Chaudhary AG, et al. Identification of De Novo and Rare Inherited Copy Number Variants in Children with Syndromic Congenital Heart Defects. Pediatr Cardiol 2018;39(5):924–40.

90. Ware SM, Peng J, Zhu L, et al. Identification and Functional Analysis of ZIC3 Mutations in Heterotaxy and Related Congenital Heart Defects. Am J Hum Genet 2004;74(1):93–105.

91. Andelfinger G, Tapper AR, Welch RC, et al. KCNJ2 mutation results in Andersen syndrome with sex-specific cardiac and skeletal muscle phenotypes. Am J Hum Genet 2002;71(3):663–8.

92. Knight Johnson A, Schaefer GB, Lee J, et al. Alu -mediated deletion of PIGL in a Patient with CHIME syndrome. Am J Med Genet Part A 2017;173(5):1378–82.

93. Nguyen TQN, Saitoh M, Trinh HT, et al. Truncation and microdeletion of EVC/ EVC2 with missense mutation of EFCAB7 in Ellis-van Creveld syndrome. Congenit Anom (Kyoto) 2016;56(5):209–16.

94. Fricke C, Schmidt V, Cramer K, et al. Characterization of Atherosclerosis by Histochemical and Immunohistochemical Methods in African Grey Parrots (Psittacus erithacus) and Amazon Parrots (Amazona spp) Published by: American Association of Avian Pathologists content in a trusted digital. Avian Dis 2009; 53(3):466–72.

95. Kleefstra T, Smidt M, Banning MJG, et al. Disruption of the gene Euchromatin Histone Methyl Transferase1 (Eu-HMTase1) is associated with the 9q34 subtelomeric deletion syndrome. J Med Genet 2005;42(4):299–306.

96. Kleefstra T, Van Zelst-Stams WA, Nillesen WM, et al. Further clinical and molecular delineation of the 9q subtelomeric deletion syndrome supports a major contribution of EHMT1 haploinsufficiency to the core phenotype. J Med Genet 2009;46(9):598–606.

97. Dimitrov BI, Ogilvie C, Wieczorek D, et al. 3p14 deletion is a rare contiguous gene syndrome: Report of 2 new patients and an overview of 14 patients. Am J Med Genet Part A 2015;167(6):1223–30.

98. Sharma A, Wasson LK, Willcox JAL, et al. GATA6 mutations in hiPSCs inform mechanisms for maldevelopment of the heart, pancreas, and diaphragm. Elife 2020;9:1–28.

99. Le Meur N, Goldenberg A, Michel-Adde C, et al. Molecular characterization of a 14q deletion in a boy with features of Holt-Oram syndrome. Am J Med Genet Part A 2005;134A(4):439–42.

100. Lei TY, Li R, Fu F, et al. Prenatal diagnosis of Smith–Magenis syndrome in two fetuses with increased nuchal translucency, mild lateral ventriculomegaly, and congenital heart defects. Taiwan J Obstet Gynecol 2016;55(6):886–90.

101. Sybert VP, Bradley CM, Salk D. Mosaicism for ring 19: a case report. Clin Genet 2008;34(6):382–5.
102. Yung J-F, Sobel DB, Hoo JJ. Origin of 46,XY/46,XY,r(19) Mosaicism. AM J Med Genet 1990;36.
103. Archer HL, Gupta S, Enoch S, et al. Distinct phenotype associated with a cryptic subtelomeric deletion of 19p13.3-pter. Am J Med Genet Part A 2005;136A(1): 38–44.

Advances in the Treatment of Pulmonary Valve Stenosis

Brian A. Scansen, DVM, MS*

KEYWORDS

- Pulmonic stenosis • Canine • Dog • Congenital heart disease
- Balloon valvuloplasty • Stent implantation

KEY POINTS

- Pulmonary valve stenosis is not easily categorized into a binary classification as dogs with this disease show variable degrees of valve fusion, valve thickening, annular hypoplasia, and fibrous adhesions at the sinotubular junction.
- Balloon pulmonary valvuloplasty remains a key treatment for pulmonary valve stenosis, though is not effective for all valve morphotypes.
- High-pressure balloon pulmonary valvuloplasty should be offered to dogs that fail to respond to conventional balloon dilation and could be considered as first-line therapy for many cases.
- Transpulmonary stent implantation is an emerging therapy for pulmonary valve stenosis which is technically more challenging than balloon pulmonary valvuloplasty but appears to be effective in dogs with valve dysplasia.

 Video content accompanies this article at http://www.vetsmall.theclinics.com.

BACKGROUND

Congenital pulmonary valve stenosis (PS) is very common dogs and seemingly becoming more common with the rise in popularity of brachycephalic breeds that have a predilection for the condition.[1,2] In several reports of congenital heart disease prevalence, PS is the most commonly encountered canine congenital heart defect,[3,4] with recent epidemiologic data from Italy suggesting it comprises 34% of all cases of congenital heart disease in dogs.[2] The male sex appears to have an increased prevalence of PS, particularly in bulldogs.[1,2]

Without therapy, dogs with PS are at risk for symptoms including exercise intolerance, syncope, sudden cardiac death, congestive heart failure, and cyanosis from a right-to-left shunt.[5–7] Effective treatment options for this condition are required given

Cardiology & Cardiac Surgery, Department of Clinical Sciences, Colorado State University, 200 West Lake Street, 1678 Campus Delivery, Fort Collins, CO 80523-1678, USA
* Corresponding author.
E-mail address: Brian.Scansen@colostate.edu

Vet Clin Small Anim 53 (2023) 1393–1414
https://doi.org/10.1016/j.cvsm.2023.05.013
0195-5616/23/© 2023 Elsevier Inc. All rights reserved.

the prevalence and severity of disease encountered in practice; unfortunately, high grade evidence in favor of any particular intervention is lacking in veterinary medicine. Although consensus guidelines are not available, the author advises intervention for dogs with PS according to the criteria in **Box 1**.

ANATOMY OF PULMONARY VALVE STENOSIS IN DOGS

Pulmonary valve stenosis in dogs has variable features, several of which likely impact the potential for a successful intervention. Unfortunately, there is a lack of consensus in the veterinary literature regarding how to classify the morphologic features of PS – some reports describe a predominance of a focal valvar obstruction, while others report that multiple levels of obstruction (valvar and supravalvar) predominate. These conflicting data may reflect geographic and breed differences, but it seems probable that different centers define the morphologic lesions of canine PS differently, leading to variability in the literature and potential confusion amongst cardiologists trained at different institutions. The following discussion of PS morphology represents the author's opinion and experience, in the absence of a consensus document.

In both humans and dogs, PS is principally a disease of the valve apparatus – including the annulus, leaflets, and sinotubular junction. While the human form of valvar PS is predominately that of commissural fusion,[8,9] the canine form is more commonly characterized by thickened, dysplastic valves.[10–12] In domed PS, there is incomplete separation of the leaflets secondary to fusion along the valve commissures, systolic bowing of the domed valve into the pulmonary trunk, and post-stenotic dilation of the pulmonary trunk itself. Dysplastic PS in the human is described as thickened leaflets with limited mobility and variable commissural fusion.[9] Other forms of pulmonary stenosis may include infundibular (subvalvar) and supravalvar pulmonary stenosis.

Early work in a beagle colony specifically bred for PS described the typical canine lesions as valve thickening, valve hypoplasia, and valve fusion; in the seminal article from this laboratory, the term pulmonary valve dysplasia was chosen to describe these lesions.[10] Bussadori and colleagues originally categorized two forms of canine PS: type A, in which there was minimal leaflet thickening, fused commissures with a central orifice, systolic doming, an aortic-to-pulmonary annulus ratio less than 1.2, and post-stenotic dilation of the pulmonary trunk; and type B, in which there was marked leaflet thickening, hypoplasia of the pulmonary annulus with an aortic:pulmonary annulus ratio greater than 1.2, severe infundibular hypertrophy, and rare or minimal post-stenotic dilation of the pulmonary trunk.[12] Using this classification, Bussadori and colleagues showed that outcomes were worse for dogs with type B morphology.[12] The same author used an expanded classification of PS morphology in an epidemiologic series,

---

Box 1
Suggested criteria favoring intervention in dogs with pulmonary valve stenosis (PS)

- Clinical signs referable to PS (syncope, exercise intolerance, poor growth)
- Echocardiographically derived peak transpulmonary pressure gradient> 64 mm Hg
- Congestive heart failure (cavitary effusion, most often ascites)
- Right-to-left shunting intracardiac defect (patent oval foramen, ventricular septal defect)
- Right ventricular systolic dysfunction
- Severe right ventricular wall thickening

including mixed and hourglass types in addition to the types A and B.[2] A large retrospective review of congenital heart disease used the type A and B terminology for canine PS, based principally upon the relative diameters of the pulmonary valve annulus compared to the aortic valve annulus.[4]

Supravalvar stenosis has been reported in the canine literature, with the suggestion that PS in the French bulldog is most often valvar and supravalvar.[13,14] It is the author's opinion that the majority of cases considered supravalvar are within the spectrum of valvar stenosis. According to the anatomist Robert Anderson, the sinotubular junction belongs to and is an integral part of the semilunar valve apparatus.[15] Therefore, it seems reasonable to consider PS cases with fibrotic adhesions to the sinotubular junction as within the spectrum of valvar stenosis. Moreover, many if not most dogs have both abnormal valve leaflets (fusion, thickening) in combination with fibrous adhesions at the sinotubular junction (**Fig. 1**). Finally, a study evaluating supravalvar PS attempted to clarify this issue in humans by defining the lesion as a narrowing of the pulmonary artery and noted considerable discrepancy between the echocardiographic diagnosis and the angiographic gold standard.[16] As in people, true supravalvar pulmonary stenosis appears to be relatively rare in the dog, is perhaps better termed pulmonary artery stenosis,[4] and should be documented as an obstruction geographically distant from (distal to) the sinotubular junction. Many cases of canine PS, the majority in the author's practice, have fibrous adhesions between the leaflet tips and the sinotubular junction or exuberant fibrous tissue within the sinuses and at the sinotubular junction. These cases are considered anatomically valvar by the author.

Subvalvar obstructions are common in all cases of PS related to dynamic obliteration of the subpulmonary infundibulum during right ventricular systole. Specific forms of subvalvar obstruction geographically distant from the valve annulus (infundibular pulmonary stenosis and double chambered right ventricle) are better considered as separate diseases and will not be discussed here. Immediate subvalve obstructions, whether muscular or fibrous, do exist in dogs and can sometimes be challenging to distinguish from annular narrowing or thickening at the base of the pulmonary valve cusps.

While it is useful to consider the morphologic features of the valve, and attractive to pursue a similar classification as is used in humans with typical and dysplastic forms,

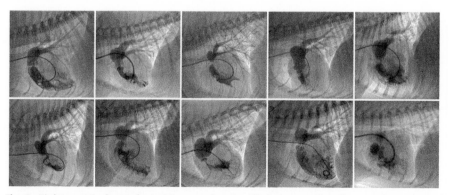

Fig. 1. Right ventriculography in 10 cases of canine PS demonstrating the complex nature of dysplastic valve morphology seen in this disease with valve thickening, valve fusion, fibrous tissue obstructing the valve sinuses, adhesions to the sinotubuluar junction, and annular hypoplasia to variable degree.

the author does not believe that canine PS fits easily into binary categories (eg, type A and type B). Rather, valve thickening, valve fusion, annular hypoplasia, fibrotic tissue at the annulus or sinotubular junction, and post-stenotic dilation of the pulmonary trunk appear to each exist along a continuum in canine PS such that some dogs are affected primarily with fusion and systolic doming of the valve, others have thick leaflets with a hypoplastic annulus, while others have a normal size annulus with exuberant fibrous tissue obstructing the sinuses and sinotubular junction. Often, the individual dog has many of the features described above (thickening, fusion, fibrous tissue, annular dimension) to variable degree. The true fused, doming valve of "typical" PS that is common in humans appears to be rare in dogs, particularly in the most affected breeds (eg, bulldogs and French bulldogs). Examples demonstrating some of the spectrum of morphology in canine PS are shown in **Fig. 1** and Video 1.

INDICATIONS FOR PULMONARY VALVE STENOSIS THERAPY

The decision to intervene in an animal with heart disease is complex. Ideally, evidence-based practice guidelines or consensus statements would guide our treatment decisions. In veterinary medicine, particularly within the field of congenital heart disease and structural heart interventions, such documents are notably absent. There are no rigorous (randomized, double-blind, placebo-controlled) trials of any therapy in canine PS. In addition to animal specific characteristics (see **Box 1**; **Box 2**), the desire of the informed client to intervene as well as their financial capacity to do so often impact whether a procedure is performed. In general, higher pressure gradients, younger age at diagnosis, and the presence of clinical signs are thought to signify more severe disease with a poorer outcome and may justify an intervention in a dog with PS.[5-7] For more than 30 years, human medicine has navigated similar challenges in determining when to intervene with balloon pulmonary valvuloplasty (BPV).[17] Currently, a physicians' decision to intervene on PS varies from the more strict criteria of a transpulmonary valve pressure gradient over 50 mm Hg,[18] to the more lenient pressure gradient of greater than 35 mm Hg with objective signs of right ventricular hypertrophy.[19] In dogs, increased cardiac mortality was observed in dogs with gradients over 80 mm Hg and this threshold has been used as a justification for intervention.[7] In a different study of 55 dogs that did not undergo BPV for their PS, a gradient over 60 mm Hg was associated with cardiac mortality.[6] While the pressure gradient is certainly a critical data

---

Box 2
Valve anatomy favoring balloon dilation versus stent implantation for dogs with pulmonary valve stenosis (PS)

Balloon Dilation Preferred	Transpulmonary Stent Implantation Preferred
• Fused, doming valve	• Moderate to severe valve thickening
• Normal size PVA (AoA:PVA < 1.1)	• Fibrotic tissue at sinotubular junction
• Trace or mild valve thickening	• Annular hypoplasia (AoA:PVA > 1.2)
• Patient age <6 mo	• Pre-pulmonary coronary artery anomaly
• Severe, primary tricuspid regurgitation	• Prior BPV – residual or recurrent stenosis
• Moderate to severe PAH	• Pulmonary artery dissection[a]

Abbreviations: AoV, aortic valve annulus; BPV, balloon pulmonary valvuloplasty; PAH, pulmonary arterial hypertension; PVA, pulmonary valve annulus.
[a] Consider covered stent implantation for pulmonary artery dissection.

point to consider when deciding whether or not to intervene, it is the author's perspective that the echocardiographically derived pressure gradient should not be the sole factor determining whether or not to pursue intervention for canine PS (see **Box 1**). If a single value for pressure gradient was to be considered as a threshold for intervention, the pressure gradient corresponding to a peak outflow velocity of 4 m/s (64 mm Hg) seems a logical starting point based on the literature and for ease of use in the clinic. The author's approach is to provide the pet family with the information we have from published studies,[5,7,11] to offer the perspective from human medicine based on a larger clinical experience and expert guidelines,[18] and to present the author's personal experience from past procedures performed in dogs with similar disease, recognizing that this latter approach falls toward the bottom of the evidence-based pyramid.[20] For some families, this will lead to a decision to intervene in a dog with a pressure gradient of 60 mm Hg and moderate right ventricular wall thickening, while another family may choose to decline intervention with a pressure gradient of 90 mm Hg in the absence of clinical signs.

THERAPEUTIC OPTIONS FOR PULMONARY VALVE STENOSIS

There are 3 primary ways to treat PS in dogs – medical therapy, transcatheter intervention, and open surgery. Medical therapy typically involves beta-blockade, with atenolol seemingly the most prescribed drug. A recent abstract comparing medical practices between physicians and veterinarians demonstrated a major difference in prescribing practices for PS, with 92% of dogs receiving beta blockade compared to only 3% of human patients.[21] The reason for this discrepancy is unclear, though may reflect earlier intervention in humans. In a study of 27 dogs with PS, atenolol decreased the echocardiographically derived transpulmonary pressure gradient compared to its baseline value, though less flow-dependent estimates of severity were not changed.[22] Finally, a short-term study evaluating dogs that received atenolol prior to BPV found no differences in perioperative complications compared to a control group that did not receive atenolol.[23] No studies have evaluated the effect of atenolol on survival or quality of life in canine PS; however, the author continues to prescribe atenolol to dogs with PS that have a moderate to severe pressure gradient (>64 mm Hg) and/or with moderate to severe right ventricular wall thickening due to the theoretic benefits of a reduced myocardial oxygen demand, potential anti-arrhythmic effects, to reduce dynamic muscular obstruction of the right ventricular outflow tract, and to limit demand ischemia associated with tachycardia. Atenolol therapy in a dog prior to and following transpulmonary stent implantation (TSI) is particularly critical to limit the compressive forces of the hypertrophied right ventricle on the stent itself and typical dosages for this purpose are 1.5 to 2.5 mg/kg PO q12 h.

Transcatheter interventions for PS have primarily focused on BPV. Balloon pulmonary valvuloplasty as it is performed today was tested first in a dog in 1980 and reported in a child in 1982.[24,25] Initial reports described a reduction in clinical signs and improved quality of life for dogs undergoing BPV, though a survival advantage was not observed.[11] A retrospective series of 81 dogs reported a 53% reduction in hazard (clinical signs or death) for dogs that underwent BPV, after adjusting for the pressure gradient, clinical signs, and age.[5] While BPV appears beneficial, it is likely of greatest benefit if a substantial reduction in the echocardiographically derived peak transpulmonary pressure gradient can be achieved. One study found that residual gradients were an independent predictor of outcome after BPV and that long-term outcome was optimal when a post-BPV pressure gradient of less than 50 mm Hg was achieved.[26] Predicting which dogs will benefit from BPV therefore seems relevant to the decision to pursue intervention. In a study of 30 dogs with valvar PS, 94% of the dogs that had a normal pulmonary annular diameter and minimal valve thickening had resolution of their clinical signs and survived more than 1 year after the procedure; however, for the dogs with marked leaflet thickening and a hypoplastic pulmonary annulus, only 66.6% had a favorable outcome and only 50% showed a resolution in their clinical signs.[12] More recently, a retrospective series of 81 dogs found progressive increase in the pressure gradient after BPV, with restenosis occurring in 18% to 38% of dogs.[27] Taken in total, while BPV can improve outcome in PS dogs, it appears that in some dogs BPV fails to provide the desired reduction in transpulmonary pressure gradient or fails to provide a durable result. Current advances in transcatheter interventions for PS have therefore focused on optimizing BPV technique, including the use of high-pressure balloons[28,29] and pre-scoring the lesion with cutting balloon dilation catheters.[30] Additional work has pursued the implantation of metallic stents across the pulmonary valve annulus to hold the dysplastic tissue to the walls of the outflow tract.[31–34] These newer transcatheter approaches will be discussed below.

Surgical options for PS palliation have existed for decades, though are minimally reported in dogs. Surgical commissurotomy in a German shepherd dog was successfully performed under hypothermic inflow occlusion as early as 1964,[35] while patch graft techniques have been reported both on and off cardiopulmonary bypass.[36–38] A series of 8 dogs with severe PS undergoing surgical palliation (closed commissurotomy or patch graft) disclosed a mean survival of 3.75 years suggesting a benefit from surgery compared to unoperated dogs.[39] Today, open surgery for PS is uncommon in dogs.

Only one study, to the author's knowledge, has retrospectively compared all therapeutic approaches to PS management though this study was only published as an abstract more than 30 years ago.[40] The study by Ewey and colleagues (1992) retrospectively reported on 72 dogs with PS that were not treated, 30 dogs that had surgery (18 commissurotomy, 12 patch graft), and 25 dogs who underwent BPV. In that cohort, survival at 2 years post-treatment was 94% for BPV, 65% for the untreated group, and approximately 30% for the combined surgical groups. The untreated dogs were reported to have a 2.1 times greater risk of death in the first 2 years as compared to dogs who underwent BPV.[40]

BALLOON PULMONARY VALVULOPLASTY

As discussed above, there is evidence that BPV improves the outcome of human and canine patients with severe PS.[5,7,11,41] The procedure is routinely performed by cardiologists with low morbidity and mortality.[42] Although effective for many patients, human and canine studies suggest that patients with valvar dysplasia and a hypoplastic annulus show less improvement following BPV than those with purely valvar fusion.[12,43] Optimizing BPV requires correct annular sizing and balloon selection, as well as an accurate inflation of the balloon centered on the stenotic valve. The full procedural steps are outside the scope of this article but can be found elsewhere.[42]

Selection of the balloon diameter is determined from measurements of the pulmonary valve annulus. A balloon-to-annulus ratio (BAR) of 1.3 to 1.5 is typically selected, with values below 1.3 not providing sufficient force to open the fused valve and ratios exceeding 1.5 being more likely to damage the valve or pulmonary artery. The pulmonary annulus diameter can be measured from transthoracic echocardiography, transesophageal echocardiography (TEE), angiography, or cardiac computed tomography (CCT) and at various phases of the cardiac cycle. The initial estimate of the pulmonary annulus diameter is made at the onset of systole from a right-parasternal short axis echocardiographic image optimized to be directly sagittal to the valve. However, if translational motion prevents an accurate measurement at the onset of systole, the end-diastolic or end-systolic frames may also be used. The measurement is repeated during CCT or TEE, if performed, and again during angiography to confirm the initial echocardiographic measurement. These different measurements are then integrated – the imaging modality with the clearest resolution that demonstrates the hinge-points of the valve diameter in a sagittal plane should be trusted. The length of the balloon is also relevant. A longer balloon provides for a smoother dilation as the valve annulus can be positioned in the middle of the balloon with greater ease; when the balloon is excessively short in length, the ejection of the right ventricle pushes the balloon into the pulmonary artery and makes "landing" the center of the balloon at the valve annulus more challenging. However, an excessively long balloon may damage the tricuspid valve chordae or the distal pulmonary artery during inflation (**Fig. 2**).

In addition to the balloon, the guidewire selected is critical to procedural success. A J-tipped exchange length guidewire (greater than 180 cm length) should be chosen of moderate to high stiffness. The J-tip (optimally a 1.5 cm J) is preferred as it will be less traumatic to the distal pulmonary artery. The guidewire is the scaffold which will help hold the balloon in position across the valve; guidewires that lack the appropriate stiffness will lead to balloon migration and prolapse of the wire, preventing an effective dilation. In general, 0.035″ super-stiff or extra-stiff guidewires are preferred for BPV. In small dogs or those with severe right ventricular hypertrophy, the super-stiff guidewires place too much pressure on the tricuspid valve and the right ventricular endocardium, particularly when they are advanced from a jugular venous approach and a standard stiffness wire should be chosen. In large dogs or when using balloon dilation catheters with a stiff shaft, super-stiff guidewires may be too flexible and ultra-stiff guidewires should be selected. For very small dogs, the chosen balloon dilation catheter may not accept an 0.035″ guidewire. In such instances, a 0.018″ or 0.025″ guidewire can be used, but such wires provide even less stability during advancement and inflation of the balloon dilation catheter and stiffer designs should be selected.

Last, a few comments on balloon inflation technique during routine BPV are relevant. Once the guidewire is positioned and the balloon dilation catheter advanced to the right ventricular outflow tract, rapid inflation should be performed with a pressure inflation device. Hand inflations are imprecise and unable to achieve the target pressure for most balloons as hand pressure on a syringe of greater than 5 mL cannot generate more than 2 to 3 atm of pressure within the balloon.[19] A pressure inflation device allows rapid filling and deflation of the balloon with knowledge of the pressure

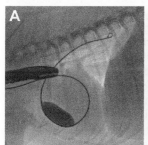 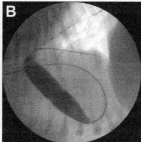 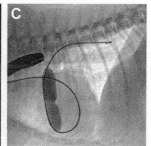

Fig. 2. Balloon lengths for balloon pulmonary valvuloplasty demonstrating a balloon that is short relative to the outflow tract (*A*), too long (*B*), and of a reasonable length to facilitate engagement of the annulus with lower risk of migration (*C*).

generated such that the nominal pressure (at which the balloon reaches labeled diameter) can be obtained and the rated burst pressure avoided. During inflation, it is helpful to have an assistant hold the balloon catheter still and to slightly push the guidewire into the catheter – this facilitates maintenance of the loop through the RV and forces the guidewire toward the cranial aspect of the outflow tract thereby stabilizing the balloon. Positioning of the guidewire in the distal pulmonary artery is important so that forward pressure on the wire stabilizes the whole system. The tendency to pull the balloon dilation catheter out of the dog if it slips distally during inflation should be avoided; a guidewire of appropriate stiffness that is well positioned distally and pushed into the catheter during inflation is the best way to maintain balloon stability. Pulling the balloon catheter out of the dog during inflation risks tightening the wire loop in the right ventricle and damaging the tricuspid valve while seldom improving the operator's ability to maintain balloon position at the annulus.

Again, more details on the precise technical aspects of BPV can be found in other sources.[19,42] Further improvement in technique may involve expanding the devices used to dilate the stenotic outflow tracts of these patients, such as high-pressure balloons, cutting balloons, or stents.

HIGH-PRESSURE BALLOON PULMONARY VALVULOPLASTY

The balloons developed for BPV in children and those that were reported in most of the case series described above in dogs have relatively low rated burst pressures (1–6 atm). Considerable advancement in balloon catheter design has occurred in the last several decades, driven by a need for the effective treatment of peripheral vascular disease in people. Dozens of balloon dilation catheters approved for percutaneous transluminal angioplasty are therefore available on the human market and can be used in an off-label manner for BPV in dogs. Specifically, human and canine patients that lack the thin, fused valve of typical PS may benefit from alternate balloon dilation catheters as studies suggest that patients with valve dysplasia and a hypoplastic annulus have less improvement following BPV, as well as a poorer prognosis with or without BPV, compared to those with predominantly valvar fusion.[12,26,43,44] High-pressure BPV, defined in one study as a balloon inflation pressure of at least 8 atm, was performed in eight humans immediately following suboptimal results from low-pressure BPV.[44] In that series, a successful outcome was achieved after high-pressure BPV for all eight children. A study of high-pressure BPV in 25 dogs demonstrated procedural success in 92% of dogs, including nine dogs considered as having type B or dysplastic valves.[29] Following that study, other authors published results of 20 dogs undergoing low-pressure BPV (defined as <4 atm) in which 60% demonstrated procedural success and no effect of valve type (A or B) was observed.[45] Currently, there is no compelling evidence to select high-pressure BPV over low-pressure BPV for canine PS. However, the high proportion of dysplastic valves in the canine population may justify a lower threshold to intervene with high pressure. Currently, the author performs high-pressure BPV for all dogs undergoing pulmonary valve dilation. The rationale for this approach is partially economical – if the valve fails to respond to low-pressure BPV a second dilation with a higher-pressure balloon would be pursued and result in twice the balloon cost. Utilizing this approach over the last 5+ years has not resulted in a recognizable increase in complications from the high-pressure balloon dilation catheters, but evidence supporting or refuting this approach is unavailable. If a valve is thin, fused, and there is no evidence of fibrous tissue complicating the obstruction then low-pressure BPV as a first line therapy is reasonable.

CUTTING-BALLOON DILATION FOR PULMONARY VALVE DYSPLASIA

Balloon dilation relieves valvar stenosis by tearing fused or thickened leaflets. The stretch achieved with balloon dilation may not be sufficient to tear very thick, fibrous tissue and relieve obstruction in dysplastic PS. There are catheters, however, that when inflated expose small microblades that incise the tissue by extending out from the balloon surface by 0.127 mm.[46] In theory, scoring the tissue with a cutting balloon may then allow a more controlled tear in resistant tissue as sequentially larger size balloons are then inflated at the same location. Cutting balloon technology to treat PS was first attempted 30 years ago when a double-blade balloon was used to dilate a stenotic pulmonary valve in a dog model, followed by its use in three children.[47] Further work in five children with dysplastic PS demonstrated apparent safety with partial relief of resistant PS in these children who failed standard BPV.[48] The author's catheterization lab reported the results of cutting balloon dilation followed by high-pressure BPV in seven dogs, with reduction in peak pressure gradient from an average of 145 mm Hg to 78 mm Hg the next day on transthoracic echocardiography.[30] Clinical improvement was reported by the clients in four of the seven dogs.

The technique of cutting balloon dilation requires additional equipment and cost compared to standard BPV. Cutting balloon dilation catheters have a guidewire lumen of 0.014″ to 0.018″, necessitating smaller wires than are used for BPV. A gradual inflation and deflation is advised (optimally 60 seconds) to properly expose and then refold the microblades during dilation[46]; this gradual deployment may not be feasible in PS as cardiac output may be compromised when the balloon is inflated. An additional challenge is the available sizes of cutting balloon dilation catheters are limited to a maximum 8 mm diameter, which may not be large enough to engage the valve in all cases of canine PS, particularly larger dogs. Finally, the small diameters of the cutting balloons mean nominal and burst pressures are reached with much less volume than typical balloons used for BPV. If the operator is not aware of this rapid inflation, burst pressure can easily be exceeded which may result in avulsion of a microblade resulting in vascular trauma.

In the author's experience, cutting balloon dilation may have value if TSI is not feasible such as in cases of mid-ventricular obstructions (double-chambered right ventricle) or subvalvar aortic stenosis. Currently, the author does not routinely perform cutting balloon dilation for PS in dogs. In nearly all cases, the valve is either amenable to high-pressure BPV alone or, if BPV is unsuccessful or presumed to lead to an inadequate result, TSI is pursued.

TRANSPULMONARY STENT IMPLANTATION

Stent implantation may provide an alternative therapeutic approach for dogs that fail to respond to BPV. The value of TSI is to physically hold the dysplastic tissue (thick valve, fibrous adhesions) to the side of the outflow tract thereby improving forward flow. In contrast to BPV, TSI leaves an implant in the patient which may be positive (preventing re-stenosis) or negative (if fractured or reactive). Stent implantation has been reported in children as a palliative strategy for cyanotic heart disease, principally tetralogy of Fallot. Nine children with unsalvageable pulmonary valves and tetralogy of Fallot had TSI performed with promising short-term results.[49] A retrospective series of 52 children who underwent TSI reported positive results for the majority of patients, with one perioperative death related to pulmonary artery perforation.[50] In recent years, TSI has evolved to be the first-line therapy for neonatal palliation of Fallot's tetralogy in children, allowing improved growth of the distal pulmonary arteries compared to surgical aortopulmonary shunt at lower morbidity compared to early primary repair.[51,52]

Stent implantation across the pulmonary valve annulus was first reported in two dogs with an initial reduction in right ventricular pressure and transpulmonary gradient, as well as reduced clinical signs.[31] However, the improvement noted in each case was short-lived, with progressive in-stent stenosis due to muscular in-growth in one case and dynamic infundibular narrowing below the stent in the other.[31] An additional report described TSI for PS in four dogs, in which one stent fractured.[33] Finally, a case series reported 15 cases of TSI, including three with a coronary artery anomaly and a prepulmonary course, which demonstrated a reduction in the median peak pressure gradient from 137 mm Hg prior to TSI to 83 mm Hg at 4 weeks post-implantation with improved clinical signs for all dogs.

In the last 5 years, the author's institution has performed 62 TSIs in dogs for congenital PS, with three separate TSI catheterizations performed in one dog. The full dataset is being reviewed prior to publication, but some preliminary results will be given here to clarify potential outcomes from TSI in dogs. Of these 64 interventions, 21 (33%) were in dogs that had previously undergone BPV, 7 (11%) had a coronary artery anomaly, and 21 (33%) were in right-sided congestive heart failure at the time of intervention. In this population, the average pre-operative peak echocardiographically derived pressure gradient was 134 ± 44 mm Hg and the average gradient the day after TSI was 53 ± 28 mm Hg for a mean reduction of 58%. These results compare favorably to BPV and perhaps are more notable in that many of these dogs had failed prior BPV or had dysplastic valves that were considered poor candidates for BPV. There are several technical aspects to be considered when performing TSI, which will be briefly addressed below.

Pre-operative Evaluation

The preferred preoperative diagnostic work-up includes a complete transthoracic echocardiography and, optimally, a CCT of the patient's right ventricular outflow tract and coronary circulation prior to cardiac catheterization.[53] A preoperative CCT is not mandatory, but has proven useful to optimize stent sizing, to improve the understanding of valve anatomy and morphologic characteristics of the PS, and to assess risk for coronary compression/occlusion at the time of stent implantation (**Fig. 3**).

Prior to catheterization, aggressive beta-blockade is advised. The right ventricular outflow tract is often problematic in these dogs. Reducing the force of right ventricular contraction (and avoiding stent implantation into the infundibulum) can help to limit risk for stent fracture and re-stenosis. An atenolol dosage of 1.5 to 2 mg/kg PO q12 hr is the target.

If a preoperative CT is not performed, careful attention should be directed to the levophase of the right ventriculogram during diagnostic angiography to evaluate the location and course of the coronary arteries. If there is a concern for coronary occlusion or compression, a test balloon inflation should be performed with concurrent coronary angiography to confirm safety of the desired stent size.[54]

Stent selection

Sizing of the stent is not well defined in human reports, but most authors report a stent diameter equal to or at most 1 to 2 mm larger than the diastolic pulmonary annular diameter.[55,56] There are many stents that could be considered. Balloon-expandable stents are relatively easy to deploy at the target site and can be post-dilated if the animal grows or a larger diameter is desired after implant. Self-expanding stents are advantageous in that they continue to exert outward radial force after implant but are more challenging to land at a distinct and narrow target zone and cannot be post-dilated. The size of the annulus also plays a role in selection. Most stents available on the human market are labeled for atherosclerotic disease of the iliofemoral system

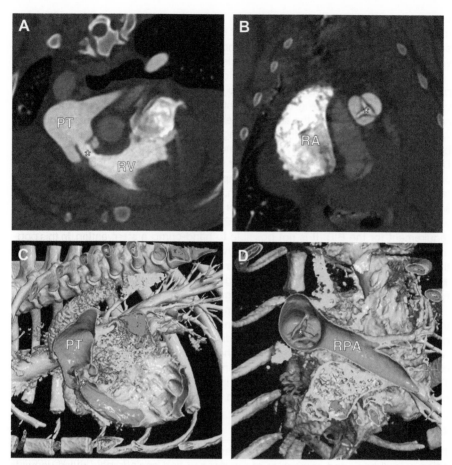

Fig. 3. Images of a cardiac computed tomography (CCT) scan from a 3-year-old Pittbull dog with severe pulmonary valve stenosis. The thickened and fused pulmonary valve leaflets (*asterisk*) can be appreciated and the outflow tract reformatted in any plane, including sagittal (*A, C*) or dorsal (*B, D*), and in a planar (*A, B*) or volume-rendered (*C, D*) format to highlight relevant anatomy and plan for transpulmonary stent implantation. PT, pulmonary trunk; RA, right atrium; RPA, right branch pulmonary artery; RV, right ventricle.

and are sized to these vessels. Biliary stents are also commonly available and of comparable size (usually 7–12 mm in diameter and of variable length). Balloon-expandable stents can be over-dilated beyond their nominal diameter, but doing so increases the risk of fracture or "napkin-ring" formation where the stent dramatically foreshortens. Bench-top testing has shown that serial dilation (expanding the stent in 2 mm increments) can limit these risks and has also demonstrated the maximal extent to which many commercially available products can be dilated.[57]

For relatively small dogs – those with a pulmonary annulus diameter up to 12 mm – a pre-mounted iliac and biliary stent[a] is a good choice and was used in 66% of the cases treated at our institution. The pre-mounted stent saves time and complexity, tracking

---

[a] Express LD Iliac and Biliary Premounted Stent System, Boston Scientific Corporation, Marlborough, MA, USA.

better through the sheath with less risk for dislodgement from the balloon. The pre-mounted stent requires vascular access of 6 to 7 Fr depending on the stent diameter selected. A long, flexible sheath[b] with a short taper on the dilator is desirable to traverse the reverse curve of the right ventricle from a jugular approach.

For dogs with a target pulmonary valve diameter larger than 12 mm, there are no pre-mounted stents of adequate diameter available in the United States and these cases require hand-crimping of a different stent.[c] Although a hand-crimped stent adds cost and complexity, the author has expanded this stent up to 20 mm diameter without fracture or excessive foreshortening. The stent is mounted onto a balloon-in-balloon (BIB) catheter[d] with an outer diameter determined by desired annular size. During crimping, the lumen of the catheter should be protected by the placement of a guidewire; the stent is then gently compressed onto the balloon using umbilical tape soaked in contrast to provide even, circumferential compression (Video 2). Most BIB catheters of this size require 10 or 11 Fr vascular access. The crimped stent will create a larger profile, typically 1 to 2 Fr sizes larger than the labeled sheath requirement for the BIB. It is not possible to hand-crimp a stent as firmly as a pre-mounted stent and the bend of the sheath as it traverses the right ventricle makes the dislodgement of the stent a concern as it is advanced into the sheath. Therefore, a sheath inner diameter that is 3 to 4 Fr larger than that labeled for the BIB is chosen, typically a 14 Fr sheath[e] for medium to large size dogs.

Cases with a pulmonary artery dissection represent a unique population.[58] The author's approach in these dogs is to implant a covered stent, also known as a stent graft. The technique is comparable to that discussed below with a pre-mounted stent, with the exception that the covered stent has a non-penetrable outer covering (typically polytetrafluoroethylene) which may limit the risk of arterial rupture during TSI. The author has implanted covered stents in three dogs, without notable differences compared to bare metal stent implantation.

Stent Implantation Procedure

The cardiac catheterization is performed as is routinely done for BPV. A diagnostic pressure pull-back and angiogram are performed and angiographic measurements of the pulmonary annulus recorded and compared to CCT and TEE. Once the desired stent size is determined from the measurements, a super-stiff or extra-stiff guidewire is advanced to the distal left pulmonary artery (typically using a balloon wedge pressure catheter). The balloon dilation catheter, stent, and pressure inflation device are prepared, and everything made ready before the long sheath is advanced into the dog. If the diagnostic catheterization was performed through a short vascular introducer, this is removed over the wire while holding pressure on the jugular access site and exchanged for the long delivery sheath (typically 7 Fr for pre-mounted stents, 14 Fr for BIB and hand-crimped stents), which is positioned with its tip in the pulmonary trunk distal to the target landing zone. The stent is then advanced over the wire within the long sheath. Advancement through the hemostatic valve can be assisted with the cut end of a short vascular introducer or an advancement device that is provided with some stents. Advancement of the stent through the long sheath should be

---

[b] Flexor High Flex Ansel Guiding Sheath, Cook Medical, Bloomington, IN, USA.

[c] IntraStent Max LD Peripheral and Biliary Stent, Medtronic, Minneapolis, MN, USA.

[d] BIB Stent Placement Balloon Catheter, Numed Inc., Hopkinton, NY, USA.

[e] Sentrant Introducer Sheath, Medtronic, Minneapolis, MN, USA.

watched under fluoroscopy, particularly when a hand-crimped stent is used, as dislodgement is possible. If dislodgement of the stent from the balloon occurs, the entire delivery system will have to be removed from the dog. Once the stent is positioned across the pulmonary annulus and centered on the primary site of obstruction, the sheath is gently retracted to uncover the stent. Contrast is injected through the side-port of the sheath to confirm proper stent position and it is helpful to have concurrent TEE to verify the landing zone. The balloon is then inflated to nominal pressure to deploy the stent. If the target diameter is not reached, the delivery balloon is removed, and serial dilation performed (optimally in 2 mm increments) up to the desired diameter. Examples of both pre-mounted (**Fig. 4**, Video 3) and hand-crimped (**Fig. 5**, Video 4) TSI procedures are provided here to demonstrate these techniques

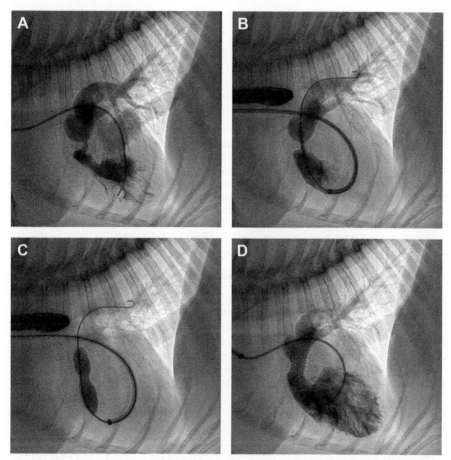

Fig. 4. Images during transpulmonary stent implantation using a pre-mounted stent in a 1-year-old French bulldog with dysplastic pulmonary valve stenosis. The initial right ventriculogram (A) demonstrates severe narrowing through the valve with exuberant cranial fibrous tissue resulting in a large filling defect. After crossing the stenosis with a wire and long 8 Fr sheath, the stent is unsheathed and a positioning angiogram performed (B). The balloon is expanded to deploy the sheath across the pulmonary valve (C). Post-stent right ventriculography demonstrates markedly improved outflow tract diameter and resolution of the stenosis (D).

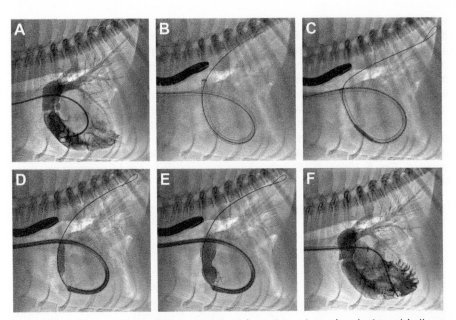

Fig. 5. Images during transpulmonary stent implantation using a hand-crimped balloon-expandable stent on a balloon-in-balloon (BIB) delivery catheter in the same dog shown in **Fig. 3**. Right ventriculography (*A*) defines the site of obstruction and a 14 Fr sheath is advanced to the pulmonary trunk over a wire positioned in the distal left branch pulmonary artery (*B*). The stent is advanced through the sheath (*C*) and the sheath retracted to expose the stent at the pulmonary annulus. A positioning angiogram is performed through the sheath and once proper position is confirmed, the stent expanded first with the inner balloon (*D*), followed by the outer balloon (*E*). Final ventriculography (*F*) confirms proper stent position and improved right ventricular outflow tract diameter.

Complications of Transpulmonary Stent Implantation

In some dogs, the annular size or selected balloon may require a sheath larger than desirable for the patient's vasculature. There are reports of front-loading stents into the sheath prior to advancement into the patient to avoid risk for stent dislodgement in a small sheath where vascular access is limited by patient size.[59] This is feasible in dogs and the author has performed a front-loaded deployment in one dog (**Fig. 6**). However, the transition of the wire to the balloon and outer sheath is not smooth when using a front-loaded stent and should only be performed as a last resort.

A common concern after TSI is the presence of severe pulmonary insufficiency (PI) and the pulmonary arterial waveform after TSI typically shows ventricularization – a sign of severe PI (**Fig. 7**). There is minimal literature on the natural history of moderate to severe PI in dogs; in humans, PI is well-tolerated often into the third or fourth decade of life where eventual right heart dilation and dysfunction develop.[60] As PI is seldom quantified in animals, it is also unknown what impact PI has after BPV in dogs. Regardless, the pulmonary vasculature has notable differences to the systemic vasculature which may negate some of the concerns of wide-open PI. That is, the normal pulmonary circulation has low resistance and high capacitance – 80% to 85% of the blood ejected from the right ventricle has diffused to the pulmonary capillary bed by the end of systole, resulting in only a small proportion of the stroke volume that remains in the pulmonary trunk.[19] Additionally, this blood is at low diastolic pressure and therefore

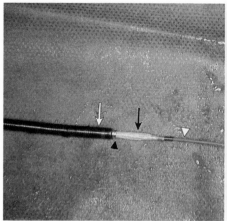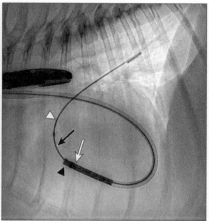

Fig. 6. Front-loading of a stent is shown when the required sheath is not large enough to accommodate advancement of a stent through its lumen. At the table, the stent is crimped onto the balloon that has been advanced through the sheath and manipulated into the end of the sheath. The system is then advanced into the patient over a guidewire that has been positioned in the distal left branch pulmonary artery. In both the photograph on the left and the fluoroscopic image on the right, the sheath can be seen (*white arrow*) with a small amount of stent exposed (*black arrowhead*) and the tip of the balloon (*black arrow*) can be seen creating a transition to the guidewire (*white arrowhead*). Once advanced to the level of the pulmonary valve, deployment proceeds as usual.

the actual volume of blood that leaks back during PI is likely to be less than what might be expected from a non-valved pathway from right ventricle to pulmonary trunk. Having performed TSI in dozens of dogs, the author has not seen clear evidence that PI is a problem unless the tricuspid valve is also severely incompetent. Such dogs are often in right-sided congestive heart failure before stenting and it is unclear how much the PI contributes to persistent congestive signs. For such patients, the resolution of right ventricular afterload probably has some benefit but the increased volume load of PI may be disadvantageous.

As discussed above, aggressive post-dilation can cause the stent to foreshorten dramatically, a so-called napkin ring effect (**Fig. 8**). This can be avoided by serial dilation in no more than 2 mm increments, use of a BIB catheter, and by correct stent size selection from the outset.

Stent migration is a potential concern, but in congenital PS migration appears to be very unlikely as there is often exuberant valve tissue present to hold the stent in position once it is expanded. If migration occurs, it typically happens within seconds after deployment and related to inaccurate sizing or deployment position. In that scenario, it is critical that wire access be maintained. So long as the wire is not lost, it is still possible to coaxially engage the stent with a balloon or second stent. It will not be feasible in most cases to retrieve the migrated stent, but it can be expanded into a branch pulmonary artery where it will be harmless or the proximal aspect can be locked in place with a second stent that extends down and more appropriately engages the pulmonary valve annulus (**Fig. 9**)

The implantation of a metal foreign body into a hypertrophied and contracting ventricle is a recipe for metal fatigue, compression, and fracture. Interestingly, fractures are commonly observed with transcatheter pulmonary valve implantation in humans, though most are incidental and not clinically relevant.[61] In the author's experience,

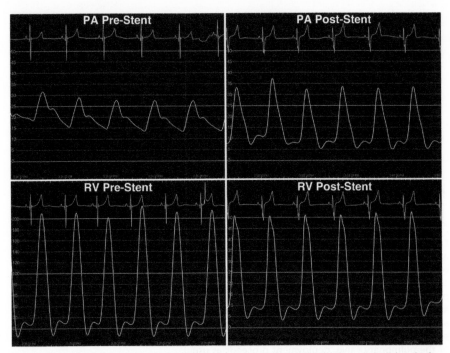

Fig. 7. Hemodynamic pressure traces measured in a 10-month-old French bulldog before and after transpulmonary stent implantation. Note the change in the appearance of the pulmonary artery (PA) waveform after stent implantation, with a drop in the diastolic pressure signifying severe pulmonary insufficiency (ventricularization of the PA pressure trace). Note also that the peak-to-peak pressure gradient across the pulmonary valve has fallen from ~180 mm Hg pre to ~15 mm Hg post-stenting.

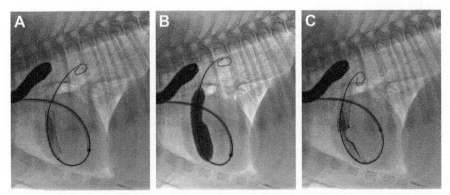

Fig. 8. Images during the post-dilation of an 8 mm diameter transpulmonary stent with a 14 mm diameter balloon in a 3-month-old Golden retriever. Note the initial length of the transpulmonary stent after deployment (A). During post-dilation, the large balloon fails to dilate the stent equally and the stent begins to foreshorten from the proximal aspect (B). In the final image (C), the degree of proximal stent foreshortening, known as napkin-ring formation, can be appreciated.

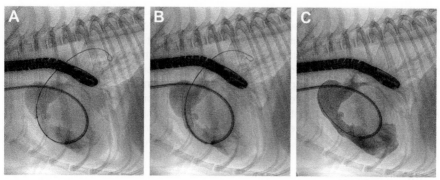

Fig. 9. Migration of a transpulmonary stent in a 4-year-old border terrier with pulmonary valve stenosis. The angiogram after deployment of the first stent (*A*) demonstrates poor positioning as the stent migrated distal to the pulmonary annulus. Maintaining coaxial wire position, a second stent is advanced into the first (*B*) and used to lock the migrated stent in place. The final angiogram (*C*) demonstrates appropriate stent position and relief of the stenosis at the level of the valve.

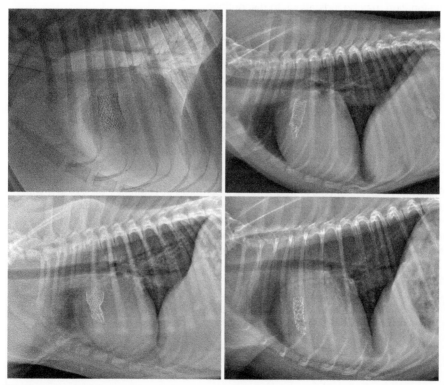

Fig. 10. Examples of stent fractures after transpulmonary stent implantation in dogs. Loss of stent integrity and recurrence of stenosis are the primary complications seen after stent fracture. Minimizing the amount of stent implanted into the right ventricle is the best mechanism to avoid this complication.

the risk of stent compression and fracture can be minimized if all or most of the stent can be implanted at and above the level of the pulmonary valve annulus. Anecdotal experience suggests that fracture is most likely when the stent is deployed within the right ventricular outflow tract, particularly one with systolic cavity obliteration (**Fig. 10**). Interestingly, the 5 to 10 mm portion of the right ventricle immediately below the pulmonary annulus seldom shows complete chamber collapse even in severely thickened right ventricles. Paying attention to this area on angiography or CT may provide a guide to where the stent can be deployed with less risk for compression. Admittedly, some cases require the stent to extend proximal to the pulmonary annulus, but in such cases the risk of compression and fracture should be clearly relayed to the family prior to intervention.

Post-Operative Care

Following stent implantation, evaluation of the pulmonary arterial and right ventricular pressures is performed as would be done for BPV assessment. Typically, a post-stent right ventriculogram is performed to assess position and location of any dynamic obstruction and verify stent position relative to the pulmonary annulus. Follow-up care thereafter is comparable to a post-BPV patient with the addition of thoracic radiographs on a once to twice per year timeframe to assess for fracture. The author's preference is to continue beta-blockade for life in most dogs after TSI, though near complete resolution of right ventricular hypertrophy or severe right ventricular dysfunction may be indications to discontinue.

Post-operative use of anti-platelet or anti-coagulant medications can be considered following TSI and is advocated by some authors. In the author's experience, these medications do not appear necessary given the high flow rate across the stent. However, if the dog has an underlying prothrombotic condition then prophylactic therapy should be pursued. Additionally, when a covered stent is implanted, the author typically prescribes clodidogrel for 6 months and apixaban for 3 months to limit any thrombotic reaction to the outer stent covering. Finally, if stasis of blood is observed (often into a partially covered valve sinus) on the post-TSI angiogram, then anti-thrombotic medications should be considered and prescribed.

SUMMARY

Pulmonary valve stenosis is frequently encountered in veterinary cardiology, with an apparent increase in prevalence due to the popularity of brachycephalic breeds in recent years. Despite this prevalence, evidence-based approaches to the care of these dogs are lacking. Current therapy involves atenolol and BPV, with an emerging consideration for TSI in dogs with dysplastic valves or those that do not respond to BPV.

CLINICS CARE POINTS

- The diagnosis of pulmonary valve stenosis should focus on more than just the peak pressure gradient as determined by echocardiography – valve morphology (valve thickness, valve fusion, fibrous adhesions, annular dimension) and secondary lesions (right ventricular wall thickness, right atrial size, concurrent tricuspid insufficiency, right ventricular systolic function, coronary artery anatomy) should also be evaluated to fully assess the dog with pulmonary stenosis.

- The optimal treatment strategy for pulmonary valve stenosis in dogs is unclear, but several transcatheter interventions are now available that may serve a greater role for the variable valve morphologies encountered than conventional balloon pulmonary valvuloplasty.

• Referral to a center capable of conventional balloon pulmonary valvuloplasty, high-pressure balloon pulmonary valvuloplasty, cutting-balloon dilation, and transpulmonary stent implantation may be helpful for a dog with pulmonary valve stenosis and complex anatomy or for a dog that has failed to respond to pulmonary valve balloon dilation.

DISCLOSURE

The author discloses no conflicts of interest relative to this work.

SUPPLEMENTARY DATA

Supplementary data related to this article can be found online at https://doi.org/10.1016/j.cvsm.2023.05.013

REFERENCES

1. Buchanan JW. Causes and prevalence of cardiovascular diseases. In: Kirk RW, Bonagura JD, editors. Current Veterinary Therapy XI: small animal practice. Philadelphia, PA: WB Saunders Co.; 1992. p. 647–54.
2. Brambilla PG, Polli M, Pradelli D, et al. Epidemiological study of congenital heart diseases in dogs: Prevalence, popularity, and volatility throughout twenty years of clinical practice. PLoS One 2020;15(7):e0230160.
3. Oliveira P, Domenech O, Silva J, et al. Retrospective review of congenital heart disease in 976 dogs. J Vet Intern Med 2011;25(3):477–83.
4. Schrope DP. Prevalence of congenital heart disease in 76,301 mixed-breed dogs and 57,025 mixed-breed cats. J Vet Cardiol 2015;17(3):192–202.
5. Johnson MS, Martin M, Edwards D, et al. Pulmonic stenosis in dogs: balloon dilation improves clinical outcome. J Vet Intern Med 2004;18(5):656–62.
6. Francis AJ, Johnson MJ, Culshaw GC, et al. Outcome in 55 dogs with pulmonic stenosis that did not undergo balloon valvuloplasty or surgery. J Small Anim Pract 2011;52(6):282–8.
7. Locatelli C, Spalla I, Domenech O, et al. Pulmonic stenosis in dogs: survival and risk factors in a retrospective cohort of patients. J Small Anim Pract 2013;54(9):445–52.
8. Waller BF, Howard J, Fess S. Pathology of pulmonic valve stenosis and pure regurgitation. Clin Cardiol 1995;18(1):45–50.
9. Fathallah M, Krasuski RA. Pulmonic Valve Disease: Review of Pathology and Current Treatment Options. Curr Cardiol Rep 2017;19(11):108.
10. Patterson DF, Haskins ME, Schnarr WR. Hereditary dysplasia of the pulmonary valve in beagle dogs. Pathologic and genetic studies. Am J Cardiol 1981;47(3):631–41.
11. Ristic J, Marin C, Baines E, et al. Congenital Pulmonic Stenosis a Retrospective study of 24 cases seen between 1990–1999. J Vet Cardiol 2001;3(2):13–9.
12. Bussadori C, DeMadron E, Santilli RA, et al. Balloon valvuloplasty in 30 dogs with pulmonic stenosis: effect of valve morphology and annular size on initial and 1-year outcome. J Vet Intern Med 2001;15(6):553–8.
13. Treseder JR, Jung S. Balloon dilation of congenital supravalvular pulmonic stenosis in a dog. J Vet Sci 2017;18(1):111–4.
14. Chetboul V, Damoiseaux C, Poissonnier C, et al. Specific features and survival of French bulldogs with congenital pulmonic stenosis: a prospective cohort study of 66 cases. J Vet Cardiol 2018;20(6):405–14.

15. Anderson RH. Anatomy. In: Wernovsky G, editor. Anderson's pediatric cardiology. 4th edition. Philadelphia, PA: Elsevier; 2020. p. 17–32.

16. Poupart S, Navarro-Castellanos I, Raboisson MJ, et al. Supravalvular and Valvular Pulmonary Stenosis: Predictive Features and Responsiveness to Percutaneous Dilation. Pediatr Cardiol 2021;42(4):814–20.

17. Lau KW, Hung JS. Controversies in percutaneous balloon pulmonary valvuloplasty: timing, patient selection and technique. J Heart Valve Dis 1993;2(3):321–5.

18. Rao PS. Percutaneous balloon pulmonary valvuloplasty: State of the art. Cathet Cardiovasc Interv 2007;69(5):747–63.

19. Mullins CE. Pulmonary valve balloon dilation. In: Cardiac catheterization in congenital heart disease: pediatric and adult. 1 edition. Malden, Massachusetts: Blackwell Publishing, Inc.; 2006. p. 430–40.

20. Masic I, Miokovic M, Muhamedagic B. Evidence based medicine - new approaches and challenges. Acta Inf Med 2008;16(4):219–25.

21. Markovic L, Scansen B, Hiremath G, et al. Comparative transcatheter treatment for pulmonary valve stenosis: Multicenter collaborative study across pediatric and ceterinary cardiology centers (Abstract). Pediatr Cardiol 2022;43(8):1969–70.

22. Nishimura S, Visser LC, Belanger C, et al. Echocardiographic evaluation of velocity ratio, velocity time integral ratio, and pulmonary valve area in dogs with pulmonary valve stenosis. J Vet Intern Med 2018;32(5):1570–8.

23. Gomart S, MacFarlane P, Payne JR, et al. Effect of preoperative administration of atenolol to dogs with pulmonic stenosis undergoing interventional procedures. J Vet Intern Med 2022;36(3):877–85.

24. Buchanan JW, Anderson JH, White RI. The 1st balloon valvuloplasty: an historical note. J Vet Intern Med 2002;16(1):116–7.

25. Kan JS, White RI Jr, Mitchell SE, et al. Percutaneous balloon valvuloplasty: a new method for treating congenital pulmonary-valve stenosis. N Engl J Med 1982; 307(9):540–2.

26. Locatelli C, Domenech O, Silva J, et al. Independent predictors of immediate and long-term results after pulmonary balloon valvuloplasty in dogs. J Vet Cardiol 2011;13(1):21–30.

27. Winter RL, Clark WA, Cutchin E, et al. Integrative echocardiographic assessment of post-operative obstruction severity and restenosis after balloon valvuloplasty in 81 dogs with pulmonary stenosis. J Vet Cardiol 2023;45:71–8.

28. Scansen BA. Interventional Cardiology: What's New? Vet Clin North Am Small Anim Pract 2017;47(5):1021–40.

29. Belanger C, Gunther-Harrington CT, Nishimura S, et al. High-pressure balloon valvuloplasty for severe pulmonary valve stenosis: a prospective observational pilot study in 25 dogs. J Vet Cardiol 2018;20(2):115–22.

30. Markovic LE, Scansen BA. A pilot study evaluating cutting and high-pressure balloon valvuloplasty for dysplastic pulmonary valve stenosis in 7 dogs. J Vet Cardiol 2019;25:61–73.

31. Scansen BA, Kent AM, Cheatham SL, et al. Stenting of the right ventricular outflow tract in 2 dogs for palliation of dysplastic pulmonary valve stenosis and right-to-left intracardiac shunting defects. J Vet Cardiol 2014;16(3):205–14.

32. Scansen BA. Cardiac Interventions in Small Animals: Areas of Uncertainty. Vet Clin North Am Small Anim Pract 2018;48(5):797–817.

33. Sosa I, Swift ST, Jones AE, et al. Stent angioplasty for treatment of canine valvular pulmonic stenosis. J Vet Cardiol 2019;21:41–8.

34. Borgeat K, Gomart S, Kilkenny E, et al. Transvalvular pulmonic stent angioplasty: procedural outcomes and complications in 15 dogs with pulmonic stenosis. J Vet Cardiol 2021;38:1–11.

35. Ott BS, Raymond BA, North RL, et al. Diagnosis and Surgical Repair of Congenital Pulmonary Stenosis in the Dog. J Am Vet Med Assoc 1964;144:851–6. Journal Article).

36. Breznock EM, Wood GL. A patch-graft technique for correction of pulmonic stenosis in dogs. J Am Vet Med Assoc 1976;169(10):1090–4.

37. Staudte KL, Gibson NR, Read RA, et al. Evaluation of closed pericardial patch grafting for management of severe pulmonic stenosis. Aust Vet J 2004;82(1–2):33–7.

38. Tanaka R, Shimizu M, Hoshi K, et al. Efficacy of open patch-grafting under cardiopulmonary bypass for pulmonic stenosis in small dogs. Aust Vet J 2009;87(3): 88–93.

39. Fingland RB, Bonagura JD, Myer CW. Pulmonic stenosis in the dog: 29 cases (1975-1984). J Am Vet Med Assoc 1986;189(2):218–26.

40. Ewey DM, Pion PD, Hird DW. Survival in treated and untreated dogs with congenital pulmonic stenosis. J Vet Intern Med 1992;6(2):114.

41. Rao PS, Galal O, Patnana M, et al. Results of three to 10 year follow up of balloon dilatation of the pulmonary valve. Heart 1998;80(6):591–5.

42. Scansen BA. Pulmonary valve stenosis. In: Weisse C, Berent A, editors. *Veterinary image-guided interventions.* Ames, IA, USA: John Wiley & Sons, Ltd; 2015. p. 575–87.

43. McCrindle BW. Independent predictors of long-term results after balloon pulmonary valvuloplasty. Valvuloplasty and Angioplasty of Congenital Anomalies (VACA) Registry Investigators. Circulation 1994;89(4):1751–9.

44. Moguillansky D, Schneider HE, Rome JJ, et al. Role of high-pressure balloon valvotomy for resistant pulmonary valve stenosis. Congenit Heart Dis 2010;5(2): 134–40.

45. Gunasekaran T, Javery E, Sanders RA. Immediate outcomes of low-pressure balloon valvuloplasty for severe pulmonary valve stenosis in 20 dogs: a retrospective, single-center case series. J Vet Cardiol 2021;36:99–104.

46. Cejna M. Cutting balloon: review on principles and background of use in peripheral arteries. Cardiovasc Intervent Radiol 2005;28(4):400–8.

47. Yang SY, Qian CC, Hsia YF, et al. Transcatheter double-blade valvotomy for the treatment of valvar pulmonary stenosis. Pediatr Cardiol 1991;12(4):224–6.

48. Gavri S, Perles Z, Golender J, et al. Cutting balloon for the treatment of resistant pulmonic valve stenosis. Intervent Cardiol 2011;3(5):543–7.

49. Dohlen G, Chaturvedi RR, Benson LN, et al. Stenting of the right ventricular outflow tract in the symptomatic infant with tetralogy of Fallot. Heart 2009;95(2): 142–7.

50. Stumper O, Ramchandani B, Noonan P, et al. Stenting of the right ventricular outflow tract. Heart 2013;99(21):1603–8.

51. Banjoko A, Seyedzenouzi G, Ashton J, et al. Tetralogy of Fallot: stent palliation or neonatal repair? Cardiol Young 2021;31(10):1658–66.

52. Pizzuto A, Cuman M, Assanta N, et al. Right Ventricular Outflow Tract Stenting as Palliation of Critical Tetralogy of Fallot: Techniques and Results. Heart 2021;2(2): 278–87.

53. Scansen BA. Cardiac Computed Tomography Imaging. Advances in Small Animal Care 2022;3(1):39–55.

54. Morgan KRS, Stauthammer C, Stewart B, et al. Coronary arterial compression testing by simultaneous balloon valvuloplasty and coronary angiography in an English bulldog with pulmonary valve stenosis. J Vet Cardiol 2021;35:124–9.

55. Steadman CD, Clift PF, Thorne SA, et al. Treatment of dynamic subvalvar muscular obstruction in the native right ventricular outflow tract by percutaneous stenting in adults. Congenit Heart Dis 2009;4(6):494–8.

56. Castleberry CD, Gudausky TM, Berger S, et al. Stenting of the Right Ventricular Outflow Tract in the High-Risk Infant With Cyanotic Teratology of Fallot. Pediatr Cardiol 2014;35(3):423–30.

57. Danon S, Gray RG, Crystal MA, et al. Expansion Characteristics of Stents Used in Congenital Heart Disease: Serial Dilation Offers Improved Expansion Potential Compared to Direct Dilation: Results from a Pediatric Interventional Cardiology Early Career Society (PICES) Investigation. Congenit Heart Dis 2016;11(6):741–50.

58. Mikulak H, Morgan KRS, Fundingsland S, et al. Pulmonary artery dissection following pulmonary balloon valvuloplasty in dogs. J Vet Cardiol 2022;44:48–56.

59. Venczelova Z, Tittel P, Masura J. First experience with AndraStent XL implantation in children and adolescents with congenital heart diseases. Cathet Cardiovasc Interv 2013;81(1):103–10.

60. Masuda M. Postoperative residua and sequelae in adults with repaired tetralogy of Fallot. General thoracic and cardiovascular surgery 2016;64(7):373–9.

61. Lurz P, Bonhoeffer P, Taylor AM. Percutaneous pulmonary valve implantation: an update. Expert Rev Cardiovasc Ther 2009;7(7):823–33.

Treating Stubborn Cardiac Arrhythmias—Looking Toward the Future

Weihow Hsue, DVM, DACVIM (Cardiology)[a],*,
Allison L. Gagnon, DVM, MS, DACVIM (Cardiology)[b],*

KEYWORDS

- Veterinary • Tachycardia • Implantable cardioverter-defibrillator • Electrophysiology
- Catheter ablation • Electroanatomical mapping
- Stereotactic arrhythmia radiotherapy

KEY POINTS

- Implantable cardioverter-defibrillator devices can cardiovert or defibrillate tachyarrhythmias via antitachycardia pacing or delivery of high-energy shocks; however, programming issues in animals are still unresolved.
- Electrophysiological studies and catheter ablation have a proven track record of eliminating tachyarrhythmias, especially accessory pathway-mediated tachycardias, focal atrial tachycardia, and atrial flutter.
- Three-dimensional electroanatomical mapping integrates anatomic and electrophysiological data into a single three-dimensional reconstruction of the heart, facilitating direct visualization of activation wave fronts, low-voltage scar regions, and paced-matched electrocardiographic morphologies.
- Stereotactic arrhythmia radiotherapy delivers high-dose external-beam radiation to noninvasively ablate tachyarrhythmias but initial application in people is still being explored.

 Video content accompanies this article at http://www.vetsmall.theclinics.com.

Antiarrhythmic medications are the current mainstay of treatment of tachyarrhythmias in veterinary medicine, but many animals develop unacceptable side effects or remain refractory despite multidrug regimens.[1] Inadequate control contributes not only to persistent clinical signs and decreased quality of life, but also to progressive deterioration in heart function leading to a dilated cardiomyopathy phenotype (ie,

---

Both authors contributed equally in their author roles.
 a Department of Clinical Sciences, College of Veterinary Medicine, Cornell University, 930 Campus Road, Ithaca, NY 14853, USA; b Department of Medicine and Epidemiology, School of Veterinary Medicine, University of California – Davis, One Shields Avenue, Davis, CA 95616, USA
* Corresponding authors.
E-mail addresses: wh446@cornell.edu (W.H.); algagnon@ucdavis.edu (A.L.G.)

tachycardia-induced or arrhythmia-induced cardiomyopathy).[1] However, even if medications can reduce arrhythmia burden and clinical signs, they may not decrease the risk for sudden death. There is no evidence from randomized controlled human trials that antiarrhythmic medications, other than β-blockers, are effective at the primary or secondary prevention of sudden death.[2,3] Although comparable studies in veterinary patients have not been performed, sudden death is still known to occur in dogs receiving antiarrhythmic medications.[4] Pacemaker implantation is considered a routine procedure for veterinary patients with medically unresponsive bradyarrhythmias[5] but device and interventional therapies for tachyarrhythmias are underutilized despite being potential first-line options.[1,3] This review will highlight background information and potential veterinary applications of implantable cardioverter-defibrillators (ICDs), electrophysiological mapping and catheter ablation, three-dimensional electroanatomical mapping (EAM), and stereotactic arrhythmia radiotherapy (STAR).

IMPLANTABLE CARDIOVERTER-DEFIBRILLATOR

ICDs are a common treatment approach for people at high risk of sudden death, particularly from ventricular tachycardia (VT) and ventricular fibrillation (VF).[2,3] These devices continuously monitor the heart rhythm and, when faced with pathologic tachyarrhythmias, can intervene in 3 possible ways: antitachycardia pacing, cardioversion, or defibrillation.[6] Antitachycardia pacing involves delivering a short series of paced beats faster than the tachycardia cycle length to disrupt reentrant VT. This maneuver is not painful and is more effective at slower VT rates. In contrast, potentially painful high-energy shocks are delivered for cardioversion (eg, if antitachycardia pacing fails) and defibrillation. The shocks in the former are synchronized to avoid delivery during the vulnerable period to cardiovert VT to sinus rhythm, whereas the shocks in the latter are unsynchronized to rapidly defibrillate lethal VF (**Fig. 1**). Diseases treated by ICDs in people include nonischemic cardiomyopathies (eg, hypertrophic, dilated, and arrhythmogenic right ventricular cardiomyopathies), congestive heart failure with reduced ejection fraction, ion channel disorders, and VT or VF without a readily reversible cause.[2] Because the shocks can be painful and repeated shocks heighten the risk of psychological disorders and decreased quality of life, the devices should be programmed to limit inappropriate shocks.[2,6,7]

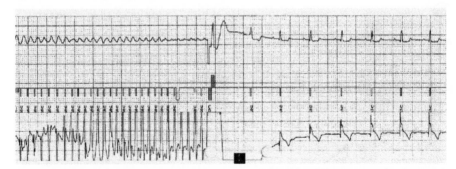

Fig. 1. Intraoperative testing of an ICD in a Boxer dog. The ventricle was rapidly paced, and then a shock was delivered on the T wave to induce VF. The top row is the surface lead II electrocardiogram, demonstrating VF initially. The bottom row illustrates intracardiac electrograms. The device successfully identified rapid ventricular sensed beats (VS) associated with VF and subsequently delivered a 30-J shock, which is indicated by the CD mark (cardioversion/defibrillation energy delivery). Sinus rhythm was restored thereafter. Paper speed: 25 mm/s. (*From* Nelson et al.[10]; with permission.)

These devices can be placed either subcutaneously or transvenously. The subcutaneous devices consist of a subcutaneous lead implanted near the sternum, which senses the underlying heart rhythm, and a pulse generator implanted in the left lateral thorax.[8] The shock is directed through the heart between the coil and the generator. These subcutaneous devices eliminate the risks associated with transvenous leads (eg, thromboembolism), but they are not able to perform antitachycardia pacing or cardiac pacing for bradyarrhythmias, which may be concurrent issues or occur after shock delivery.[8] The transvenous leads are placed in the heart and consist of an active or passive fixation tip with either 1 (single) or 2 (dual) defibrillation coils.[9] The shock can be directed between the coil and the generator or between the 2 coils in dual defibrillation coil devices.[9]

The use of ICD devices has been investigated experimentally in dogs for many years, with the first successful test in a dog occurring in 1969.[10,11] Although ICDs are not routinely placed in veterinary medicine, several case reports have investigated their use in client-owned dogs.[10,12,13] The ICD lead and generator have typically been implanted transvenously in the right ventricle and in the thoracic wall to allow for the current to travel across the heart.[10,13] Placement of the generator in the cervical region, as is typical for transvenous pacemakers, did not allow for successful defibrillation in at least one case.[13]

Unfortunately, programming issues have limited the efficacy of ICDs in dogs. First, although a 10 J safety margin above the tested defibrillation threshold (DFT) is recommended to ensure reliable shocks, all reported cases in dogs required programming to the maximum possible DFT.[10,12,13] This led to a Doberman dying due to failure of the device to terminate unstable VT despite delivering 6 high-energy shocks.[12] Because of this, another study evaluated different shock waveform configurations in 10 research dogs to see if one may lower the required DFT in healthy dogs to accommodate a safety margin. However, there was no statistically significant difference in mean DFT or the mean differences in voltage, energy, and impedance at the DFT for fixed-pulse or fixed-tilt configurations.[12] Newer ICDs can deliver higher energy shocks and thus may achieve appropriate safety margins, but this has not yet been investigated in dogs. Second, the delivery of inappropriate shocks has been reported to cause intense vocalization and distress in dogs.[10,13] Monitoring of the heart rhythm is dictated by human-based algorithms, so inappropriate shocks are easier to trigger in dogs because dogs have faster sinus rates and their QRS complexes and T waves are more similar in amplitude (and thus double counting of the T wave frequently occurs).[10,13] In order to reduce this risk, it is recommended to place the lead in an area where there is a 3-times difference between the R wave and T wave amplitudes.[10,13] However, despite adhering to these recommendations, sympathetic stimulation can lead to increases in T wave amplitude along with heart rate, which have led to inappropriate shocks being delivered during exercise.[10,13] These dogs have required multiple reprogrammings, and in one case, the owner elected to disable high-energy shock deliveries while retaining antitachycardia pacing capabilities because the shocks were so distressing.[10,13] Finally, dogs are at risk of infection of the device. Dogs in 2 reported cases developed septic inflammation that warranted the removal of the device.[10,13] Therefore, permanent reduction of tachyarrhythmias are preferred for dogs.

ELECTROPHYSIOLOGICAL STUDIES AND CATHETER ABLATION

Cardiac electrophysiology studies, in which catheters are inserted into the heart to record intracardiac electrograms, were first reported in dogs in 1993.[14] Unlike electrocardiograms that reflect whole surface electrical activity of the heart, intracardiac electrograms represent local electrical signals at a pinpoint site. Using fluoroscopy, catheters are placed in varied locations in the heart to record from multiple sites.[1] After induction of tachyarrhythmia, these recordings would allow the clinician to deduce the activation path based on the sequence in which intracardiac electrograms appear, which may reflect a focal origin or a macroreentry circuit.[1] This, along with additional strategies such as evaluation of electrogram morphology and pacing maneuvers, can be used to identify critical sites that originate and/or propagate the tachyarrhythmia. These sites are then targeted with radiofrequency catheter ablation.[1,15] Radiofrequency energy is delivered between the catheter tip and an indifferent electrode, usually an electrocautery-type grounding pad. Because energy in the radiofrequency portion of the energy spectrum is poorly conducted by cardiac tissue, radiofrequency energy causes resistive heating of the tissue at the catheter tip, resulting in irreversible cellular damage at high temperatures (ie, coagulation necrosis). This eliminates electrical activity at the target site and can terminate arrhythmias that depend on that site.[1] This technique has been successfully used for a variety of supraventricular tachycardias in dogs, including orthodromic atrioventricular reciprocating tachycardia (ie, accessory pathway-mediated tachycardia),[16,17] permanent junctional reciprocating tachycardia,[18] typical and atypical atrial flutter,[19–21] and focal atrial tachycardia.[22] In patients with atrial fibrillation that are refractory to rate-control medications, catheter ablation of the atrioventricular node with simultaneous placement of a permanent pacemaker is a palliative option to obtain rate control.[23] Successful use is more limited for ventricular arrhythmias, but it has been beneficial in English bulldogs with a focal area of aneurysmal tissue in the right ventricular outflow tract.[24]

Orthodromic atrioventricular reciprocating tachycardia has been the most common tachyarrhythmia treated by catheter ablation in dogs.[16,17] The reported long-term success rate with catheter ablation is high at ~97% to 98%.[16,17] Recurrence occurred in 3% to 8% of dogs, but these cases were successfully treated with a second procedure.[16,17] There is a low rate of major complications (5%–7%),[16,17] which included death during induction of general anesthesia, VF, and third-degree atrioventricular block. Minor complications include self-limiting hematoma at the femoral vein access site and transient first-degree and second-degree atrioventricular blocks. At this time, information on the treatment of the other tachyarrhythmias in dogs is mainly limited to small case series or case reports.

The major disadvantage of conventional electrophysiological studies is their reliance on fluoroscopy for anatomic positioning and catheter visualization. Because fluoroscopy captures the 3-dimensional shape of the heart onto a 2-dimensional image, it is difficult to determine the precise location of an intracardiac electrogram within the heart and returning to a previously investigated site depends on operator recall. Therefore, conventional mapping may be time-consuming and require large amounts of radiation exposure as catheters are continuously repositioned. Although conventional mapping is highly successful especially in guiding catheter ablation of discrete target sites, application in tachyarrhythmias with complex circuits, anatomy, and/or substrates proves more challenging.

THREE-DIMENSIONAL ELECTROANATOMICAL MAPPING

Three-dimensional EAM allows nonfluoroscopic integration of both anatomic and electrophysiological data into a single 3-dimensional reconstruction of the heart, combining precise geometry of heart chambers, display of electrical activation sequences and voltages of tissues, and real-time position and movement of intracardiac catheters. This technology has resulted in improved clinical outcomes in people with anatomically or electrically complex tachyarrhythmias.[25] Feasibility, safety, and potential complications have been documented in isolated reports involving laboratory dogs,[26] client-owned dogs,[27–29] and horses.[30,31]

Commercially available EAM systems include CARTO 3 (Biosense Webster, Diamond Bar, California), EnSite Precision and X (Abbott, Chicago, Illinois), and Rhythmia HDx (Boston Scientific, Cambridge, Massachusetts), all of which use a combination of magnetic-based and impedance-based technologies to achieve localization accuracy within a 1-mm margin of error.[25] The CARTO 3 system consists of a location pad (containing 3 low-level magnetic-field-emitting coils arranged as a triangle) placed under the patient table and 6 electrode patches positioned on the thorax (3 ventrally and 3 dorsally). A location sensor is embedded in the tip of specialized mapping catheters that can detect the magnetic field strength from each coil. Because the distance between the sensor and a coil is inversely proportional to the measured magnetic field strength, the distances between each of the 3 coils can be calculated to triangulate the position of the catheter.[32] Additionally, the system sends a small current across the catheter electrode and each of the 6 patch electrodes with distinct frequencies, creating a unique current ratio for each location in the heart. This impedance-based modality augments the accuracy of magnetic localization and enables respiratory motion compensation.[33] EnSite X is the newest EAM platform set to replace its predecessor, EnSite Precision. For impedance-based tracking, the EnSite systems uses 3 pairs of skin patches (positioned on the sides of the patient for the x-axis, on the chest and back for the y-axis, and the back of the neck and inner left thigh for the z-axis) and a system reference patch. The electrical current transmitted between the skin patches through the thorax causes a drop in voltage across the heart. Intracardiac catheters can then read the relative voltages and calculate an impedance gradient in relation to the reference electrode for localization. The Precision system later added 2 sensors and a magnetic field frame to incorporate magnetic-based tracking,[34] with the EnSite X continuing to use both technologies. For Rhythmia HDx, the magnetic tracking feature requires one sensor-coil-embedded back patch and a magnetic field generator under the patient's table, whereas the impedance field is generated by applying currents to the back patch, patches for the electrocardiographic limb leads, and the V_1, V_3, and V_6 chest leads.[35]

The value of EAM is its ability to portray electrophysiological data in a color-coded manner on an anatomic shell. This shell is constructed by aggregating all electrode locations associated with accepted beats, with the locations of the outermost electrodes defining the endocardial surface of a chamber. Additionally, anatomic data from computed tomography, MRI, and intracardiac echocardiography can be incorporated for more accurate and vivid anatomic descriptions (**Fig. 2**).[36] The electroanatomical maps include activation maps, voltage maps, and pace maps. Entrainment mapping is also commonly performed to delineate reentrant tachyarrhythmias and definitively locate the isthmus (slowly conductive myocardial tissue bordered by nonconductive tissue that represent a key site for perpetuation, and hence ablation, of a tachyarrhythmia), although the sites of interest are typically annotated onto activation maps.

Activation mapping displays the electrical activation sequence of a heart rhythm across the anatomic shell. At the mapping catheter tip, the steepest negative slope of the unipolar intracardiac electrogram and the first sharp peak of the bipolar intracardiac electrogram seem to correlate best with local depolarization.[37] The difference in time between these features and a fixed reference (time = 0 ms) is the local activation time (LAT); the reference can be derived from a surface electrocardiographic feature or an invariable intracardiac electrogram (eg, from a decapolar catheter wedged into the

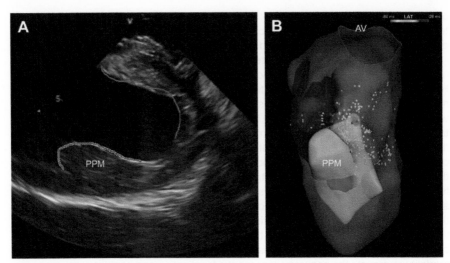

Fig. 2. Integration of intracardiac echocardiography to outline the posterior papillary muscle (PPM). (*A*) A long-axis image of the left ventricle obtained from intracardiac echocardiography is displayed in the CartoSound module on the CARTO 3 system. The PPM is traced and converted into an anatomic shell by the software; intracavitary structures are not normally seen on EAM because anatomic shells are derived from points obtained from the outermost surfaces of a cavity. (*B*) Anatomic shells of the left ventricle and the PPM are shown. The left ventricle is displayed from the posterior aspect and made 25% transparent. Each individual point signifies the LAT of an intracardiac electrogram, color-coded from red (≤-84 ms) to purple (≥-28 ms); the reference time was selected from a distinct notch on the surface QRS complexes (not shown). There is evidence of centrifugal activation starting from the tip of the PPM. Radiofrequency ablation targeting near the early activation eventually resulted in termination of the patient's frequent ventricular premature complexes. AV; aortic valve.

coronary sinus).[29] The EAM system can then graphically represent all the LATs by a static color-coded map or a video portraying a moving wave front of activation, facilitating visualization of the origin and/or path of tachyarrhythmias. A focal tachyarrhythmia is diagnosed when centrifugal spread occurs from a circumscribed site of early activation, and ablation is targeted to this earliest site of activation (see **Fig. 2**B and **Fig. 3**A). In contrast, a macroreentrant tachyarrhythmia is diagnosed when continuous activation, occurring throughout the cycle length, circles around conduction barriers to return to the earliest site of activation; ablation is then targeted at a vulnerable isthmus within the circuit (**Fig. 3**B; Video 1).[38] The main limitation of activation mapping is the requirement for ongoing hemodynamically tolerable tachyarrhythmia with a stable cycle length and morphology. General anesthesia may suppress arrhythmogenicity, so appropriate anesthetic drug selection is paramount to ensure inducibility of clinical arrhythmias.[39] VT in the context of structural heart disease and compromised heart function is particularly challenging because patient stability may preclude completion of activation maps.

Tachyarrhythmias, especially VT, in ischemic and nonischemic cardiomyopathies are usually caused by myocardial reentry in areas of patchy scar or at scar borders, where anisotropic conduction and unidirectional block frequently occur.[40] Substrate mapping assumes that surrogates for a reentrant isthmus, produced in the context of fixed barriers of inexcitable scar, can be recognized during sinus rhythm. Because

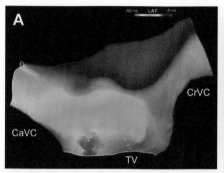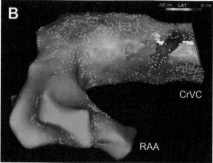

Fig. 3. Three-dimensional activation maps illustrating a focal rhythm and a reentrant rhythm in the right atrium. (*A*) The right atrium is seen from the right lateral aspect, with the cranial vena cava (CrVC), caudal vena cava (CaVC), and tricuspid valve (TV) orifice delineated. Each individual point signifies the LAT of an intracardiac electrogram, color-coded from red (≤ -52 ms) to purple (≥ -3 ms); the reference time was selected as the peak positive deflection on a coronary sinus intracardiac electrogram from a separate decapolar catheter (not shown). There is evidence of centrifugal activation from the posterolateral aspect of the right atrium bordering the tricuspid valve annulus. After ruling out atrioventricular accessory pathways, this was interpreted as focal atrial tachycardia. (From Hsue, et al.[29]; with permission.). (*B*) The right atrium is seen from the right lateral aspect, with the CrVC and right atrial appendage delineated. The higher density of points was acquired from multielectrode mapping as opposed to point-by-point mapping. The ranges of color encompass the entire cycle length (~ 180 ms). Again, the reference time was selected as the peak positive deflection on a coronary sinus intracardiac electrogram from a separate decapolar catheter (not shown). There is evidence of early-meets-late (red-meets-purple) activation, which is characteristic of reentry circuits. This is diagnostic of CrVC flutter.

this modality is not dependent on inducibility of sustained tachyarrhythmia, modern ablation strategies in people are increasingly reliant on substrate modification. Substrate mapping may involve identification of late or split potentials indicative of abnormal signal propagation and slow conduction[41] but it typically signifies voltage mapping (**Fig. 4**).[27] Scar is electrically inert and does not have a voltage. Rather, the admixture between collagen and surviving tissue is reflected as low-voltage areas; very low voltages represent dense scar with the greatest concentration and confluence of fibrosis. This was first validated in porcine postinfarction models and in human controls, where bipolar amplitudes less than 1.5 mV corresponded with gross anatomic scar in the ventricles.[42,43] The thresholds from these studies, where dense scar was defined as less than 0.5 mV and the border zone was defined as 0.5 to 1.5 mV, are universally implemented to represent scar regions in human clinical cases. Substrate mapping can also be applied to the atria; bipolar amplitudes of 0.2 to 0.45 mV correlate with scar in people who had undergone an earlier atrial fibrillation ablation.[44] However, substrate mapping has limitations. First, the exact voltage cutoffs in dogs are not described. Furthermore, electrogram voltages can be influenced by a variety of factors, including conduction velocity, fiber orientation and curvature, the relationship of fiber orientation to the propagating wave front, tissue contact, and characteristics of the recording catheter.[41] Finally, tachyarrhythmias may not always emanate from scar tissue even in those with structural heart disease. Therefore, other mapping techniques are ideally incorporated to further characterize the low-voltage scar regions.

Pace mapping is another modality that can circumvent the requirement for sustained tachyarrhythmias. It involves stimulating different endocardial sites and evaluating the

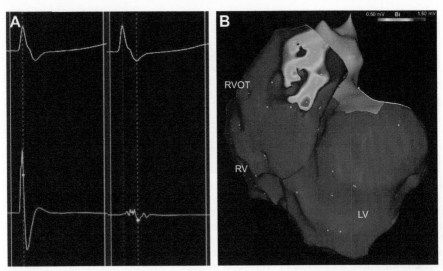

Fig. 4. Three-dimensional bipolar voltage map of the right and left ventricles in a Boxer. (A) The left and right panels contain a surface V$_2$ lead tracing on the top and a corresponding intracardiac ventricular electrogram on the bottom; the red and yellow dotted line represent annotations for LATs. The left panel demonstrates a normal bipolar (Bi) intracardiac electrogram. Note the sharp signals with ample amplitude, consistent with rapid and uniformly conducting myocardium. The right panel demonstrates a fractionated Bi electrogram. Note the diminished amplitude and multicomponent signals, consistent with both decreased number of conducting myocytes and multidirectional conduction characteristic of scar tissue. (B) The anterior surfaces of the right ventricle (RV) and left ventricle (LV) are shown. Each individual point on the heart signifies the Bi voltage amplitude of an intracardiac electrogram acquired during sinus rhythm, color-coded from red (≤0.5 mV) to purple (≥1.5 mV). This Boxer had suspected electroanatomic scar (Bi voltage areas <1.5 mV) at the anterior endocardial surface of the right ventricular outflow tract (RVOT), suggestive of arrhythmogenic right ventricular cardiomyopathy. (*From* Crooks et al.[27]).

resulting surface electrocardiographic morphologies, where the probability of obtaining an exact match with the clinical tachyarrhythmia morphology is inversely correlated with the distance between the paced site and the site of the focal arrhythmic origin (ie, a perfect match suggests that the paced site is the ideal ablation site). This is usually applied to VT as matching P′ wave morphologies for atrial tachycardias is more challenging. Computerized algorithms (eg, the PASO [PAce mapping SOftware] module on CARTO) allow quantification of the concordance between paced and spontaneous ventricular ectopic morphologies and the generation of "pace maps" with precise spatial localization, which can dramatically improve the precision of pace mapping **(Fig. 5)**.[28,45] However, it is important to recognize that concordance of QRS morphologies may be affected by pacing settings and structural limitations. For example, high pacing outputs may capture both "near" and "far" myocardium, altering the QRS morphology; the lowest possible output is thus recommended. Pacing at the VT cycle length is also advised as different rates may alter functional properties and the conduction profile. Additionally, origins in deep muscle may not be faithfully reproduced with endocardial pace mapping. Finally, QRS morphologies can differ in the presence of pathologic scar because radial impulse propagation from the catheter tip may not mimic a wave front emerging from an exit site, myocardial fusion of 2 or more wave

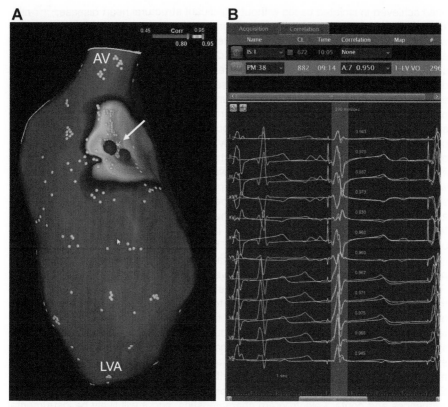

Fig. 5. Three-dimensional pace map of the left ventricle. (*A*) The left ventricle is shown from the right anterior surface. The color represents the percentage of correlation (correlation index or Corr) between ventricular complex morphologies of local paced-mapped signals (PM) and intrinsic ventricular premature complex signals (IS), ranging from purple (≤80%) to red (≥95%). The large red points symbolize the 2 ablation sites that resulted in the termination of the underlying ventricular arrhythmia. The white arrow points to the location (marked by an asterisk) with the highest correlation. (*B*) The PASO module, an automated template matching program associated with the CARTO 3 mapping system, has calculated a correlation index for the marked point in (*A*). Here, the morphologies of the 38th PM (PM:38, illustrated in green in the 12-lead electrocardiogram) and the 1st IS (IS:1, illustrated in yellow) are compared, with individual correlations calculated for each lead. The overall correlation is 0.950 or 95%. AV: aortic valve; LVA: left ventricular apex. (*From* Hsue et al.[28]; with permission.)

fronts from different exit sites may occur, or areas of functional block that facilitate reentry may be absent during pace mapping.[46]

Although 3D EAM has been used in human medicine for the last 2 decades, experience in companion animals is limited. The accuracy of EAM maps is not clinically validated in companion animals. Patient size is also a major limiting factor, as both the standard ablation catheters and the high-density mapping catheters of the major EAM systems are 7 to 8 French in size. Nevertheless, Hellemans and colleagues successfully mapped all 4 chambers during sinus rhythm using the CARTO system in 8 healthy beagles (11.2–15.7 kg), demonstrating that EAM can still be used for medium-sized dogs.[26] However, although resolution of the clinical arrhythmia has been achieved in isolated cases without significant structural heart disease,[28,29] clinical benefit in dogs with structural heart disease, the population most often presenting with significant tachyarrhythmias, is ultimately unknown. In 5 Boxers with symptomatic VT, only the number of VT runs showed consistent improvement following EAM and catheter ablation, whereas the total ventricular ectopic burden did not always decrease.[27] Additionally, structural heart diseases are often progressive and the benefits of these interventions on long-term survival are unclear. Importantly, the safety profile and possible complications of the procedures are not fully defined, given the small number of published cases. Most documented complications relate to intraoperative or immediate postoperative arrhythmias including tachyarrhythmias and even third-degree atrioventricular block, which were all self-limiting.[26,27] Pericardial effusion necessitating pericardiocentesis was observed in one case, although this was likely related to the atrial transseptal procedure performed.[26] Vascular access site bleeding and even an episode of retroperitoneal hemorrhage were documented, although this was likely contributed by the perioperative anticoagulants administered.[27] However, persistent pelvic limb lameness and new aortic regurgitation observed in one dog were complications that had more lasting consequences.[27] Nevertheless, no intraoperative or immediate postoperative deaths have been reported thus far, and safety will likely improve as more experience is accumulated.

Although EAM can increase spatial understanding of tachyarrhythmias in relation to the anatomy, it is still paramount to adhere to basic electrophysiological principles to navigate the limitations of each mapping technique. Integrating multiple mapping techniques will also compensate for individual weaknesses. For example, the origin sites of focal tachyarrhythmias are often characterized by fractionated electrograms even in the absence of structural heart disease,[22] and pursuing these characteristics may further refine potential target sites identified on activation mapping. Nevertheless, EAM facilitates visualization and intuitive comprehension of intracardiac electrogram sequences and contact electrogram characteristics, and it will likely be instrumental in successful ablation of anatomically and electrically complex arrhythmias.

STEREOTACTIC ARRHYTHMIA RADIOTHERAPY

Noninvasive ablation of VT secondary to structural heart disease using stereotactic body radiation therapy has been gaining traction in human medicine.[47,48] STAR delivers precise high-dose external-beam radiation to the underlying arrhythmogenic substrate while minimizing damage to normal adjacent tissue. It can overcome inherent limitations of catheter ablation, particularly if the arrhythmogenic site is located deep within the myocardium or on the epicardial surface where endocardial ablation is difficult to reach. Preclinical evidence suggests that clinical radiation doses (namely 25 Gy) increase electrical coupling and conduction velocity in the heart by enhancing conduction protein function and expression (eg, sodium channels and gap junctions).[49] As such, restoration of electrical conduction may represent a new paradigm in antiarrhythmic treatment.

Although STAR is appealing because of its noninvasive nature, many technical aspects are not established in veterinary medicine. The biggest challenges are as follows: (1) how to precisely define the target sites and (2) how to accurately deliver radiation therapy in relation to cardiac and respiratory motions. In humans, multiple modalities are used to delineate the arrhythmogenic substrate, both structurally and electrically. Because scar-related reentry is the major mechanism for VT secondary to ischemic and nonischemic cardiomyopathies, structural scar is the main target and can be outlined using radionuclide imaging, computed tomography, and/or

MRI.[47,48] Because not all scar tissue is arrhythmogenic, refining the electrical substrate within the scar is accomplished using minimally invasive EAM or noninvasive electrocardiographic imaging. Electrocardiographic imaging uses body surface electrodes to map epicardial potentials, electrograms, and activation sequences onto a cardiac computed tomography scan.[50] However, none of these diagnostics is routine in veterinary medicine. Furthermore, compensation for both cardiac and respiratory motions is not often performed for existing stereotactic body radiation therapies in veterinary practice. In summary, although significant technical gaps need to be addressed, STAR has become a promising novel treatment of refractory VT in humans and may offer the same for veterinary species.

SUMMARY

Device and interventional therapies are available for veterinary patients that cannot tolerate or are refractory to antiarrhythmic medications. Implantable cardioverter-defibrillators can reduce the likelihood of sudden death, although improvements in shock delivery and programming are needed. Catheter ablation has been successful in eliminating tachyarrhythmias in veterinary patients, and EAM may further improve visualization and treatment of complex tachyarrhythmias. Stereotactic arrhythmia radiotherapy may promise noninvasive termination of tachyarrhythmias, but this is just beginning to be investigated in people.

DISCLOSURE

Authors declare no conflict of interest.

ACKNOWLEDGMENTS

The authors would like to thank Drs Cory Tschabrunn, Anna Gelzer, and Roberto Santilli for their indispensable roles in obtaining the 3-dimensional EAM images.

SUPPLEMENTARY DATA

Supplementary data related to this article can be found online at https://doi.org/10.1016/j.cvsm.2023.06.003.

REFERENCES

1. Wright KN, Knilans TK, Irvin HM. When, why, and how to perform cardiac radio-frequency catheter ablation. J Vet Cardiol 2006;8(2):95–107.
2. Passman R, Kadish A. Sudden death prevention with implantable devices. Circulation 2007;116(5):561–71.
3. Al-Khatib SM, Stevenson WG, Ackerman MJ, et al. 2017 AHA/ACC/HRS guideline for management of patients with ventricular arrhythmias and the prevention of sudden cardiac death: A report of the American College of Cardiology/American Heart Association Task Force on Clinical Practice Guidelines and the Heart Rhythm Society. J Am Coll Cardiol 2018;72(14):e91–220.
4. Santilli R, Saponaro V, Carlucci L, et al. Heart rhythm characterization during sudden cardiac death in dogs. J Vet Cardiol 2021;38:18–30.
5. Santilli RA, Giacomazzi F, Porteiro Vázquez DM, et al. Indications for permanent pacing in dogs and cats. J Vet Cardiol 2019;22:20–39.
6. Miller JD, Yousuf O, Berger RD. The implantable cardioverter-defibrillator: An update. Trends Cardiovasc Med 2015;25(7):606–11.

7. Sears SF, Hauf JD, Kirian K, et al. Posttraumatic stress and the implantable cardioverter-defibrillator patient what the electrophysiologist needs to know. Circ Arrhythm Electrophysiol 2011;4(2):242–50.

8. Schukro C, Santer D, Prenner G, et al. State-of-the-art consensus on non-transvenous implantable cardioverter-defibrillator therapy. Clin Cardiol 2020; 43(10):1084–92.

9. Borne RT, Varosy P, Lan Z, et al. Trends in use of single- vs. dual-chamber implantable cardioverter-defibrillators among patients without a pacing indication, 2010-2018. JAMA Netw Open 2022;5(3):e223429.

10. Nelson OL, Lahmers S, Schneider T, et al. The use of an implantable cardioverter defibrillator in a Boxer dog to control clinical signs of arrhythmogenic right ventricular cardiomyopathy. J Vet Intern Med 2006;20(5):1232–7.

11. Mower MM. Implantable cardioverter defibrillator therapy: 15 years experience and future expectations. In the beginning: from dogs to humans. Pacing Clin Electrophysiol 1995;18(3 Pt 2):506–11.

12. Pariaut R, Saelinger C, Vila J, et al. Evaluation of shock waveform configuration on the defibrillation capacity of implantable cardioverter defibrillators in dogs. J Vet Cardiol 2012;14(3):389–98.

13. Pariaut R, Saelinger C, Queiroz-Williams P, et al. Implantable cardioverter-defibrillator in a German shepherd dog with ventricular arrhythmias. J Vet Cardiol 2011;13(3):203–10.

14. Scherlag BJ, Wang X, Nakagawa H, et al. Radiofrequency ablation of a concealed accessory pathway as treatment for incessant supraventricular tachycardia in a dog. J Am Vet Med Assoc 1993;203(8):1147–52.

15. Wright KN. Interventional catheterization for tachyarrhythmias. Vet Clin North Am Small Anim Pract 2004;34(5):1171–85.

16. Santilli RA, Mateos Pañero M, Porteiro Vázquez DM, et al. Radiofrequency catheter ablation of accessory pathways in the dog: the Italian experience (2008–2016). J Vet Cardiol 2018;20(5):384–97.

17. Wright KN, Connor CE, Irvin HM, et al. Atrioventricular accessory pathways in 89 dogs: Clinical features and outcome after radiofrequency catheter ablation. J Vet Intern Med 2018;32(5):1517–29.

18. Santilli RA, Santos LFN, Perego M. Permanent junctional reciprocating tachycardia in a dog. J Vet Cardiol 2013;15(3):225–30.

19. Santilli RA, Ramera L, Perego M, et al. Radiofrequency catheter ablation of atypical atrial flutter in dogs. J Vet Cardiol 2014;16(1):9–17.

20. Battaia S, Perego M, Santilli R. Radiofrequency catheter ablation of cranial vena cava flutter in four dogs. J Vet Cardiol 2021;36:123–30.

21. Santilli RA, Perego M, Perini A, et al. Radiofrequency catheter ablation of cavotricuspid isthmus as treatment of atrial flutter in two dogs. J Vet Cardiol 2010; 12(1):59–66.

22. Santilli RA, Perego M, Perini A, et al. Electrophysiologic characteristics and topographic distribution of focal atrial tachycardias in dogs. J Vet Intern Med 2010; 24(3):539–45.

23. Wright KN, Bright JM, Cox JW, et al. Transcatheter modification of the atrioventricular node in dogs, using radiofrequency energy. Am J Vet Res 1996;57(2): 229–35.

24. Santilli RA, Bontempi LV, Perego M. Ventricular tachycardia in English bulldogs with localised right ventricular outflow tract enlargement. J Small Anim Pract 2011;52(11):574–80.

25. Kim YH, Chen SA, Ernst S, et al. 2019 APHRS expert consensus statement on three-dimensional mapping systems for tachycardia developed in collaboration with HRS, EHRA, and LAHRS. J Arrhythm 2020;36(2):215–70.

26. Hellemans A, Van Steenkiste G, Boussy T, et al. Feasibility and safety of three-dimensional electroanatomical cardiac mapping, mapping-guided biopsy and transseptal puncture in dogs. J Vet Cardiol 2022;44:23–37.

27. Crooks AV, Hsue W, Tschabrunn CM, et al. Feasibility of electroanatomic mapping and radiofrequency catheter ablation in Boxer dogs with symptomatic ventricular tachycardia. J Vet Intern Med 2022;36(3):886–96.

28. Hsue W, Huh T, Gelzer AR, et al. Three-dimensional electroanatomic mapping and radiofrequency catheter ablation of ventricular arrhythmia in a dog without structural heart disease. J Vet Cardiol 2022;39:14–21.

29. Hsue W, Gelzer AR, Tschabrunn CM. Three-dimensional activation maps of sinus rhythm and focal atrial tachycardia in a dog. J Vet Cardiol 2022;44:43–7.

30. Van Steenkiste G, De Clercq D, Boussy T, et al. Three dimensional ultra-high-density electro-anatomical cardiac mapping in horses: methodology. Equine Vet J 2020;52(5):765–72.

31. Van Steenkiste G, Boussy T, Duytschaever M, et al. Detection of the origin of atrial tachycardia by 3D electro-anatomical mapping and treatment by radiofrequency catheter ablation in horses. J Vet Intern Med 2022;36(4):1481–90.

32. Gepstein L, Hayam G, Ben-Haim SA. A novel method for nonfluoroscopic catheter-based electroanatomical mapping of the heart. Circulation 1997;95(6):1611–22.

33. Jiang Y, Farina D, Bar-Tal M, et al. An impedance-based catheter positioning system for cardiac mapping and navigation. IEEE Trans Biomed Eng 2009;56(8):1963–70.

34. Lin C, Pehrson S, Jacobsen PK, et al. Initial experience of a novel mapping system combined with remote magnetic navigation in the catheter ablation of atrial fibrillation. J Cardiovasc Electrophysiol 2017;28(12):1387–92.

35. Nakagawa H, Ikeda A, Sharma T, et al. Rapid high resolution electroanatomical mapping evaluation of a new system in a canine atrial linear lesion model. Circ Arrhythm Electrophysiol 2012;5(2):417–24.

36. Finlay MC, Hunter RJ, Baker V, et al. A randomised comparison of Cartomerge vs. NavX fusion in the catheter ablation of atrial fibrillation: The CAVERN trial. J Interv Card Electrophysiol 2012;33(2):161–9.

37. Paul T, Moak JP, Morris C, et al. Epicardial mapping: How to measure local activation? Pacing Clin Electrophysiol 1990;13(3):285–92.

38. Shah DC, Jaïs P, Haïssaguerre M, et al. Three-dimensional mapping of the common atrial flutter circuit in the right atrium. Circulation 1997;96(11):3904–12.

39. Vladinov G, Fermin L, Longini R, et al. Choosing the anesthetic and sedative drugs for supraventricular tachycardia ablations: A focused review. Pacing Clin Electrophysiol 2018;41(11):1555–63.

40. Ciaccio EJ, Ashikaga H, Kaba RA, et al. Model of reentrant ventricular tachycardia based on infarct border zone geometry predicts reentrant circuit features as determined by activation mapping. Heart Rhythm 2007;4(8):1034–45.

41. Josephson ME, Anter E. Substrate mapping for ventricular tachycardia Assumptions and misconceptions. JACC Clin Electrophysiol 2015;1(5):341–52.

42. Callans DJ, Ren JF, Michele J, et al. Electroanatomic left ventricular mapping in the porcine model of healed anterior myocardial infarction: Correlation with intracardiac echocardiography and pathological analysis. Circulation 1999;100(6):1744–50.

43. Marchlinski FE, Callans DJ, Gottlieb CD, et al. Linear ablation lesions for control of unmappable ventricular tachycardia in patients with ischemic and. nonischemic cardiomyopathy 2000;101(11):1288–96.

44. Kapa S, Desjardins B, Callans DJ, et al. Contact electroanatomic mapping derived voltage criteria for characterizing left atrial scar in patients undergoing ablation for atrial fibrillation. J Cardiovasc Electrophysiol 2014;25(10):1044–52.

45. Moak JP, Sumihara K, Swink J, et al. Ablation of the vanishing PVC, facilitated by quantitative morphology-matching software. Pacing Clin Electrophysiol 2017; 40(11):1227–33.

46. Tung R, Mathuria N, Michowitz Y, et al. Functional pace-mapping responses for identification of targets for catheter ablation of scar-mediated ventricular tachycardia. Circ Arrhythm Electrophysiol 2012;5(2):264–72.

47. Robinson CG, Samson PP, Moore KMS, et al. Phase I/II trial of electrophysiology-guided noninvasive cardiac radioablation for ventricular tachycardia. Circulation 2019;139(3):313–21.

48. Carbucicchio C, Andreini D, Piperno G, et al. Stereotactic radioablation for the treatment of ventricular tachycardia: preliminary data and insights from the STRA-MI-VT phase Ib/II study. J Interv Card Electrophysiol 2021;62(2):427–39.

49. Zhang DM, Navara R, Yin T, et al. Cardiac radiotherapy induces electrical conduction reprogramming in the absence of transmural fibrosis. Nat Commun 2021;12(1):5558.

50. Cluitmans MJM, Bonizzi P, Karel JMH, et al. In vivo validation of electrocardiographic imaging. JACC Clin Electrophysiol 2017;3(3):232–42.

The Role of Point-of-Care Ultrasound in Managing Cardiac Emergencies

Jessica L. Ward, DVM, DACVIM (Cardiology)[a],*,
Teresa C. DeFrancesco, DVM, DACVIM (Cardiology), DACVECC[b]

KEYWORDS

- Echocardiography • Congestive heart failure • Respiratory distress
- Pulmonary edema • Ascites • Pleural effusion • Pericardial effusion
- Cardiac tamponade

KEY POINTS

- In a dog with respiratory distress, point-of-care ultrasound (POCUS) findings of diffuse B-lines and severe left atrial enlargement provide corroborative evidence for left-sided congestive heart failure (CHF).
- In a cat with respiratory distress, POCUS findings of severe left atrial enlargement along with diffuse B-lines, pleural effusion, or pericardial effusion are supportive of CHF.
- In a dog with ascites, the POCUS findings of a distended, nonfluctuating caudal vena cava and right heart enlargement provide corroborative evidence for right-sided CHF. POCUS findings of severe right heart enlargement and hypertrophy are indicative of right heart pressure overload, possibly related to pulmonary hypertension.
- POCUS is useful in the diagnosis, treatment, and monitoring of pericardial effusion and cardiac tamponade. The finding of an anechoic ring of fluid around the heart, right atrial collapse, and a distended nonfluctuating caudal vena cava is diagnostic for pericardial effusion with cardiac tamponade and an indication for a therapeutic pericardiocentesis.
- POCUS can be used to monitor resolution (and detect recurrence) of CHF by tracking presence and extent of B-lines or cavitary effusion.

INTRODUCTION

Point-of-care ultrasound (POCUS) is commonly used in emergency settings[1] to expedite the diagnosis and treatment of cardiac emergencies and is usually performed by providers who are not imaging specialists.[2–4] Unlike complete echocardiography or

[a] Department of Veterinary Clinical Sciences, College of Veterinary Medicine, Iowa State University, 1809 South Riverside Drive, Ames, IA 50010, USA; [b] Department of Clinical Sciences, College of Veterinary Medicine, North Carolina State University, 1052 William Moore Drive, Raleigh, NC 27607, USA
* Corresponding author.
E-mail address: jward@iastate.edu

Vet Clin Small Anim 53 (2023) 1429–1443
https://doi.org/10.1016/j.cvsm.2023.05.017
0195-5616/23/© 2023 Elsevier Inc. All rights reserved.

abdominal ultrasonography, POCUS is a time-sensitive examination involving a select subset of targeted views to identify severe abnormalities relevant to a patient's current clinical status. Thoracic POCUS for cardiac emergencies includes interrogation of the heart, lungs, pleural space, and caudal vena cava (CVC). The goal is to identify cardiovascular disease severe enough to cause emergent clinical signs (dyspnea, tachypnea, syncope, and cavitary effusions), and to use this information in combination with signalment, history, and physical examination to prioritize relevant differential diagnoses and expedite emergency treatment. In small animals, POCUS is most helpful in the diagnosis and monitoring of left-sided or right-sided congestive heart failure (L-CHF or R-CHF) and pericardial effusion with cardiac tamponade.

Studies in humans have shown that the use of POCUS in acutely decompensated heart failure allowed earlier directed therapy (18 hours on average) and reduced length of hospital stay.[5] There is good evidence to suggest that identification of several conditions by POCUS techniques is easy to learn with good repeatability. With minimal didactic and hands-on ultrasound training, noncardiologist and nonradiologist veterinarians can achieve proficiency in identifying pleural and pericardial effusions and detecting the presence of left atrial enlargement.[6] Thoracic POCUS is also less stressful than thoracic radiography for an animal in respiratory distress. Animals can be provided flow-by oxygen and maintained in sternal recumbency during the POCUS examination. Portable ultrasound has essentially become an extension of the triage examination in emergency settings. Improved diagnostic accuracy compared to the cardiac physical examination alone is the reason why POCUS has been coined the "visual stethoscope of the 21st century."[7]

IMAGE ACQUISITION AND RECOGNIZING NORMAL ANATOMY

Ultrasound machines used for POCUS imaging in cardiac emergency settings are typically smaller, portable devices ranging in size from hand-held devices (with limited technical capabilities) to small cart-based ultrasound platforms (usually with some advanced imaging options). Major differences between complete echocardiography and thoracic POCUS are patient positioning (sternal or standing are often safer for dogs and cats in a triage setting) and transducer selection (microconvex is often more available for POCUS). Although thoracic POCUS provides useful information in many emergency patients that can be immediately integrated into a clinical picture, technical factors related to patient size and body condition, suboptimal image enhancement, and limited artifact reduction capabilities may limit the ability to acquire clinically useful images.[8] For example, it would be challenging to image an obese Rottweiler in respiratory distress using a standard midrange frequency microconvex probe. Awareness of the limitations of portable ultrasound machines is important.

Several acoustic windows facilitate key standard views of the heart, lungs, pleural space, and pericardium. For imaging of the heart, the right parasternal acoustic window (located on the right hemithorax where the apex heartbeat is palpated) is used to obtain a short-axis view of the left ventricle (LV) just below the mitral valve (mushroom view), a short-axis view at the level of the heart base (left atrium [LA] to aorta [Ao], or LA:Ao view), and a long-axis view of all 4 heart chambers (4-chamber view). These standard cardiac views are important for qualitative evaluation of cardiac chamber size and function. For lung ultrasound, several different protocols have been described, including Vet BLUE (4 sites on each hemithorax, corresponding to radiographic lung quadrants),[9–11] a vertical sliding scanning approach through 6 intercostal spaces (18 sites on each hemithorax),[12] and modifications thereof.[13] Sites for lung ultrasound imaging are also interrogated for pleural or pericardial effusions, as described in the traditional thoracic focused assessment with sonography for trauma protocol in dogs and cats.[14] The subxiphoid window facilitates the imaging of the CVC [15,16] and provides an additional opportunity to assess possible pericardial or pleural effusions.

Table 1 lists expected findings in standard thoracic POCUS views of the heart, lung, and pleural and pericardial spaces. Examples of standard POCUS cardiac views from normal dogs are shown in **Fig. 1**. The primary goals of POCUS for cardiac emergencies are qualitative ("eyeball") assessments of the presence or absence of pericardial and pleural effusion, presence or absence of abnormal lung ultrasound artifacts, subjective size and function of cardiac chambers, and subjective size and collapsibility of the CVC.

SEVERE LEFT HEART DISEASE AND LEFT-SIDED CONGESTIVE HEART FAILURE IN DOGS

L-CHF in dogs occurs most commonly secondary to myxomatous mitral valve disease (MMVD) or dilated cardiomyopathy (DCM). In dogs, L-CHF manifests almost exclusively as pulmonary edema (fluid accumulation within the lungs), which is visible on lung ultrasound as B-line artifacts. B-lines result from the juxtaposition of air with small fluid-filled alveoli (less than ultrasound resolution threshold) and provide evidence for alveolar-interstitial syndromes such as cardiogenic pulmonary edema.[17,18] B-lines are visible ultrasonographically as discrete narrow-based vertical hyperechoic artifacts that extend from the pleural-pulmonary interface to the far aspect of the ultrasound screen without fading, and more synchronously with respiration.[9,11] An example lung ultrasound image showing B-lines is shown in **Fig. 2**.

Findings on POCUS that support a diagnosis of L-CHF include (1) evidence of severe left heart disease and (2) numerous and multifocal B-lines on lung ultrasound (see **Fig. 2**, **Table 2**). Generally, dogs with L-CHF will have severe LA dilation visible on right parasternal short-axis heart base views (with LA:Ao ratio usually >2:1). Dogs with clinical signs of L-CHF typically have multiple sites with numerous B-lines per intercostal space (termed "strong positive" sites), often with diffuse distribution of infinite coalescing B-lines at all lung ultrasound sites.[11,19]

Additional POCUS findings supportive of L-CHF will differ based on the underlying cardiac disease. Advanced MMVD is most common in older small-breed dogs; additional POCUS features include LV volume overload (eccentric hypertrophy) with normal to hyperdynamic LV systolic function.[20] DCM is more common in middle-aged large breed dogs or dogs with history of nontraditional diet consumption[21,22]; the most salient additional POCUS features are severe LV dilation with severely decreased LV systolic function.[23,24]

POCUS findings should always be integrated with patient signalment, history, and physical examination findings when considering a diagnosis of L-CHF. A small breed dog presenting for acute tachypnea with a loud left apical systolic heart murmur whose POCUS reveals severe LA enlargement and multifocal B-lines can be confidently treated for L-CHF (presumed MMVD). A small breed dog without a heart murmur is *highly unlikely* to have L-CHF, regardless of POCUS findings. A dog with normal respiratory rate and effort and no B-lines on POCUS is *highly unlikely* to have L-CHF, regardless of severity of LA dilation.

SEVERE HEART DISEASE AND CONGESTIVE HEART FAILURE IN CATS

Cats in CHF can be challenging to diagnosis because their physical examination and radiographic findings are nonspecific and variable.[25,26] Additionally, cats in respiratory distress can be extremely fragile, which limits the diagnostic evaluation. The POCUS

Table 1
Transducer sites and cardiac views for point-of-care ultrasound in dogs and cats, structures evaluated at each view, and normal cardiac anatomy to recognize

Site + View or Technique	Structures Evaluated	Normal Structure and Function
Right parasternal short-axis at the level of LV just below the mitral valve (mushroom view)	LV size LV wall thickness LV systolic function RV size	LV size in diastole: subjective or weight-based normal values LV wall thickness: subjective LV systolic function: subjective RV should be small crescent shape Interventricular septum should be rounded (not flattened)
Right parasternal short-axis at the heart base (LA:Ao view)	LA size MPA size	LA:Ao ≈ 1:1 (severe dilation if > 2:1) MPA:Ao ≈ 1:1
Right parasternal long-axis 4-chamber (4-chamber view)	RA and RV size LA and LV size LV systolic function	LA ≈ RA size with neutral interatrial septum position LV 3-4× size and thickness of RV LV should be bullet-shaped (not round) LV systolic function: subjective
Lung and pleural space (various protocols)	Pulmonary-pleural interface Lung ultrasound artifacts Presence of pericardial or pleural effusion	Intact pulmonary-pleural interface; glide sign with respiration A-lines; single isolated B-line can be normal No evidence of pericardial or pleural effusion
Subxiphoid sagittal CVC	CVC size CVC collapsibility Hepatic veins	CVC maximal diameter (compared with weight-based normal values) $CVC_{max}:Ao < 0.6$ CVC collapsibility >30% Hepatic veins should not be prominent

Abbreviations: Ao, aorta; CVC, caudal vena cava; LA, left atrium; LV, left ventricle; MPA, main pulmonary artery; RA, right atrium; RV, right ventricle.

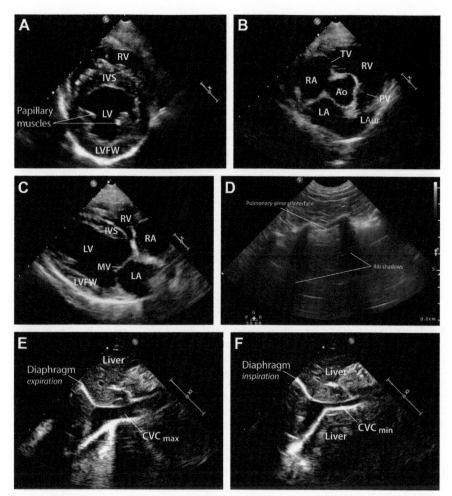

Fig. 1. POCUS images in normal dogs. (*A*) Right parasternal short-axis LV (mushroom) view. (*B*) Right parasternal short-axis image at the heart base (LA:Ao view). (*C*) Right parasternal long-axis (4-chamber) view. (*D*) Lung ultrasound from the left middle Vet BLUE site. (*E*) Subxiphoid CVC image of a normal dog on expiration, demonstrating maximal CVC diameter. (*F*) Subxiphoid CVC image of a normal dog on inspiration, demonstrating minimum CVC diameter. Ao, aorta; CVC, caudal vena cava; IVS, interventricular septum; LA, left atrium; LAur, left auricle; LV, left ventricle; LVFW, left ventricular free wall; MV, mitral valve; PV, pulmonic valve; RA, right atrium; RV, right ventricle; RV, right ventricle; TV, tricuspid valve.

examination provides a low-stress and extremely helpful diagnostic tool for the diagnosis of CHF in cats. Regardless of the underlying cause, CHF in cats can manifest as any combination of pulmonary edema, pleural effusion, pericardial and, to a lesser extent, peritoneal effusion. Several studies suggest that in cats with respiratory signs, an increased LA size identified by ultrasound (even subjectively assessed) strongly suggests a diagnosis of CHF.[27–29] In an ER setting, most cats with CHF will have a markedly enlarged LA:Ao ratio (>2:1) (**Fig. 3**). However, some cats with CHF may only have a mildly to moderately enlarged LA, especially if CHF was precipitated by a stressful event.

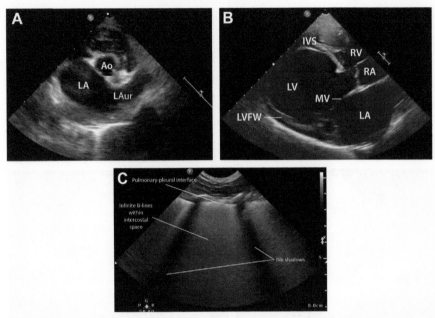

Fig. 2. POCUS images of dogs with severe left heart disease and L-CHF. (*A*) Right parasternal short-axis image at the heart base (LA:Ao view) in a dog with L-CHF secondary to severe MMVD, demonstrating severe left atrial enlargement. (*B*) Right parasternal long-axis 4-chamber image in a dog with severe MMVD, demonstrating severe left atrial and left ventricular dilation. (*C*) Lung ultrasound of the left middle lung lobe site in a dog with L-CHF demonstrating coalescing infinite B-lines between rib shadows within each intercostal space. Ao, aorta; IVS, interventricular septum; LA, left atrium; LAur, left auricle; LV, left ventricle; LVFW, left ventricular free wall; RV, right ventricle.

POCUS findings that would corroborate CHF in a symptomatic cat with an enlarged LA include the presence of B-lines or cavitary effusions, especially pericardial effusion (see **Fig. 3**). In one study of cats with respiratory distress, even a small amount of pericardial effusion was 100% specific for a diagnosis of CHF,[27] and CHF is the most common cause of pericardial effusion in cats.[30] Pleural effusion is common in cats with CHF, in contrast to dogs. The appearance of pleural effusion in CHF is typically anechoic angular spaces surrounding the heart and lungs. Fluid is visualized between the lung lobes often with fibrin strands floating within the fluid. The space in the ventral thorax caudal to the heart and cranial to the liver (see **Fig. 3**) is a particularly useful area to scan for pleural effusion, given that effusion depends on gravity. In large volume pleural effusion, the lung lobes are often compressed by the fluid causing consolidation of the lung. In the previously mentioned POCUS study of cats in respiratory distress,[27] nearly 80% of cats in CHF had some degree of pleural effusion, ranging from scant to large volume requiring a therapeutic thoracocentesis. POCUS is helpful to assess the volume of pleural effusion and subsequently the risk versus benefit of performing centesis. Similar to dogs, B-lines are also often present in cats with CHF. As described previously, B-lines are suggestive of fluid within the pulmonary interstitium or alveoli and are highly suggestive of pulmonary edema when integrated with the other clinical data. The distribution of strongly positive B-line sites is usually diffuse if the cat's main manifestation of CHF is pulmonary edema. However, if there is large volume pleural effusion, then the distribution of B-lines can vary.

Table 2
Point-of-care ultrasound findings supportive of cardiovascular disease as the cause of emergent clinical signs in dogs and cats

Cardiovascular Disease	Compatible Clinical Signs	Supportive POCUS Findings	Differential Diagnoses
Left-sided congestive heart failure (dogs)	• Dyspnea • Tachypnea • Syncope	• Severe left atrial dilation • Strong positive B-line sites on lung ultrasound • ± Severe left ventricular dilation • ± Severe left ventricular systolic dysfunction	• MMVD • DCM
Congestive heart failure (cats)	• Dyspnea • Tachypnea	• Severe left atrial dilation • ± Left ventricular concentric hypertrophy • Strong positive B-lines on lung ultrasound and/or • Pleural effusion and/or • Small-volume pericardial effusion	• HCM
Right-sided congestive heart failure (dogs and cats)	• Cavitary effusions (ascites > pleural effusion) • Syncope	• Severe right atrial/ventricular dilation • Distended CVC with decreased collapsibility • ± Right ventricular hypertrophy • ± Interventricular septal flattening	• Pulmonary arterial hypertension (see next row) • Tricuspid valve dysplasia • Pulmonic stenosis • Myxomatous tricuspid valve disease
Pulmonary arterial hypertension (dogs)	• Dyspnea • Tachypnea • Syncope	• Right ventricular dilation and hypertrophy • Interventricular septal flattening • Main pulmonary artery dilation • ± Distended caudal vena cava with decreased collapsibility	• Heartworm disease • Pulmonary thromboembolism • Chronic bronchopulmonary disease
Pericardial effusion and tamponade (dogs)	• Syncope/collapse • ± Ascites	• Variable volume pericardial effusion • Right atrial/ventricular diastolic collapse • Distended CVC with decreased collapsibility • ± Ascites • ± Gallbladder halo sign	• Cardiac neoplasia (right atrium/auricle or heart base) • Idiopathic pericarditis • Left atrial rupture

Abbreviations: CVC, caudal vena cava; DCM, dilated cardiomyopathy; HCM, hypertrophic cardiomyopathy; MMVD, myxomatous mitral valve disease.

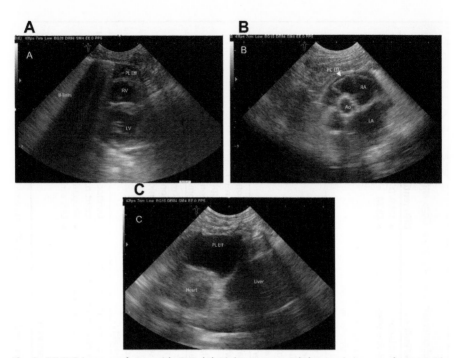

Fig. 3. POCUS images of cats with CHF. (*A*) Right parasternal short-axis image of a cat with CHF secondary to HCM, demonstrating segmental left ventricular hypertrophy, small volume pleural effusion, and B-lines representing cardiogenic pulmonary edema. (*B*) Right parasternal short-axis image at the level of the heart base in a cat with CHF demonstrating an increased LA:Ao ratio and scant pericardial effusion (*arrowhead*). (*C*) Ultrasound view from the right caudoventral thorax fanning dorsally in a cat with CHF, demonstrating a moderate volume of pleural effusion. Ao, aorta; LA, left atrium; LV, left ventricle; PC Eff, pericardial effusion; PL Eff, pleural effusion; RA, right atrium; RV, right ventricle.

In a cat with CHF secondary to hypertrophic cardiomyopathy (HCM), LV concentric hypertrophy will be seen together with an enlarged LA. An LV diastolic wall thickness of greater than 6 mm is generally defined as LV hypertrophy.[31] If present, LV hypertrophy can be either diffuse or segmental. Some cats with end-stage HCM may experience wall thinning over time.

Cats with cardiomyopathy and severe LA dilation are also at risk for thrombus formation and arterial thromboembolism. The POCUS examination may identify spontaneous echocontrast (smoke) or a thrombus within the enlarged LA of a cat with severe cardiomyopathy or CHF. Thrombi are most commonly seen in the left auricle and can be adhered to the atrial wall or freely mobile. Shadow artifacts can often be overinterpreted as thrombi; thrombi typically have sharply defined borders. The finding of an LA thrombus worsens the cat's prognosis.

SEVERE RIGHT HEART DISEASE AND RIGHT-SIDED CONGESTIVE HEART FAILURE

R-CHF in dogs is less common that L-CHF and can occur secondary to pulmonary arterial hypertension (PAH), congenital heart disease (pulmonic stenosis, tricuspid valve dysplasia), myxomatous (degenerative) tricuspid valve disease, or neoplasia. Additionally, although most dogs with DCM or MMVD progress to L-CHF, some may manifest with right-sided or biventricular CHF, particularly dogs with concurrent atrial fibrillation or PAH.[20,23,32] The most common manifestation of R-CHF in dogs is ascites; other locations of fluid accumulation (which can occur in combination) are pleural effusion, small volume pericardial effusion (without tamponade), and rarely peripheral edema.[32,33] R-CHF is uncommon in cats but can occur secondary to congenital heart diseases or cardiomyopathies that preferentially affect the right ventricle. As noted above, cats can develop pleural or pericardial effusion as a manifestation of CHF regardless of cause; however, the presence of ascites in a cat with CHF would specifically suggest an underlying right heart disease.

Findings on POCUS that support a diagnosis of R-CHF include (1) evidence of severe right heart disease, (2) cavitary effusion(s), and (3) evidence of elevated systemic venous pressure such as CVC or hepatic venous distension (**Fig. 4**, see **Table 2**). Dogs and cats with severe right heart disease will typically have severe RA and RV dilation, with right parasternal long-axis views showing the RA and RV being the same size or larger than the LA and LV, respectively. RV dilation may also be seen on right parasternal short-axis views, with the RV being larger than the "mushroom" LV. Subxiphoid views will reveal CVC distension and decreased collapsibility of the CVC with respiration , as well as hepatic venous distension.[34] In addition to assisting with the diagnosis of R-CHF, POCUS can also be used to guide cavitary centesis.

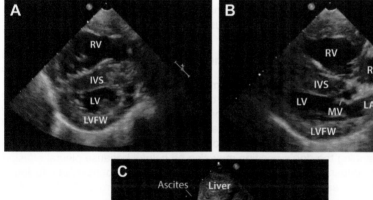

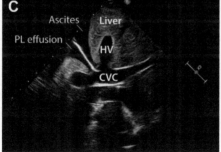

Fig. 4. POCUS images of dogs with severe right heart disease and R-CHF. (*A*) Right parasternal short-axis image at the level of the LV in a dog with R-CHF secondary to severe pulmonary arterial hypertension, demonstrating severe right ventricular enlargement and flattening of the IVS. (*B*) Right parasternal long-axis image (4-chamber view) in a dog with R-CHF secondary to severe pulmonary arterial hypertension, demonstrating severe right atrial and right ventricular enlargement and hypertrophy. (*C*) Subxiphoid image of a dog with R-CHF demonstrating an enlarged CVC and hepatic veins (HV). Ao, aorta; CVC, caudal vena cava; HV, hepatic veins; LA, left atrium; LAur, left auricle; PA, main pulmonary artery; PL, pleural; PV, pulmonic valve; RA, right atrium; RV, right ventricle; TV, tricuspid valve.

Dogs with severe PAH represent a specific clinical scenario with distinct recognizable POCUS features (see **Table 2**). Because PAH results in RV systolic pressure overload, right parasternal long-axis and short-axis views will reveal RV concentric hypertrophy (thickening) as well as enlargement, with RV wall thickness similar to or greater than the LV; the LV will often seem small and volume underloaded. RV pressure overload will also result in flattening of the interventricular septum on right parasternal short-axis views of the LV, giving a flattened "top" to the mushroom appearance of the LV. Severe PAH will also result in main pulmonary artery enlargement, with pulmonary artery diameter being larger than the Ao in right parasternal short-axis heart base views. Clinical and POCUS suspicion for severe PAH should prompt a diagnostic investigation for the underlying cause of PAH (such as heartworm disease, chronic bronchopulmonary disease, or pulmonary thromboembolic disease).[35,36] POCUS cannot differentiate these underlying causes of PAH; however, in dogs with severe heartworm disease, heartworms can sometimes be seen as double-lined (railroad-track) structures within the pulmonary artery, or even within the heart (RV or RA) in cases of heartworm caval syndrome.

As in cases of suspected L-CHF, POCUS findings should always be integrated with patient signalment, history, and physical examination findings when considering a diagnosis of R-CHF. A small breed dog presenting for acute dyspnea with a soft right-sided systolic heart murmur for whom POCUS shows RV enlargement and septal flattening with normal LA size should be treated for PAH, *not* L-CHF. Almost all dogs with R-CHF have ascites as part of their manifestation of cavitary effusion; isolated pleural effusion in dogs is almost never caused by R-CHF.

PERICARDIAL EFFUSION AND CARDIAC TAMPONADE

POCUS is an extremely useful tool for the timely and accurate diagnosis of pericardial effusion and cardiac tamponade. In normal dogs and cats, there is no visible pericardial effusion on POCUS examination. The sonographic appearance of pericardial effusion is a variable amount of (typically) anechoic fluid encircling the heart on right parasternal and subxiphoid POCUS windows.[37] Observing the fluid from multiple views and changing the dog's position may also be helpful because pleural effusion is more gravity dependent and will displace ventrally, whereas pericardial effusion is contained within its sac and more fixed in position. When pericardial effusion is identified, the operator should look for evidence of cardiac tamponade, which develops when the pressure in the pericardial space exceeds that of the right heart. Note that cardiac tamponade can develop with either large or small volume effusions depending on the time course in which the effusion develops. The POCUS criterion for cardiac tamponade is diastolic collapse of the right atrium (and possibly right ventricle) with a distended CVC with decreased collapsibility (**Fig. 5**). In some dogs with cardiac tamponade, the gallbladder may become thickened and edematous with a hypoechoic rim (gall bladder halo sign).[38]

POCUS is also helpful when performing pericardiocentesis. The ultrasound can be used to guide the centesis in real-time (termed "ultrasound-guided"), or the ultrasound can be used to simply identify the optimal site for the centesis (termed "ultrasound-assisted"). In people, ultrasound guidance has been shown to improve the safety of pericardiocentesis.[39] If there is concern for a possible intracardiac puncture during the pericardiocentesis, a small infusion of agitated saline can be helpful to confirm placement of the needle or catheter. Bubbles will appear within the cardiac chamber with an intracardiac puncture.[40]

In some situations, POCUS can also help determine the cause of the pericardial effusion. The most common cause of pericardial effusion in older dogs is cardiac

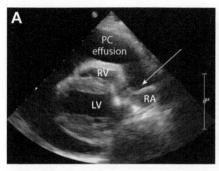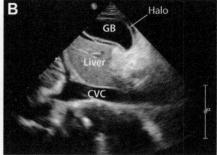

Fig. 5. POCUS images demonstrating pericardial effusion and cardiac tamponade. (*A*) Right parasternal long-axis view from a dog with large volume pericardial effusion demonstrating a collapsed right atrium (*arrow*) indicative of cardiac tamponade. (*B*) Subxiphoid view from a dog with pericardial effusion and cardiac tamponade, demonstrating a distended CVC and edematous gallbladder wall (halo sign). CVC, caudal vena cava; GB, gallbladder; LV, left ventricle; PC, pericardial; RA, right atrium; RV, right ventricle.

neoplasia, most commonly right atrial hemangiosarcoma in large-breed dogs or che-modectoma (heart base tumor) in brachycephalic dogs.[41,42] These neoplastic masses are often quite large and might be visible when imaging the right atrium or heart base. Caution should be used when interpreting small or equivocal mass lesions using POCUS, as epicardial fat (particularly near the atrioventricular junction) can be mistaken for a mass. If no mass is identified, benign idiopathic pericardial effusion is possible but concern for occult neoplasia remains. After pericardiocentesis and patient stabilization, a diagnostic echocardiogram performed by a specialist and a cardiac troponin I are recommended to confirm or refute a suspected mass lesion in a dog with pericardial effusion.[43,44] Another important cause of pericardial effusion in an older small-breed dog with MMVD is an LA rupture. In these cases, a hyperechoic tubular-shaped thrombus is visible surrounding the heart within (usually) small volume pericardial effusion. Whenever POCUS images are used to make decisions regarding treatment versus euthanasia in an emergency context, archiving of ultrasound images is advised for later review.

Note that differential diagnoses for pericardial effusion differ significantly between cats and dogs. In cats, the most common cause of pericardial effusion is CHF (see section "Severe heart disease and congestive heart failure in cats") and is usually small volume. Other causes of pericardial effusion in cats include lymphoma and feline infectious peritonitis. Cardiac tamponade requiring therapeutic pericardiocentesis in cats is rare.

USING POINT-OF-CARE ULTRASOUND TO MONITOR CARDIAC EMERGENCIES

In addition to aiding the diagnosis of cardiac emergencies, POCUS also has utility in monitoring these patients during hospitalization. Serial POCUS can be used to monitor for resolution or recurrence of cavitary effusions, particularly following centesis. This is perhaps most clinically important when monitoring for recurrence of pericardial effusion and cardiac tamponade following pericardiocentesis in dogs.

In dogs and cats diagnosed with L-CHF, POCUS can be useful to monitor for resolution of B-lines during treatment. In people, B-lines decrease within hours and resolve within days of diuretic treatment.[45,46] In one study of dogs with L-CHF, number of B-lines and strong positive sites decreased significantly from diagnosis to hospital discharge less than 24 hours later.[47] Repeating POCUS every 6 to 8 hours in hospitalized patients with CHF can provide guidance regarding aggressiveness of diuresis or identify nonresponders that might require additional diagnostic investigation.

SUMMARY

Point-of-care thoracic ultrasound is a rapid triage examination of the heart, lungs, pleural space, and great vessels that can aid the diagnosis and monitoring of cardiac emergencies in dogs and cats, including L-CHF, R-CHF, and pericardial effusion with cardiac tamponade. In combination with clinical information, POCUS provides clinicians with useful data to make immediate treatment decisions, prioritize subsequent diagnostic testing, and monitor patients during hospitalization. Cageside POCUS examinations should guide and augment clinical decision-making, ideally confirming preexamination clinical suspicions, and should not be relied on in lieu of further confirmatory diagnostic testing.

CLINICS CARE POINTS

- Use POCUS to increase or decrease index of suspicion for CHF as the cause of respiratory distress or cavitary effusion.
- Use POCUS as an extension of your triage examination to screen for severe cardiac disease as the cause of circulatory shock, arrhythmias, or syncope/collapse.
- Repeat the POCUS examination as needed during patient hospitalization to monitor for resolution or worsening of sonographic abnormalities.
- Always interpret POCUS findings in the context of patient signalment, history, and physical examination findings.

DISCLOSURE

The authors have no conflicts of interest to disclose.

REFERENCES

1. Aitken J, Freeman L, Leicester D, et al. Questionnaire on cardiovascular point-of-care ultrasound application in first opinion emergency settings in the United Kingdom. J Vet Emerg Crit Care 2019;29:S2–50.
2. Boysen S, Lisciandro G. The use of ultrasound for dogs and cats in the emergency room: AFAST and TFAST. Vet Clin North Am Small Anim Pract 2013;43: 773–97.
3. McMurray J, Boysen S, Chalhoub S. Focused assessment with sonography in nontraumatized dogs and cats in the emergency and critical care setting. J Vet Emerg Crit Care 2016;26:64–73.
4. Hezzell MJ, Ostroski C, Oyama MA, et al. Investigation of focused cardiac ultrasound in the emergency room for differentiation of respiratory and cardiac causes of respiratory distress in dogs. J Vet Emerg Crit Care 2020;30:159–64.
5. Razi R, Estrada J, Doll J, et al. Bedside hand-carried ultrasound by internal medicine residents versus traditional clinical assessment for the identification of systolic dysfunction in patients admitted with decompensated heart failure. J Am Soc Echocardiogr 2011;24:1319–24.

6. Tse YC, Rush JE, Cunningham SM, et al. Evaluation of a training course in focused echocardiography for noncardiology house officers. J Vet Emerg Crit Care 2013;23:268–73.

7. Gillman LM, Kirkpatrick AW. Portable bedside ultrasound: The visual stethoscope of the 21st century. Scand J Trauma Resusc Emerg Med 2012;20:18.

8. Via G, Hussain A, Wells M, et al. International Liaison Committee on Focused Cardiac UltraSound (ILC-FoCUS); International Conference on Focused Cardiac UltraSound (IC-FoCUS). International evidence-based recommendations for focused cardiac ultrasound. J Am Soc Echocardiogr 2014;27:683.e1–33.

9. Lisciandro GR, Fosgate GT, Fulton RM. Frequency and number of ultrasound lung rockets (B-Lines) using a regionally based lung ultrasound examination named Vet BLUE (Veterinary Bedside Lung Ultrasound Exam) in dogs with radiographically normal lung findings. Vet Radiol Ultrasound 2014;55:315–22.

10. Cole L, Pivetta M, Humm K. Diagnostic accuracy of a lung ultrasound protocol (Vet BLUE) for detection of pleural fluid, pneumothorax and lung pathology in dogs and cats. J Small Anim Pract 2021;62:178–86.

11. Ward JL, Lisciandro GR, Keene BW, et al. Accuracy of point-of-care lung ultrasonography for the diagnosis of cardiogenic pulmonary edema in dogs and cats with acute dyspnea. J Am Vet Med Assoc 2017;250:666–75.

12. Armenise A, Boysen RS, Rudloff E, et al. Veterinary-focused assessment with sonography for trauma-airway, breathing, circulation, disability and exposure: a prospective observational study in 64 canine trauma patients. J Small Anim Pract 2018;60:173–82.

13. Boysen S, McMurray J, Gommeren K. Abnormal curtain signs identified with a novel lung ultrasound protocol in six dogs with pneumothorax. Front Vet Sci 2019;6:291.

14. Lisciandro GR. Abdominal and thoracic focused assessment with sonography for trauma, triage, and monitoring in small animals. J Vet Emerg Crit Care 2011;21(2):104–22.

15. Chou YY, Ward JL, Barron LZ, et al. Focused ultrasound of the caudal vena cava in dogs with cavitary effusions or congestive heart failure: A prospective, observational study. PLoS One 2021;16:e0252544.

16. Elodie D, Soren B, Anne-Christine M, et al. Establishment of reference values of the caudal vena cava by fast-ultrasonography through different views in healthy dogs. J Vet Intern Med 2018;32:1208–18.

17. Volpicelli G, Elbarbary M, Blaivas M, et al. International evidence-based recommendations for point-of-care lung ultrasound. Intensive Care Med 2012;38:577–91.

18. Jambrik Z, Monti S, Coppola V, et al. Usefulness of ultrasound lung comets as a nonradiologic sign of extravascular lung water. Am J Cardiol 2004;93:1265–70.

19. Ward JL, Lisciandro GR, DeFrancesco TC. Distribution of alveolar-interstitial syndrome in dogs and cats with respiratory distress as assessed by lung ultrasound versus thoracic radiographs. J Vet Emerg Crit Care 2018;28:415–28.

20. Keene BW, Atkins CE, Bonagura JD, et al. ACVIM consensus guidelines for the diagnosis and treatment of myxomatous mitral valve disease in dogs. J Vet Intern Med 2019;33:1127–40.

21. Freeman L, Stern J, Fries R, et al. Diet-associated dilated cardiomyopathy in dogs: what do we know? J Am Vet Med Assoc 2018;253:1390–4.

22. Atkins C, DeFrancesco TC, Adin D, et al. Echocardiographic phenotype of canine dilated cardiomyopathy differs based on diet type. J Vet Cardiol 2018;21:1–9.

23. Borgarelli M, Santilli RA, Chiavegato D, et al. Prognostic indicators for dogs with dilated cardiomyopathy. J Vet Intern Med 2006;20:104–10.

24. Tidholm A, Häggström J, Borgarelli M, et al. Canine idiopathic dilated cardiomy-opathy. Part I: Aetiology, clinical characteristics, epidemiology and pathology. Vet J 2001;162:92–107.

25. Schober KE, Wetli E, Drost WT. Radiographic and echocardiographic assess-ment of left atrial aize in 100 cats with acute left-sided congestive heart failure. Vet Radiol Ultrasound 2014;55:359–67.

26. Guglielmini C, Diana A. Thoracic radiography in the cat: Identification of cardio-megaly and congestive heart failure. J Vet Cardiol 2015;17:S87–101.

27. Ward JL, Lisciandro GR, Ware WA, et al. Evaluation of point-of-care thoracic ul-trasound and NT-proBNP for the diagnosis of congestive heart failure in cats with respiratory distress. J Vet Intern Med 2018;32:1530–40.

28. Smith S, Dukes-McEwan J. Clinical signs and left atrial size in cats with cardio-vascular disease in general practice. J Small Anim Pract 2012;53(1):27–33.

29. Janson CO, Hezzell MJ, Oyama MA, et al. Focused cardiac ultrasound and point-of-care NT-proBNP assay in the emergency room for differentiation of cardiac and noncardiac causes of respiratory distress in cats. J Vet Emerg Crit Care 2020;30:376–83.

30. Hall DJ, Shofer F, Meier CK. Pericardial effusion in cats: a retrospective study of clinical findings and outcome in 146 cats. J Vet Intern Med 2007;21(5):1002–7.

31. Luis Fuentes V, Abbott J, Chetboul V, et al. ACVIM consensus statement guide-lines for the classification, diagnosis, and management of cardiomyopathies in cats. J Vet Intern Med 2020;34:1062–77.

32. Ward J, Ware W, Viall A. Association between atrial fibrillation and right-sided manifestations of congestive heart failure in dogs with degenerative mitral valve disease or dilated cardiomyopathy. J Vet Cardiol 2019;21:18–27.

33. Brewster RD, Benjamin SA, Thomassen RW. Spontaneous cor pulmonale in lab-oratory beagles. Lab Anim Sci 1983;33:299–302.

34. Barron LZ, DeFrancesco T, Chou YY, et al. Echocardiographic caudal vena cava measurements in normal cats and cats with congestive heart failure and noncar-diac causes of cavitary effusions. J Vet Cardiol 2023;48:7–18.

35. Kellihan HB, Stepien RL. Pulmonary hypertension in dogs: diagnosis and therapy. Vet Clin North Am Small Anim Pract 2010;40:623–41.

36. Reinero C, Visser LC, Kellihan HB, et al. ACVIM consensus statement guidelines for the diagnosis, classification, treatment, and monitoring of pulmonary hyper-tension in dogs. J Vet Intern Med 2020;34:549–73.

37. Lisciandro GR. The use of the diaphragmatico-hepatic (DH) views of the abdom-inal and thoracic focused assessment with sonography for triage (AFAST/TFAST) examinations for the detection of pericardial effusion in 24 dogs (2011-2012). J Vet Emerg Crit Care 2016;26:125–31.

38. Lisciandro GR, Gambino JM, Lisciandro SC. Thirteen dogs and a cat with ultra-sonographically detected gallbladder wall edema associated with cardiac dis-ease. J Vet Intern Med 2021;35:1342–6.

39. Tsang T, El-Najdawi E, Seward J, et al. Percutaneous echocardiographically guided pericardiocentesis in pediatric patients: evaluation of safety and efficacy. J Am Soc Echocardiogr 1998;11:1072–7.

40. Ainsworth C, Salehein O. Echo-guided pericardiocentesis: let the bubbles show the way. Circulation 2011;123:e210–1.

41. MacDonald KA, Cagney O, Magne ML. Echocardiographic and clinicopathologic characterization of pericardial effusion in dogs: 107 cases (1985–2006). J Am Vet Med Assoc 2009;235:1456–61.

42. Stafford Johnson M, Martin M, Binns S, et al. A retrospective study of clinical findings, treatment and outcome in 143 dogs with pericardial effusion. J Small Anim Pr 2004;45:546–52.

43. Shaw SP, Rozanski EA, Rush JE. Cardiac troponins I and T in dogs with pericardial effusion. J Vet Intern Med 2004;18:322–4.

44. Chun R, Kellihan HB, Henik RA, et al. Comparison of plasma cardiac troponin I concentrations among dogs with cardiac hemangiosarcoma, noncardiac hemangiosarcoma, other neoplasms, and pericardial effusion of non-hemangiosarcoma origin. J Am Vet Med Assoc 2010;237:806–11.

45. Liteplo AS, Murray AF, Kimberly HH, et al. Real-time resolution of sonographic B-lines in a patient with pulmonary edema on continuous positive airway pressure. Am J Emerg Med 2010;28:5–8.

46. Volpicelli G, Caramello V, Cardinale L, et al. Bedside ultrasound of the lung for the monitoring of acute decompensated heart failure. Am J Emerg Med 2008;26:585–91.

47. Murphy SD, Ward JL, Viall AK, et al. Utility of point-of-care lung ultrasound for monitoring cardiogenic pulmonary edema in dogs. J Vet Intern Med 2021;35:68–77.

UNITED STATES POSTAL SERVICE® Statement of Ownership, Management, and Circulation (All Periodicals Publications Except Requester Publications)

1. Publication Title	2. Publication Number	3. Filing Date
VETERINARY CLINICS OF NORTH AMERICA: SMALL ANIMAL PRACTICE	003 – 150	9/18/2023

4. Issue Frequency	5. Number of Issues Published Annually	6. Annual Subscription Price
JAN, MAR, MAY, JUL, SEP, NOV	6	$387.00

7. Complete Mailing Address of Known Office of Publication (Not printer) (Street, city, county, state, and ZIP+4®)

ELSEVIER INC.
230 Park Avenue, Suite 800
New York, NY 10169

Contact Person
Malathi Samayan

Telephone (Include area code)
91-44-4299-4507

8. Complete Mailing Address of Headquarters or General Business Office of Publisher (Not printer)

ELSEVIER INC.
230 Park Avenue, Suite 800
New York, NY 10169

9. Full Names and Complete Mailing Addresses of Publisher, Editor, and Managing Editor (Do not leave blank)

Publisher (Name and complete mailing address)

Dolores Meloni, ELSEVIER INC.
1600 JOHN F KENNEDY BLVD. SUITE 1600
PHILADELPHIA, PA 19103-2899

Editor (Name and complete mailing address)

STACY EASTMAN, ELSEVIER INC.
1600 JOHN F KENNEDY BLVD. SUITE 1600
PHILADELPHIA, PA 19103-2899

Managing Editor (Name and complete mailing address)

PATRICK MANLEY, ELSEVIER INC.
1600 JOHN F KENNEDY BLVD. SUITE 1600
PHILADELPHIA, PA 19103-2899

10. Owner (Do not leave blank. If the publication is owned by a corporation, give the name and address of the corporation immediately followed by the names and addresses of all stockholders owning or holding 1 percent or more of the total amount of stock. If not owned by a corporation, give the names and addresses of the individual owners. If owned by a partnership or other unincorporated firm, give its name and address as well as those of each individual owner. If the publication is published by a nonprofit organization, give its name and address.)

Full Name	Complete Mailing Address
WHOLLY OWNED SUBSIDIARY OF REED/ELSEVIER, US HOLDINGS	1600 JOHN F KENNEDY BLVD. SUITE 1600 PHILADELPHIA, PA 19103-2899

11. Known Bondholders, Mortgagees, and Other Security Holders Owning or Holding 1 Percent or More of Total Amount of Bonds, Mortgages, or Other Securities. If none, check box ▶ ☐ None

Full Name	Complete Mailing Address
N/A	

12. Tax Status (For completion by nonprofit organizations authorized to mail at nonprofit rates) (Check one)
The purpose, function, and nonprofit status of this organization and the exempt status for federal income tax purposes:
☐ Has Not Changed During Preceding 12 Months
☐ Has Changed During Preceding 12 Months (Publisher must submit explanation of change with this statement)

PS Form **3526**, July 2014 [Page 1 of 4 (see instructions page 4)] PSN: 7530-01-000-9931   PRIVACY NOTICE: See our privacy policy on www.usps.com.

---

13. Publication Title	14. Issue Date for Circulation Data Below
VETERINARY CLINICS OF NORTH AMERICA: SMALL ANIMAL PRACTICE	JULY 2023

15. Extent and Nature of Circulation

			Average No. Copies Each Issue During Preceding 12 Months	No. Copies of Single Issue Published Nearest to Filing Date
a. Total Number of Copies (Net press run)			425	405
b. Paid Circulation (By Mail and Outside the Mail)	(1)	Mailed Outside-County Paid Subscriptions Stated on PS Form 3541 (Include paid distribution above nominal rate, advertiser's proof copies, and exchange copies)	271	266
	(2)	Mailed In-County Paid Subscriptions Stated on PS Form 3541 (Include paid distribution above nominal rate, advertiser's proof copies, and exchange copies)	0	0
	(3)	Paid Distribution Outside the Mails Including Sales Through Dealers and Carriers, Street Vendors, Counter Sales, and Other Paid Distribution Outside USPS®	138	126
	(4)	Paid Distribution by Other Classes of Mail Through the USPS (e.g., First-Class Mail®)	7	6
c. Total Paid Distribution (Sum of 15b (1), (2), (3), and (4))			418	398
d. Free or Nominal Rate Distribution (By Mail and Outside the Mail)	(1)	Free or Nominal Rate Outside-County Copies included on PS Form 3541	6	6
	(2)	Free or Nominal Rate In-County Copies Included on PS Form 3541	0	0
	(3)	Free or Nominal Rate Copies Mailed at Other Classes Through the USPS (e.g., First-Class Mail)	0	0
	(4)	Free or Nominal Rate Distribution Outside the Mail (Carriers or other means)	1	1
e. Total Free or Nominal Rate Distribution (Sum of 15d (1), (2), (3) and (4))			7	7
f. Total Distribution (Sum of 15c and 15e)			425	405
g. Copies not Distributed (See Instructions to Publishers #4 (page #3))			0	0
h. Total (Sum of 15f and g)			425	405
i. Percent Paid (15c divided by 15f times 100)			98.4%	98.27%

* If you are claiming electronic copies, go to line 16 on page 3. If you are not claiming electronic copies, skip to line 17 on page 3.

16. Electronic Copy Circulation		Average No. Copies Each Issue During Preceding 12 Months	No. Copies of Single Issue Published Nearest to Filing Date
a. Paid Electronic Copies	▶		
b. Total Paid Print Copies (Line 15c) + Paid Electronic Copies (Line 16a)	▶		
c. Total Print Distribution (Line 15f) + Paid Electronic Copies (Line 16a)	▶		
d. Percent Paid (Both Print & Electronic Copies) (16b divided by 16c × 100)	▶		

☒ I certify that 85% of all my distributed copies (electronic and print) are paid above a nominal price.

17. Publication of Statement of Ownership

☒ If the publication is a general publication, publication of this statement is required. Will be printed in the NOVEMBER 2023 issue of this publication.   ☐ Publication not required.

18. Signature and Title of Editor, Publisher, Business Manager, or Owner	Date
Malathi Samayan - Distribution Controller *Malathi Samayan*	9/18/2023

I certify that all information furnished on this form is true and complete. I understand that anyone who furnishes false or misleading information on this form or who omits material or information requested on the form may be subject to criminal sanctions (including fines and imprisonment) and/or civil sanctions (including civil penalties).

PS Form **3526**, July 2014 (Page 3 of 4)   PRIVACY NOTICE: See our privacy policy on www.usps.com

Moving?

Make sure your subscription moves with you!

To notify us of your new address, find your **Clinics Account Number** (located on your mailing label above your name), and contact customer service at:

Email: journalscustomerservice-usa@elsevier.com

800-654-2452 (subscribers in the U.S. & Canada)
314-447-8871 (subscribers outside of the U.S. & Canada)

Fax number: 314-447-8029

Elsevier Health Sciences Division
Subscription Customer Service
3251 Riverport Lane
Maryland Heights, MO 63043

*To ensure uninterrupted delivery of your subscription, please notify us at least 4 weeks in advance of move.

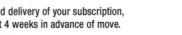

Printed and bound by CPI Group (UK) Ltd, Croydon, CR0 4YY

03/10/2024

01040476-0016